Optimum Sports Nutrition

Optimum Sports Nutrition

Your Competitive Edge

Dr Michael Colgan

Advanced
Research Press
New York 1993

For information contact: Advanced Research Press, 2120 Smithtown Avenue, Ronkonkoma, NY 11779

FIRST EDITION

Library of Congress Cataloging-in-Publication Data
Colgan, Michael, 1939-
Optimum Sports Nutrition

Bibliography:p
Includes index.
1. Sports Nutrition 2. Physical Fitness 3. Health.
I. Title.

ISBN 0-9624840-4-0 (cloth)
ISBN 0-9624840-5-9 (pbk)

Printed in the United States of America

To Tammy,
my youngest princess

Also by Dr. Michael Colgan:

Your Personal Vitamin Profile
Prevent Cancer Now
The Power Program

Forewords

"Listen to this man. He's the best in sports nutrition."
Arthur Lydiard
New Zealand Olympic Coach

*"**Optimum Sports Nutrition** is easy reading and a well researched guide to sports nutrition and improving overall physical performance and well being."*
Lee Haney
8-time Mr. Olympia

"A great nutrition program. Helped me win big."
Rick Roberts
National Sub-Masters Powerlifting Champion

*"If you are serious about your athletics **Optimum Sports Nutrition** is a must."*
Julie Moss
Triathlon Champion

"Consumate counsel on sports nutrition. I owe a strong debt of gratitude."
Doug Benbow
Bodybuilding Champion
Owner, Benbow Performance Centers

"For me the results have been excellent. Thanks Michael for helping to keep me young."
Kathy Keeton
President, Omni and Longevity magazines

"Dr Michael Colgan has systematically and brilliantly compiled the research you need to move yourself into a new era of vitality."
Dr Bernard Rimland
Director of Special Programs
Department of the Navy, San Diego

"The work of The Colgan Institute is an especially valuable contribution to human knowledge."
Dr Andrew Strigner
Harley St, London

"We tried to entice Mike Colgan back to Australia. He was teaching too many American athletes how to win."
Dr Richard Telford
Director of Sport Science
Australian Institute of Sport

"Dr Colgan is one of the world's top nutrition scientists."
Dr Donald Whittaker
Christian Television Network

"Michael Colgan's work is brilliant, irreverent, ahead of its time."
Dr Carl Pfeiffer
Director, Princeton Brain Bio Center

"Dr Colgan, your program has made a difference!"
Bobby Czyz
World Champion Boxer

"Required reading, an absolute must for the novice and world class athlete alike."
Vic Lee
Owner, Frogs Gyms

"There is no hype with Michael Colgan. Thanks for giving me back the edge!"
Gary Owen
Masters Karate Champion

"As usual the Doctor tells it like it is. Straight to the point information like this is sorely needed in the sports community."
Jim Heflin
Owner, Beverly International

"Without your advice my success in the Western States 100 Mile Race would be just a dream."
James Bond
Champion Ultra Distance Runner

"Couldn't have done it without you."
Jeff Smullen
Champion Bodybuilder
Winner: Tournament of Champions

"After I went on the Colgan Program my training really picked up."
Howard Dorfling
Five times California State Cycling Champion
Member, U.S. Cycling Team

Acknowledgments

So many great people have helped me along the road to this book, it is impossible to name them all. In thanking a few, I extend my thanks equally to everyone.

Stuart Slater, my mentor at Victoria University in New Zealand gave me the ability to analyze evidence, so as to extract the gold from the dross. Michael Brines, my friend at Rockefeller University, showed me how to become a real scientist. Rene Dubos at Rockefeller tolerated my theories and taught me how the force of human will can utterly change the body.

Linus Pauling, Jonas Salk, Carl Pfeiffer, Hans Selye, Bernie Rimland, Joe Beasley, all supported and gently criticised my early work. Arthur Lydiard taught me more than anyone about athletics. Roger Williams taught me more than anyone about nutrition. And each of the hundreds of athletes I have worked with over the last 18 years helped shape my hand and my knowledge.

Throughout the writing, Steve Blechman, Jim Bie, Herb Boynton, Brian Liebowitz and many others, tirelessly plied me with all the latest studies in sports nutrition.

And my wife and fellow scientist, Lesley encouraged and supported and helped beyond measure to bring this book to fruition.

The work is really the product of them all. But for the words herein that describe it, I take sole responsibility.

Introduction

I began my research on sports nutrition at the University of Auckland in New Zealand in 1974. Since then I have worked hands-on with many hundreds of fine athletes in almost every sport, from recreational to Olympic status. My training as a research scientist has given me an edge in analyzing the evidence from scientific research and assessing the implications of that evidence for athletes.

The information in this book is an analysis of the evidence that specific, precise nutrition, exercise, and lifestyle strategies, can improve the human body far beyond the level usually achieved by even the best sports training.

I urge you to consult the scientific and medical references given herein, to decide for yourself the merits of my analysis. You should also pursue other references, as this is only a single book, covering only a tiny fraction of the research. I have done my best to ensure that it covers the most representative work, that it gives you the correct trends in science that will most benefit your performance.

Some of the practices described herein, such as the taking of large amounts of certain nutrients, are still highly experimental. If you choose to pursue them, you do so upon your own responsiblity. No one should take large doses of vitamins or minerals or amino acids without consulting a physician trained in sports nutrition. Some people can be adversely affected by nutrients, and nutrients can adversely affect some prescribed medications.

Because of such complications, your approach to sports nutrition should always be careful and informed. Nevertheless, hundreds of athletes have used these programs at the Colgan Institute with winning results. Properly applied, the programs have turned genetic limitations into talents, and limited talents into champions. You have within you the seeds of greatness. This book provides the fertile soil wherein they can grow to match your dreams.

Michael Colgan,
San Diego, CA.
November 1992.

Contents

Part I

Ground Rules

Never believe you have insufficient time for the attention to detail that is essential to excellence. You have exactly the same 24 hours every day as Carl Lewis, Magic Johnson and Evander Holyfield.

Michael Colgan, Lecture Series, 1989

Chapter 1

Nutrition Basics

Every greedy business day you are bombarded by a conflicting mass of nutrition facts, marketing hokum, bold-faced lies, hogwash, and flapdoodle, all claiming to be the best in sports nutrition. When big-name athletes are seduced by the dead smell of money to prostitute fat and sugar loaded candy bars as official foods of the Olympic Games, who the hell can you trust?

The only source of unbiased information left to us is the research presented in peer-reviewed scientific journals. That's the precise and accurate science that gave you every facet of modern life, from the car that you drive to the fillings in your teeth. Our task at the Colgan Institute for the past 18 years, has been to analyze the science of sports nutrition and present the facts to athletes in understandable and usable form.

Some sports medicine folk still claim that nutrition is no magic bullet, and that all an athlete needs is three square meals a day equally selected from the four food groups; meats, dairy foods, fruits and vegetables, and grains. This false idea has been carefully promoted by the meat and dairy industries through the media, and through health and sports organizations for the last 50 years. It contradicts everything modern science has discovered about human nutrition. Champion Masters runner Bill Robinson said it best:

Putting meats and dairy foods on a par with other nutrients is one big reason why development of athletics in America has not kept pace with other countries.

Not an exaggeration. Take the sad state of the marathon for example. Steve Spence's third place finish at the World Championships in 1991 is the first American medal in international competition since 1976. The world record for the marathon has now improved to 2:06:50. But no American has ever beaten Alberto Salazar's time of 2:08:52 set in 1982. The 1992 Olympic Trials marathon was won by Steve Spence in a slow 2:12:43, giving him little chance at the Olympics. In Barcelona he came 12th. O.K., we are doing better in some other events. But with our vast pool of athletes and resources, we should be world dominant in every sport.

I am writing this book because many of our athletes are not getting the truth about nutrition. And the rest of the world is starting to leave us behind. Look at the Barcelona Games. U.S. television tended to show events where America won a medal, so most people got a false idea of results. Our highly acclaimed cycling team, for example, didn't win any of the 10 golds or silvers, and took a total of only 2 bronzes. Lance Armstrong, praised by U.S. journalists as the world's best road racer, came 13th.[25]

In track and field, where America is often cited as the best, we did have some great wins in the sprints. And Carl Lewis in the long jump, and Jackie Joyner Kersee in the heptathlon were superb. But U.S. men won 8 of 23 golds and U.S. women won only 4 of 19 golds.[26] Of course it's not all poor nutrition. But I'll say this only once: with optimal nutrition results would have been a lot different. If the Olympic talent we have now use the principles in this book to prepare for '96, they will clean the world's clock.

Building Materials

Optimal bodily function, especially in athletes who are always pushing the limits, cannot occur without daily ingestion of a precise mix of 59 substances. Some you need a lot of, some you need only infinitesimal amounts. But they all have to be provided in the *correct* amounts. The first five, **oxygen, hydrogen, carbon, nitrogen, and sulfur,** we need in large amounts. They are widely

Table 1. Vitamins and co-factors, essential elements, essential fatty acids and amino acids required for the human body.*

Elements required in large amounts daily
Oxygen   Hydrogen   Nitrogen   Carbon   Sulfur

Elements required in medium amounts daily

Calcium	Magnesium	Potassium
Phosphorus	Sodium	Chloride

Elements required in small amounts daily

Iron	Zinc	Copper	Manganese
Silicon	Cobalt	Chromium	Selenium
Iodine	Fluoride	Molybdenum	Nickel
Arsenic	Boron	Tin**	Germanium**

    **Probable essential elements

Vitamins and co-factors (common form names)

A (retinol)	B_1 (thiamin)	B_2 (riboflavin)
B_3 (niacin)	B_5 (pantothenic acid)	B6 (pyridoxine)
B_{12} (cobalamin)	Folic Acid	Biotin
C (ascorbic acid)	D (calciferol)	E (d-alpha-
K (phylloquinone)		tocopherol)

Co-factors

Choline   Inositol   Bioflavonoids
Para-amino-benzoic acid (PABA)
Coenzyme Q10   Pyrroloquinoline quinione (PQQ)

Essential Amino Acids

Isoleucine	Leucine	Lysine	Methionine
Phenylalanine	Threonine	Tryptophan	Valine
Arginine†	Histidine†	Taurine†	

    †Conditionally essential

Essential fatty acids

    Linoleic acid   Linolenic acid

*Sources: Colgan Institute, San Diego, CA, also References 3 & 4.

dispersed in foods and in the air we breathe, so supply is not often a problem. The remaining 54 nutrients we need in medium or small amounts, but they are less plentiful in the environment and may be deficient or entirely absent in any particular food.

As of May 1992, 13 vitamins, 22 minerals, 6 co-factors (helper substances), 8 amino acids (plus 3 more in certain circumstances), and 2 essential fatty acids are recognized as essential to the human system (see Table 1). All these essential substances interact with each other in precise synergy to produce, maintain, and renew your body. If even one is missing, or in short supply, then the functions of all the others are impaired.[1]

Although the essentiality of co-factors is still controversial, I have included them because recent evidence all points in that direction. In science jargon, the word "essential" means;

    (a) the nutrients have to be present in adequate amounts or function is impaired;

    (b) the body cannot make the nutrients or cannot make enough of them for normal tissue function;

    (c) you have to get them from your diet.

Commercially spawned ideas of food groups take little account of the scarcity and irregular supply of essential nutrients in many foods, or of the principle of **synergy**, now widely accepted as the basis of nutrition science.[1, 2] Athletes who follow anyone who preaches the four food groups, condemn themselves to an inferior level of performance, way inferior to what they can achieve with optimal nutrition.

Adherents to obsolete ideas of nutrition might try to persuade you that my criticisms are not in the mainstream of science. To save you from the clutches of these people, whose minds are filled more with job security and the next research grant than what is best for athletes, here are some examples that indicate we are on the right track.

On 9 April 1991, the Physicians Committee for Responsible Nutrition, a Washington lobby representing 3,000 physicians, asked the US Department of Agriculture (USDA) to abandon the four food groups and to reclassify meats and dairy products as "optional foods." Dr T. Colin Campbell, Professor of Nutritional Biochemistry at Cornell University, presented evidence that the excess intakes of meat and dairy products in America are now strongly linked with our high rates of cancer, heart disease, diabetes, obesity, and osteoporosis. If these foods disrupt bodily function so much that they cause major disease, don't believe anyone who tells you that they can improve bodily function for athletic performance.

It's a long awaited pleasure to report that on 27 April 1992, the USDA issued a food pyramid emphasizing whole grains, then vegetables, then fruits, as the basis for nutrition, with meats and dairy products as minor foods. This pyramid buries the arrant nonsense of the four food groups forever. In its place, I will give you the latest science on sports nutrition. When you apply this science, you will find that nutrition *is* a magic bullet that will help you more than you ever dreamed to achieve your athletic goals.

The Most Complex Machine

To apply nutrition properly, first you need to grasp just how much you can be affected by what you put in your mouth. Over three million years, evolution developed the human body to convert a mix of certain compounds that occur in Nature into muscles, bones, organs, glands, and brain. The hairy bags of salty chemical soup that we call human beings *are* the interactions of these nutrient compounds. Every time you screw around with them, they will screw around with you.

Athletes who scarf down fat-loaded burgers and nutrient-poor fries, do not understand how much they are disturbing the exquisite precision of nutrient use by their bodies. Let's use a couple of examples to illustrate how that precision makes the engine of a Masserati look like a child's toy.

Vitamin B_{12} is a good one. You require only a few micrograms (millionths of a gram) of B_{12} each day: the RDA is only 2 micrograms.[4] Your blood contains only about 5 nanograms (billionths of a gram) per liter, less than a speck of dust. You couldn't see that amount even under a microscope. It represents less than one part per *trillion* of your bodyweight. Yet if you lack that infinitesimal speck, your whole body declines into the serious disease of pernicious anemia, which gradually destroys the myelin sheaths protecting your nerves, leading to blindness, insanity, and death.[5]

A second example is iodine. About 50 micrograms per day is considered sufficient for most people.[4] This is still an amount so tiny that you could not see it on the head of a pin. Every day your body separates out the few molecules of iodine that occur in different foods with a precision far beyond the most advanced computer, and transports them straight to the thyroid gland. There they convert an inert chemical called thyronine into powerful thyroid hormones. These hormones then control your energy supply, your mood, and even how well you can think.[3]

The same applies to other micronutrients. It is still a mystery to science how such minute amounts of these substances can hold the keys to health, to sanity, even to life itself. But they do! If you own a sports car, a power boat, or any highly tuned machine, you know to be v-e-r-r-r-y careful what you feed it. Yet these are simple devices compared with the human body. If you want optimum sports performance the first rule is: **Don't put junk fuel in your Masserati.**

Synergy

Synergy of nutrients is the first principle of modern nutrition. In your body, nutrients operate only by multiple interactions with each other. Prior to 1980, many silly experiments were done with single vitamins and minerals *in vitro* (in the test tube), on which many silly recommendations were made for human nutrition. The human test tube is quite different from the laboratory flask.

Vitamin D in the test tube, for example, has little effect on human cells. But most people who know a little nutrition, are aware that vitamin D in the human body plays a controlling role in the metabolism of calcium and phosphorus.[6] Most athletes have also heard that the B vitamins work only in synergy with each other.[7] But even among sports nutrition folk, many are still unaware of the interactions between vitamin E and vitamin B12,[8] calcium and magnesium,[9] vitamin C and iron, or vitamin A and zinc.[10] The list of established first-order interactions between nutrients increases every year.

Complex multiple interactions have also been established. Vitamin E, for example, interacts with both copper and zinc. Vitamin E deficiency reduces bodily levels of zinc, because the two nutrients interact to protect membranes against damage by free radicals (lipid peroxidation). When E is deficient, more zinc is used by the body to pinch-hit for the missing nutrient. This action has the added effect of increasing body levels of copper.[11]

Another example of multiple interactions is vitamin C. Use of vitamin C to inhibit colds, for example, depends as much on the other nutrients that interact with vitamin C as on the vitamin itself. The recently established interactions of vitamin C, show that use of large doses to stop a cold also requires increased intake of vitamin B6, vitamin B12, zinc, folic acid, and choline. [12]

Unfortunately, many health professionals and the general public are still operating with erroneous single nutrient information. We know now that there is never a deficiency of just one nutrient. There is never any nutrient activity by itself. **It is the multiple interactions of nutrients that is the basis of their biological function.**

I will take one more example from my practice in sports nutrition. In the early 1970s, athletes were often referred to our clinic for psychosomatic disorders. "Psychosomatic" is medical jargon for, "there is something wrong with this guy but we don't know what. Could be psychological but maybe not." Some of these athletes showed symptoms that looked like incipient pellagra, gastrointestinal disturbances, loss of appetite, intermittent diarrhea, and a beef-red, shiny tongue.

Pellagra is commonly believed to be a vitamin B_3 deficiency. But these athletes did not respond to a vitamin B_3 supplement. So, initially we thought we were wrong, and pellagra was not involved. We quickly learned better. We learned that well before pellagra appears, vitamin B_2, vitamin B_6, and the amino acid tryptophan are also likely to be deficient, in addition to vitamin B_3. The research on this problem is reviewed in my book, **Your Personal Vitamin Profile.**[13]

Because of the principle of synergy, these deficiencies also affected other nutrients. B_2 deficiency impairs B_{12} metabolism, which then impairs folic-acid metabolism. Folic acid dysfunction then affects vitamin C metabolism. The resultant depletion of the body's vitamin C impairs iron absorption. Impaired iron absorption encourages excessive copper absorption, which then impairs zinc metabolism. And on and on and on.[1]

These impaired functions did not make the athletes really ill, or even stop their training. But performance was way below expectations. It took individually designed nutrition programs, adequate in all nutrients, which permitted all the synergistic interactions to take place, to restore these young men to good health.

Biochemical Individuality

Notice that I said, "individually designed nutrition programs." That leads us into the second principle of nutrition: **biochemical individuality.** Because of genetic variations, individual bodies are biochemically different from each other. Some people have fat feet. Others have skinny feet, or short feet or long feet, or high-arched feet, or flat feet. The range of individual differences in feet is enormous. Making one size of shoe to fit everyone would be rank stupidity. Yet that is exactly what happens in most sports nutrition.

Sports magazines and health food stores all promote dozens of different brands of one-size-fits-all supplements as if they are exactly what your individual body needs. You don't have to do complex tests to know just how wrong they are. Just look at your training partner. Your body differs radically from his, from the shape of your nose and toes, to the patterns of fingerprints, the texture of hair, the range of movement of limbs, even the sound of your voice. Inside is just as different. Your muscles, glands, organs, nerves, and brain are different from his in size, shape, and function right down to the molecular function of individual cells. For optimal performance your body clearly requires different nutrition than his. To be effective, a sports nutrition program has to fit your individual form and function at least as well as your shoes fit your feet.

This biochemical individuality is well established in medical science. Over forty years ago, at the University of Texas, Professor Roger Williams began to patiently document the huge difference in individual needs for nutrients. He showed that, for optimal growth, some animals require 20 times the vitamin C of others. And the difference in bodily usage of vitamin A varies 40-fold.[14,15] Wide individual differences in nutrient requirements are now established for a variety of vitamins, minerals, and amino acids. [16,17]

One example from my own laboratory is vitamin C. At the Colgan Institute we routinely measure excretion of vitamin C and its metabolites in the urine of athletes. Excretion of vitamin C is a normal function that helps protect the urinary tract. Increases in excretion rates are often used to measure at what level the body tissues become saturated with a vitamin. When they are saturated, the excess spills into the urine and you can measure it. The amount that stays in the body gives the saturation level.

Over a series of studies, we found that some people could take 5,000 mg of vitamin C and show only a little increase in excretion. [13] All that vitamin C was being used by their bodies in the hundreds of biological functions vitamin C is known to have.[18] Other people showed a large increase in excretion of vitamin C after taking only 1,000 mg. We found that the biochemical individuality in use of vitamin C is at least 10-fold.

If anyone tells you that a particular program of foods and supplements will fit everyone on your team -- don't believe him. Ask him why they can't all wear one size shoe.

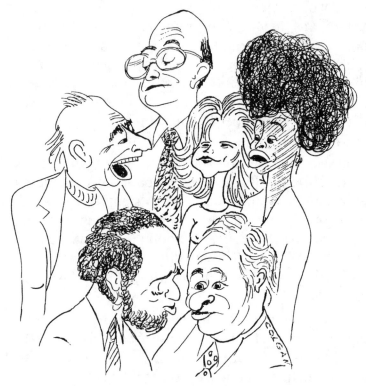

"Biochemical individuality balderdash!
Everyone is exactly the same."

Ditch the RDAs

If this biochemical individuality is so well established, why do some sports medicine folk still flog one-size-fits-all nutrition, and the single-point figures of the Recommended Dietary Allowances (RDAs). Unfortunately, the RDAs have been so misused by medical professionals and the food industry as a standard for individual nutrition, that the error became nationally accepted and gave rise to numerous general recommendations on nutrition that are supposed to fit everyone. They fit no one, because the RDAs were never meant for individuals. The 1980 RDA handbook states prominently on page 1:

> RDA are recommendations for the average daily amounts of nutrients that population groups should consume over a period of time. RDA should not be confused with requirements for a specific individual.[19]

Dr A.E. Harper, former Chairman of the RDA Committee, emphasized this further by stating that RDAs "are not recommendations for the ideal diet." He went on that the term "recommended allowance" was adopted "to avoid any implication of finality or...optimal requirements".[20] If you use the RDAs to plan your nutrition, you will *never, never* reach your athletic potential.

Lifestyle Dynamics

It would be easy to design individual nutrition programs if biochemical individuality alone determined your personal need for nutrients. Unfortunately, your lifestyle and environment radically affect your needs also. Nutritional requirements vary with **lifestyle dynamics** such as food quality, smoking, alcohol, pollution, medication, occupation, training, age, and a zillion other factors.

Training is a good example. Athletes who are on decent nutrition programs that keep them in top form at a particular training intensity, can quickly show evidence of physiological decline when they begin a more intense training program.

Decline in hematological (red blood) status, which determines your capacity to use oxygen, is a common problem. It can be reasonably assessed by measuring blood levels of three variables, hemoglobin, the red pigment that carries oxygen, hematocrit, the proportion of your blood composed of red blood cells, and red blood cell count (RBC), the number of red cells in your blood.

Figure 1 shows some results of a study on 12 male marathon runners who about doubled their usual training distance. Instead of an average of 8 miles per day, they ran 312 miles over a 20-day period, averaging 17 miles a day. Although the required running speed was not stressful (8.5 min/mile), all subjects showed large reductions in hemoglobin from excellent to marginal. They showed similar reductions in hematocrit, and RBC count.[21] Over the three weeks, their usual nutrition was unable to maintain the blood components essential to carry oxygen to their tissues.

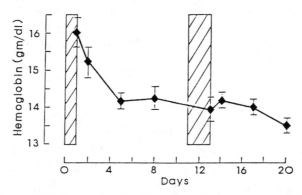

Figure 1. Hemoglobin levels declined from excellent to marginal in 12 marathon runners over a 20-day, 312-mile run that doubled their usual training mileage. Hatched areas are rest periods. Redrawn from Dressendorfer, Reference 21.

The principal nutrients involved in making red blood cells are iron, zinc, folic acid, vitamin B_6, vitamin B_{12}, and vitamin C.[22] In a double-blind crossover trial, the Colgan Institute fed athletes increased levels of these nutrients over a 12-week period, during which they increased their training levels. Compared with a control group given 100% of the RDAs for all nutrients, the athletes given additional nutrients maintained their red blood status, increased their VO_2 max (the maximum amount of oxygen they could use), and improved their performance.[22]

The vital lesson from these studies is that your individual

lifestyle dynamics, be it changes in training, drinking alcohol, air pollution, work, medications, or other variables, radically affect your nutritional needs. Unless your nutrition program is matched to your lifestyle, you cannot expect optimum performance.

Precision

The most common objection to the need for individual nutrition programs matched to biochemical individuality and individual lifestyle is, "Why can't I just take a handful of one-a-day vitamins or a pill of each nutrient, so that I get a mega-dose of all the nutrients? The body will sort out what it needs and eliminate the excess."

To do so violates the principle of **precision**. Each individual has a particular range of intake of each nutrient that will yield optimum function. Figure 2 illustrates that, below this range, function becomes sub-optimal because of deficiency. Above this range, function becomes sub-optimal because of toxicity. To optimize athletic performance you need a program that puts all your nutrition in the optimal range.

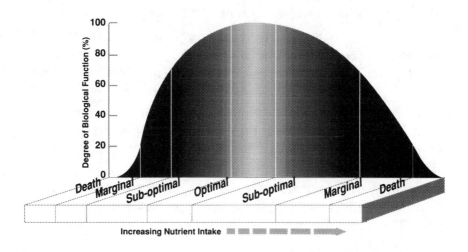

Figure 2. Percentage of optimal function with increasing nutrient intake. There is a narrow range of dietary intake of each nutrient that will produce optimum biological function. Inadequate intake produces sub-optimal function because of deficiency. Overdose produces sub-optimal function because of toxicity.

Taking arbitrary mega-doses of nutrients into the toxic range as many athletes do, disrupts performance in four ways. First, some vitamins and minerals are toxic at only 5-10 times the RDA. The minimum toxic dose of vitamin A, for example, is 25,000 IU. [23] One-a-day vitamins commonly contain 10,000 IU. A handful of these pills would subject you every day to subclinical vitamin A poisoning. The same applies to selenium, chromium, fluoride, iron, and vitamin K.

Second, the interaction between nutrients change radically when some of them are taken to excess. Excess zinc, for example, interferes with iron metabolism, excess essential fatty acids deplete the body of vitamin E, excess iron disrupts copper metabolism. [1]

Third, mega-doses of nutrients determined by guess-work are not in correct ratios to each other. Folic acid, for example, which may be low in a one-a-day supplement, has to be present in adequate amounts for iron to make hemoglobin, the red blood pigment that carries your oxygen. Vitamin B_6 has to be present in adequate amounts for the body to absorb vitamin B_{12}. Many other essential interactions require nutrients to be eaten in the correct ratios to each other for optimal function to occur.

Fourth, individuals vary in their needs for nutrients in ways that cannot be covered by mega-doses, not only because of individual genetics but also because of activity and lifestyle. As we will see in later chapters, a person who exercises regularly, for example, has increased requirements for certain nutrients such as vitamin E and chromium, but not for others. A person who lives in a smog-polluted area, has an increased requirement for vitamin A and other antioxidants that would be an overdose for people living in clean air. There are hundreds of such factors determining nutritional needs that cannot be covered by arbitrary mega-dosing. The only answer is an individually designed personal nutrient program.

Physiological Dynamics

The final principle of nutrition you need to know is **physiological dynamics**. Unlike drugs, nutrients do not have rapid effects. No quick fix. The business of nutrition is to build a better body. That has to wait on Nature to turn over body cells. A blood cell lasts 60-120 days. In 3-4 months your whole blood supply is completely replaced. In 6 months almost all the proteins in your body die and are replaced, even the DNA of your genes. In a year all your bones and even the enamel of your teeth is replaced, constructed entirely out of the nutrients that you eat.

This time course is well illustrated by the course of deficiency diseases. If I remove all the vitamin C from your diet, within 4 weeks blood vitamin C will drop to zero. But you will see no symptoms of disease at 4 weeks. You have to wait until enough of the healthy cells have been replaced by unhealthy cells. It is another 12 weeks before symptoms of scurvy start to ravage your body.

So when you implement an optimum nutrition program, don't expect rapid results. In one of our studies at the Colgan Institute, runners were supplemented to try to improve their hemoglobin, hematocrit, and red blood cell count. But after one month of supplementation, there was no improvement at all. After 6 months, however, all three indices were signficantly increased. [24]

Think of it this way. If you take a neglected house plant and start feeding and watering it, the leaves may perk up a bit from the improved nutrition. But you have to wait for the old leaves to die off and new leaves to grow before you get a really healthy plant. It is the same with the human body. When you start feeding it better, you have to wait on the physiological dynamics of the body to grow new improved cells in the improved nutrient medium. After 18 years in sports nutrition, the shortest program we will give any athlete is six months.

First Principles

1. **Synergy**. Nutrients do not function singly. They function only by interdependent interactions with each other.

2. **Completeness**. The corollary of synergy is that even if one essential nutrient is in short supply, none of the others can function properly.

3. **Biochemical Individuality**. Nutritional needs of individuals differ as much as their genetically given faces and finger-prints. Each athlete requires an individual nutrition program.

4. **Lifestyle Dynamics**. Lifestyle choices such as the choice of training level, or the choice of living in a polluted urban environment, dramatically affect nutritional needs.

5. **Precision**. There is only a narrow range of intake of each nutrient that will produce optimum function.

6. **Physiological Dynamics**. Improved nutrition must wait on nature to renew whole bodily systems before its effects can show.

These principles give us the correct perspective to investigate the combinations and actions of nutrients that will improve your athletic performance. Let's get to it!

Chapter 2

A Hairy Bag Of Water

Even your bones are a quarter water. The muscles that drive your performance are three-quarters water. The brain that steers your limbs is 76% water. The blood that carries your nutrients is 82% water. And the lungs that provide your oxygen are near 90% water.[1] These basic facts of biochemistry emphasize the first nutrient in your quest for optimum performance. **The most important nutrient in your body is plain water.**

The quality of your tissues, their performance, and their resistance to injury, is absolutely dependent on the quality and quantity of the water you drink. And you have to drink it constantly. Light exercise in a temperate climate uses half a gallon of water a day in breath, sweat, and urine. Athletes in heavy training use over two gallons a day. A 165 lb athlete (75 kg) is mainly composed of 50 quarts of water. In heavy training, he has to replace all of it every six days.[2,3]

You can replace your body water with any beverage. They are all mainly water, including milk, fruit juices, coffee, tea, even the thickest soup, even whole fruits and vegetables. But if you fail to do so, performance suffers immediately. Dehydrate a muscle by only 3% and you cause about a 10% loss of contractile strength, and an 8% loss of speed. Performance literally dries up.[4,5]

At the famous Human Performance Laboratory at Ball State University, Indiana, Dr David Costill and colleagues dehydrated athletes by just 2-3%. That's 3-5 lb for a 165 lb man. Many athletes consider such a loss no big deal, because losses of 7-10 lb are common during marathons, even with regular drinking along the way. But when these lightly dehydrated athletes were made to run time trials at 1,500 meters, 5K, and 10K, their performance bombed.[6] Even at the 1,500, a distance not usually thought to be affected by body water, they were 3% slower.

In the 10K, performance declined by a whopping 7%. For an elite athlete who can do this distance in under 30 minutes, that adds a huge 2 minutes to his time. At national level 10K competition, that would move you from winning to dead last. So if you want optimum performance, the unbreakable rule is: **Continually top up your water**.

And Not A Drop To Drink

But, and it's a big but, you have to drink it clean. Clean water is a scarce commodity. Most faucet water in America is badly polluted. Yet many athletes who are very careful what food they put into their bodies, are careless about water. They will drink from public water fountains, from faucets at home and gym, or from gym coolers filtered only through a cheap carbon filter to make the water taste better.

Biochemical analyses of some of these athletes, done at the Colgan Institute, show they have been ingesting polluted fluids, thereby polluting muscles, organs, and brain. If you do the same, don't expect to reach your potential. No high performance machine can operate at optimum with dirty lubricants.

Think I'm exaggerating? Today we tested the San Diego faucet water from our lab faucet (we test it each week). It registered 562 parts per million of contaminants. That's about average. Some cities are a bit cleaner, some a lot dirtier. Environmental Protection Agency figures show that about 85% of faucet water in America is now contaminated.

This contamination is beyond help. More than 55,000 of the *regulated* chemical dumps across the nation are leaking into the ground water.[7] Even the best of these regulated dumps are leaking. At Los Alamos, for example, with every type of control you can think of, radioactive wastes have now migrated into the ground water, and have spread two miles from their dump.[8]

If that's the best that regulation can achieve, imagine the state of the estimated 200,000 illegal, unregulated dumps. Each year the EPA regulates disposal of 50-60 million tons of toxic wastes. Yet the federal watchdog, the Office of Technology Assessment, reports that over 250 million tons are generated annually.[9] Where do you think the bulk of that toxic waste is going?

No secret. You can't incinerate it or dump it at sea -- too visible. You can't fire it into space -- too expensive. Most of it is dumped illegally in pits, holes, and hollows, where it leaks deep into the aquifers to pollute the ground water for hundreds of miles around. If you drink any of it, don't expect to excel at sports.

They Can't Clean The Water

Don't believe that water treatment authorities can protect you. In response to a critical article by the Colgan Institute that got wide publicity, our local authority sent us a thick wad of computer readouts showing negligible levels of 35 different chemicals that they tested for. I hated to remind them that there are more than 60,000 chemical contaminants of water. Any municipal water supply is likely to harbor at least a thousand. The Office of Technology Assessment reports a test of the water supplies of 954 cities, showing that almost 30% of them are "seriously contaminated".[10]

Water authorities do what they can, but it is far too expensive to make our tap water healthy enough to drink. Only a tiny fraction is drunk in any case. Most goes down the plug in bathroom, laundry, and kitchen.

So our tap water is treated only to minimum standards, by sedimentation, filtration, chemical conditioning, and disinfection with chlorine. The toxic metals, pesticides, industrial chemicals, *they are all still in there* when it comes out of your tap. So are the 50 or so chemicals used in the water treatment. So are the dead bacteria killed by the chlorine. So are the carcinogenic trihalomethanes from the chlorine itself, that are known to cause liver and colorectal cancers.[11] Oh, tap water will not kill you, or even make you obviously sick, but there is no way your body can function properly on poisons.

One telling example is a runner we were training for the last Olympics. After good training progress all winter in San Diego, in spring he moved to the altitude of Denver, to gain those extra oxygen carrying blood cells that come from training above 4,000 feet. After a couple months, training bombed.

His health was good and all blood tests were normal. But his hair showed arsenic levels of 11.4 ppm. Normal arsenic levels in hair run less than 2 ppm. We finally traced it to the tap water which came from a local "deep, pure" well. The well was slightly polluted with arsenic, probably from weedkiller runoff from adjacent farm land.

His daily dose of arsenic was tiny, but effects on performance were profound. We switched him to bottled distilled water and he slowly returned to top form. But not in time for the Olympic Trials. By dint of dirty water, he missed his shot. Don't let it happen to you.

Buying Clean Water

Bottled water is booming, with 350 American companies producing 425 brands. Imports add another 35 brands. Most people believe that the Food and Drug Administration carefully regulates this industry because it sells the most important nutrient in the human body. No way! Beyond simple hygiene, the bottled water industry is almost entirely self-regulated.

Why? Because most bottled water is simply tap water put through minimal conditioning filters to make it taste better.[12] That's why it's so profitable. Brands called "Mineral Waters" may have a modicum of minerals added. And "Sparkling Mineral

Waters", seltzers, and club sodas also have carbonation added. But they are all just tap water with most of its contaminants still in there. Brands labelled "Spring Water" legally have to be from a spring, unless the words are a brand name, or part of a brand name. Then they are just tap water.

There is nothing intrinsically wonderful about springs anyway. They are never pure water. Springs contain all kinds of organic matter and often some very toxic minerals. I know several springs in the Grand Canyon National Park that look as pure as new snow, but contain enough natural arsenic to kill you outright. Not a far-fetched example. Dr Joseph Weissman at UCLA Medical School reports a test of bottled Appollinaris water imported from West Germany, showing excessive levels of selenium and cobalt, and a level of arsenic that exceeded the EPA standards by 6000%.[13]

FDA regulations do not require water bottlers to test their wares for many minerals, or for the huge variety of other toxic contaminants likely to be present. Remember the Perrier fiasco? Perrier voluntarily withdrew its whole American stock, 72 million bottles, because traces of benzene got into one batch from a faulty filter. The company acted very responsibly, but the public was appalled. Benzene in drinking water!

I have news for you. The FDA does not require bottled water companies even to test for benzene, or for a variety of other solvent hydrocarbons that may be in the water. One bottling plant I toured two years ago, began each morning bottling cycle without any testing to see whether the solvents used to clean the system the night before had been properly flushed out. That company has since been cited for selling contaminated water.

Bottled distilled waters are the only clean bottled source. Virtually everything is removed from the water by steam distillation. Seven brands we have tested run from 2-12 ppm contaminants. That's about as clean as you can get.

Contrast those figures with typical faucet water at 350 - 1000 ppm contaminants. Whenever you drink the usual run of bottled water (essentially faucet water), these contaminants build into every cell of your body. If you aim to achieve top performance, stick to distilled.

Clean Your Own Water

The uncertainties and cost of bottled water have persuaded many sensible people to clean their faucet water at home. But most systems sold in this lucrative market by supermarkets, mail order, or pyramid marketing schemes, are pretty well useless. Those we have tested at the Colgan Institute remove only some of the larger particles, above 5 microns in diameter (1/5000th of an inch). The molecules of many chemicals, pesticides, and toxic metals are much smaller than that, and pass through the filter as if it wasn't there.

A big advance is the new four-step reverse osmosis system, using Kodak's cellulose triacetate (CTA) membranes. They can remove up to 97% of contaminants. The Colgan Institute has tested one of these systems for more than a year. For water that starts at 500 ppm contaminants (a common level for city water), the system produces water at 20-40 ppm contaminants.

Seeing the growing market for its membranes, Kodak itself has now entered the water cleaning business. It has just introduced an undersink system, linked to your water line, that feeds up to 25 gallons of purified water per day to a custom faucet. It is rated to remove 95% of contaminants, and sells for about $600.

But reverse osmosis is not the best method. Far and away the cleanest water is produced by the new home distillers. Unlike the older models that required frequent cleaning and manual attention, and lasted only 2-3 years, the latest distillers are no more trouble than your house furnace, and give constant clean water to faucets placed wherever you need them. They are built to last at least a decade.

One of the best is the Pure Water A-12 system produced by Pure Water Inc of Lincoln, Nebraska (402) 467-9300. We have been running and testing one of them continuously for over a year, producing 12 gallons of clean water per day. With entry water of 500 ppm contaminants, it yields water of 10-12 ppm. That's whistle clean H_2O.

Some folk object to this purity, complaining that the very emptiness of clean water causes it to leach minerals from the body. They have no understanding of basic biochemistry. As soon as you drink it, water becomes a soupy mixture with all the contents of your gut. On absorption through the intestinal wall, the mixture immediately blends with your body fluids and becomes part of you. There is no physiological way it can suck minerals out.

Other folk claim that, although it may not leach minerals, distilled water does not contain the essential minerals found in ground water. They point to studies showing lower rates of heart disease in areas with hard water, that is, water with lots of minerals. They are dead wrong. It is not the water people drink in those areas that prevents heart disease, it is the food they eat that is grown there.

If you relied on water for your minerals, you would be sadly lacking. It is the growing produce that takes up the water and concentrates its minerals, that provides most of your mineral requirements. The calcium content of a one-cup serving of pumpkin, for example, is about 80 mg if the pumpkin is grown in an area with 60 ppm calcium in the water. The calcium content of a cupful of the water itself is less than 10 mg. World authority on minerals Dr Eric Underwood of the University of Western Australia, states it plainly, "Plant materials provide the main source of minerals to animals and to most members of the human race." [14]

So use pure water simply for what it is, the main component of your body. What you need to know next, is how much water to use for peak performance, and when. That's all in Chapter 3.

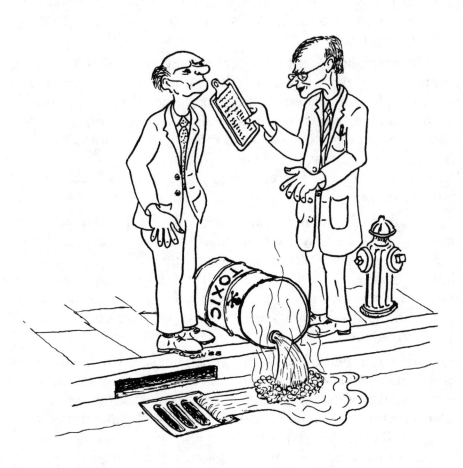

"Relax George. The City ought to give us a medal.
This stuff will kill every rat in the sewers".

Chapter 3

Play It Cool

Whenever your body is short of water, performance bombs. The three big factors involved are overheating, disruption of chemical balances, and dehydration. The biggest problem is overheating.

Exercise increases body temperature in direct proportion to the exercise load. Your body tries to maintain its resting temperature of 98.6°F, by moving the extra heat to the skin via the blood. There it dissipates into the air, mainly by evaporation of sweat. But your blood must also carry oxygen and nutrients to the muscles, and remove the wastes of muscle metabolism. Available blood is shared between all these tasks. The higher your core temperature rises, the more blood is used for cooling, and the less is available for the muscles. So the cooler you stay during exercise, short of being cold, the better your muscle function.

Outside the narrow range of 98-100°F, your body will always sacrifice muscle function for temperature regulation, because a decline in muscle function, even to complete immobility, is not life threatening. But if body core temperature rises a mere 9°F, normal biochemistry ceases and you die.[1]

Heavy exercise can increase heat production in muscles to more than 20 times their resting rate. Even with optimum hydration and a cool environment, this heat load can raise your core temperature to 103°F within 15 minutes. Studies by Dr David Costill and colleagues at Ball State University, Indiana, show that you can still perform well at this temperature, though probably not at your best.[2]

But when temperature rises above 104°F, your physiology starts to disintegrate. A large volume of blood is shunted to the skin for emergency cooling, causing blood pressure and cardiac output to fall, and depriving muscles of oxygen.[3] The usual symptoms are a feeling of overheating in the face, throbbing temples, and a chill over chest and trunk.

Many athletes continue to press under these conditions, driving core temperature over 105°F. At that level, you become dizzy, weak, and disoriented, and risk heat stroke. Alberto Salazar, former world record holder in the marathon, was notorious for forcing himself to run into the heat stroke zone, and celebrated several victorious races in the hospital. You have to admire his guts, but the long-term effects on his body were disastrous, and were a prominent factor in the premature end to his brilliant winning career.

The 70/70 Rule

One purpose of this book is to give you a long career, because it takes 12-15 years to develop the skills required to compete at an elite level in almost any sport. Another purpose is to inhibit the age decline in performance that usually begins by age 35. As a masters athlete myself, I want to see all us old toots continue to kick butt into extreme old age. It can be done with the right nutrition and training, but you also have to stay cool. Aim to keep your exercising temperature below 104°F.

Air temperature and humidity are important, and experienced athletes praise overcast skies and a few spits of cooling drizzle. A good rule of thumb is the 70/70, 80/60 rule. That is, when external temperature (°F) and humidity (%) both exceed 70, or when either exceeds 80 with the other over 60, do everything to stay cool.

Drink all liquids as cold as you can stand them, to give a reservoir of cold in the gut. Do warm up, but only enough to just break a sweat. Wear light and light colored clothing, and as little as possible. And stay out of the sun. Multi-time winner of the Boston marathon, Bill Rodgers, used to lie on the stone floor in a local church basement before the start of the race. World triathlon champion, Mark Allen, also takes cool comfort (and spiritual enlightenment) in churches.

Expose all the skin you can, to maximize heat loss by evaporation of sweat. Don't believe the ads that this or that type of cloth will "wick away" the sweat, leaving you cool and comfortable. Even the best wicking sports shirt creates a mini high humidity environment over every inch it covers. Humidity kills evaporation.

At the Colgan Institute, we tested various materials on athletes running at 6.5 minutes per mile on a flat course, in ambient temperatures of 70 - 75°F with humidity of 70 -80%. The coolest shirt was a skimpy mesh and tricot running top. But rectal temperature at the end of the run, was almost a degree higher than after the same run done in just shoes and shorts. Unlike the ancient Greeks, our social conventions prohibit sports in the buff; but from the point of view of temperature control, it's a pretty good idea.

Drink Big!

As a member of the American College of Sports Medicine, I support their recommendation[4] that endurance events longer than 10 miles (equivalent to sports of more than about one hour continuous duration) should not be held when the ambient temperature exceeds 82.4°F (28°C). Unfortunately, the weather often doesn't cooperate. But even in real hot conditions, if you follow the cool rules above, and also maintain hydration, body temperature usually plateaus below 104°F.

If dehydration sets in, however, temperature jumps sharply again, blood is diverted to the skin for emergency cooling, and muscles and brain are left short of oxygen. Energy metabolism also shifts and starts gobbling your glycogen store.[5,6] The science is technical and boring, but the implication is clear. To avoid overheating and sustain performance, you must drink enough water to sweat like a hog.

Yet athletes often object they don't feel thirsty during competition. True. Thirst sensors in throat and gut are inhibited during strenuous exercise,[7] even though you are losing water fast. So don't be fooled by lack of thirst. With our marathon runners, triathletes and any event beyond five minutes duration, we do everything possible to boost hydration. You should too.

Load Carbohydrates

Your first step to maintain hydration is to load carbohydrates in the six days before competition, because they are also a great source of water. After digestion, carbohydrates are converted to glycogen, and stored in your muscles and liver for use as fuel. But in order to store each gram of glycogen, the body also has to store 2.7 grams of water. Basic biochemistry, but great news for athletes.

Careful carbohydrate loading can double your usual glycogen store. How to do it right is explained in Chapter 10. In a 150 lb athlete, total stored glycogen increases from about 400 grams (14 oz.) to about 800 grams (28 oz.). The extra glycogen pulls in 400 x 2.7 grams of extra water (36 oz.), more than two pints.

Then the metabolism of glycogen during exercise forms another 0.6 grams of water per gram of glycogen used for energy.[8,9] So using the extra 400 grams you have loaded, yields a further 10 oz. of water. That yields a total of 46 oz. of extra water, making carbohydrate loading as important to fluid status as it is to glycogen status.

Prehydrate

The second step is prehydration. Numerous studies support our findings at the Colgan Institute that pre-event water loading yields lower performance temperatures, and smaller weight losses.[10,11] The rule is: drink extra water for two days before the event. Then, between four hours and one hour before competition, drink an 8 oz. glass every 10-15 minutes.

Drink another two glasses between 30 minutes and 20 minutes before the start. Then gain bladder comfort again. Drink nothing during the 20 minutes before you start, because your stomach requires that much time to nearly empty. Otherwise you will start with a lot of water sloshing about, which is uncomfortable and may cause cramps or inhibit breathing. Don't worry about a call to urinate during performance. With heavy exercise the kidneys almost shut down urine production.

Don't wait for the big event to prehydrate. Practice it during training. Athletes differ in their capacity to water-load. Some even get diarrhea. It improves with practice.

The amount of extra water you retain from drinking extra for two days before the event, varies widely with individuals, and with the amount of sodium and other nutrients in the diet. You do retain some of it. However, the water-loading on competition day is the more important source. In the four hours prior to competition, you can drink 80-100 oz. of water. You will lose 40-60 oz. in urine, leaving a net prehydration of perhaps 40 oz. So with carbohydrate loading yielding 46 oz., and water-loading yielding 40 oz., you have at least 86 oz. of extra water available for sweating. You will need every drop.

Drink During Performance

Some athletes tough it out without water during events, thereby avoiding time loss, disruption of rhythm, loss of concentration, and other bogeys. Several elite runners used to race "dry" before coming to the Colgan Institute. Yet they would lose over 5% bodyweight, indicating a big deficit of body water, with all its multiple effects in reducing performance.

Even if you take water at every opportunity during a race, it's never enough. In the marathon and ultra-distance events, we have measured bodyweight losses of 5-6% in athletes who drink copiously throughout competition. In the marathon, for example, say you drink at miles 4, 7, 10, 13, 16, 19, and 22, seven drinks in all. You get a paper cup with, hopefully, 5-6 ounces of water. Total drunk is about 40 oz., if you don't spill any. But sweat loss at best, marathon effort can be as high as 8 oz. per mile.[12] A common sweat rate is 6 oz. a mile, a total of 160 oz. for the race. Subtract the 40 oz. drunk while running and you get a huge 120 oz. deficit.

Dr David Costill ran subjects on the treadmill for two hours, some with no water and some given 3 1/2 oz. every five minutes for the first 100 minutes, 70 oz. in all. Despite the heavy intake, the water group still *lost* an average of 4 lbs bodyweight. So their total loss, including the water drunk was over 8 lbs. Without the drinks, they would have been severely dehydrated.

The water group finished in much better condition. Both water-loaded and water-deprived subjects showed an initial rise in temperature to 101.8°F in the first 60 minutes. Thereafter, temperature remained almost constant for the water group at around 102°F (39°C), a comfortable running heat. Temperatures of the water-deprived group continued to rise the whole two hours.[2]

The message from this research is pretty clear. Even if you are water-loaded before competition, you should take all the plain cold water you can during any long event. In running races beyond 1,500 meters, aim to grab two cups at each aid station. In triathlons, put three water bottles on your bike. In tennis, football, baseball, even weight training and karate, sip at every stop.

To return to the marathon example, say you have success-fully pre-loaded with 90 oz. of water (plus carbohydrate) and you also take 40 oz. of water on the run. Then you have a total extra water of 130 oz. on top of your normal bodyweight. On average, in temperate weather, at best marathon pace, a 150 lb runner loses about 160 oz. of water. So water-loaded runners should finish only 30 oz. light, less than 2% bodyweight.

That's the theory, but it doesn't quite work. They still lose 2-4% of bodyweight. Part is fat loss, but most is from faster sweating, therefore better cooling. When water intake matches sweat loss, temperature rises the least.[13] Loaded athletes initially have water to spare. So they can run harder. They therefore generate more sweat and lose more water than they would if they were not water-loaded.

Racing a marathon without preloading water or drinking on the run can raise temperature above 105°F.[16] That not only crucifies your biochemistry, it's also a great way to do permanent damage. Cool, comfortable and less dehydrated by comparison, the loaded athlete can run nearer maximum effort. Performance has to be better.

At the Colgan Institute, we measured 23 marathoners, 18 males and 5 females, with and without water-loading. Ages ranged from 21 to 47, and marathon times from 2 hours 21 minutes to 3 hours 38 minutes. With water-loading, *every one* of them did better marathon times, recovered faster, and felt better. We used the results of this study to calculate a rule of thumb estimate of improvement with water-loading. For a three hour marathoner, it yields about 9 minutes, that is 20 seconds per mile. Worth every drop.

Maximize Absorption

Drinking the water is easy: getting the body to absorb it may not be. Our tests agree with David Costill's laboratory that cold water, below 50°F (10°C), is absorbed faster than room temperature water.[15] As a bonus it supplies a reservoir of cold in the stomach that will absorb considerable body heat. Sip, don't gulp. Gulping swallows air which disturbs stomach function and slows absorption. The same applies to carbonated drinks. The gas slows absorption. Avoid them.

Almost anything added to water slows absorption. The walls of your intestines are semi-permeable membranes like very fine mesh. Water passes through easily but most particles do not.

So pure water, containing no particles, is absorbed rapidly. As soon as you dissolve anything in it, say sugar, absorption slows. In addition, dissolved particles make it harder for water to pass from the stomach to the small intestine, where it is absorbed.

Many commercial sports drinks contain high levels of glucose or sucrose or similar simple sugars. They inhibit absorption. Don't use them during exercise. Soft drinks and sodas are worse. Typically, they are over 10% simple sugars. If you drink 12 oz. of plain water, 8 oz. of it will empty from your stomach within 15 minutes. If you drink 12 oz. of a 10% sugar solution, less than 1 oz. will empty in the same period.[15]

But a lesser level of sugar can be helpful. Simple glucose at 1-5% hardly inhibits stomach emptying at all, and does provide a boost to blood glucose.[16] Fructose at 2% *enhances* stomach emptying and preferentially restores hepatic (liver) glycogen.[17] And **polymerized glucose** (made by chaining simple glucose molecules) also allows rapid emptying. In 1983, Dr Robert Sieple and colleagues at Ohio State University, confirmed earlier studies that a solution of 2% fructose plus 5% polymerized glucose empties from the stomach only a mite slower than plain water.[18]

Getting fluid from the stomach to the intestines is only half the story. It still has to be absorbed. Recent studies by Dr Mark Davis and colleagues at the University of South Carolina, showed little difference in absorption rates for glucose, fructose, and glucose polymers, when the solutions are at low concentration (5-7%).[19] So the *form* of sugar taken during exercise makes little difference to absorption. Fructose, however, causes less of a insulin burst than glucose, and is also superior at replacing hepatic (liver) glycogen.[20, 21]

Despite the research, heavy soft drinks and sucrose-based sports drinks still lead the market, because they have an inbuilt motivator: the sugar rush caused by their high sugar content creates a false feeling of increased energy. For fluid replacement during exercise, forego the feeling and stick by the science. Both your water and fuel stores will run a lot better on it.

A number of companies have followed the research to produce sports drinks that work well to maintain hydration. The Colgan Institute makes a fructose/glucose polymer drink "Crux", which is specially buffered for our research on reducing the stomach acidity of long endurance events. Crux has become popular on Everest expeditions, and other high altitude activities, where both dehydration and acid gut are pervasive problems.

An excellent brand that is widely available, is Hydra Fuel by TwinLab. Its 7% carbohydrate profile matches the latest research findings, and also includes small amounts of potassium, magnesium, chromium, phosphate and sodium, now shown to enhance fluid absorption.[22,23]

These drinks are especially important for the late stages of races, tennis matches, ball games, and ultra-distance events, because they permit you to maintain hydration while also absorbing carbohydrate, thus giving the body added fuel. We deal with the new discoveries for refueling on the run in Chapter 9.

Rehydrate

You have just finished a tough endurance event. How do you get your body back to normal? First, and most important you are dehydrated. Second, your stomach is in a highly acid condition and almost empty. Third, your muscles are loaded with the debris of metabolism. Fourth, your glycogen reserves are depleted. Fifth, and least important, you are in electrolyte *overload*, because the percentage of body water lost is much greater than the percentage of body minerals lost.

Rehydrate immediately by drinking plain cold water. Sip, don't gulp. Coax yourself, because the thirst response is still inhibited after performance.[24] Avoid juices, especially citrus juices, which inhibit rehydration because of their high sugar content, and only add to stomach acidity, promoting cramps and nausea. Plain water is the only story.

Until you are four large glasses ahead, avoid sodas, beer, fruit, yogurt, candy bars, muffins, and all other sugary, fatty comestibles proffered after races for the intestinal torture of the uninformed. If you have a sensitive gut, a quarter-teaspoon of bicarbonate of soda in your water, or two capsules of a sports buffering supplement, such as TwinLab Phos Fuel, can do wonders. Once your stomach is bathed with water, then all the sponsored goodies are fair game.

Don't sit down or lie down right after an event, no matter how tough. Muscle cramps and post-event injuries often occur because insufficient blood gets to the fatigued muscles to remove wastes. A lot of the force for blood circulation comes not from the heart, but from working muscles. Keep drinking and walking.

Continue drinking extra for the next twelve hours. A common problem among endurance athletes is chronic partial dehydration. They never drink enough to completely rehydrate. Usually they are back to training the day after competition, depleting their body water again. Remember if you are 100 oz. of water short, then counting losses in urine, it will take about twenty 8 oz. glasses over the next 12 hours to rehydrate you.

Carbohydrates are equally important. You want to replace muscle glycogen fast. So after four glasses of water, eat any easily digested complex carbohydrate, such as whole grain pancakes or whole grain pasta. Oatmeal and "Kashi" cereals are good; and carbohydrate loading drinks, such as TwinLab Ultra Fuel, also work well. Some fruits, such as bananas and apples are good, others, especially citrus are too acid. Cookies can be good or bad, and ice-cream fair to terrible. Confused? Don't be. The right carbohydrates for sport are detailed in Chapter 9.

Chapter 4

Real Food

Until the 1940s, most farmers returned essential minerals to the soil by mulching, manuring, and crop rotation. These methods have been used to maintain soil quality since agriculture began. Then, at the end of the Second World War, drug conglomerates making nitrates and phosphates for explosives, were suddenly left with few buyers for their stockpiles of chemicals. Frantic for new markets, they began selling nitrate/phosphate/potassium (NPK) fertilizers at fire sale prices that made traditional farming methods uneconomic.

By the 1960s, 97% of American farms had become totally dependent on NPK fertilizers to make a living.[1] Mixtures of nitrogen phosphorus and potassium will grow fine-*looking* produce. But as each succeeding crop soaked up the other minerals in the soil, and only N, P, and K were replaced, soil quality was decimated. Many essential minerals declined virtually to zero. The latest RDA handbook, for example, reviews studies indicating a direct correlation between the growth of NPK fertilization and declining magnesium levels in our food supply.[2]

Human bodies are not vegetables. They cannot grow on NPK alone. Bodies also require selenium, chromium, calcium, magnesium, iron, copper, iodine, molybdenum, zinc, cobalt, boron, and vanadium.[2] Bodies cannot make minerals. If they are not in the soil, they are not in the produce, and they are not in you. Without consuming every one of the essential minerals in adequate amounts, no athlete can expect top performance. From the soils we have today and the produce and food animals that grow on them, that is an impossible task.

Nutrient Losses in Processing

Soil degradation is only the first problem with our food. Further nutrients are lost in ripening, storing, drying, cooking, freezing, blanching, pasteurization, hydrogenation, ultrafiltration, and multiple other practices of modern food processing. The RDA handbook reviews hundreds of studies, showing that the already degraded crops of today, may lose even their meager supply of nutrients between harvesting and your table.[2]

The handbook states, "the tocopherol [vitamin E] content of foods varies greatly depending on processing, storage, and preparation procedures during which large losses may occur" (p.101). Vitamin C can be "considerably lower because of destruction by heat and oxygen" (p.117). Vitamin B6: 50-70% is lost in processing meats, and 50-90% is lost in milling cereals (p.144). Folic acid: "as much as 50%...may be destroyed during household preparation, food processing, and storage" (p.150).

For magnesium, the mineral essential for all cell growth and replacement, the RDA handbook states, "more than 80% is lost by removal of the germ and outer layers of cereal grains" (p.189). Next time you eat a slice of bread, remember that the germ and outer layers of grains are removed in the making of all white and so-called "enriched" flours.

These facts don't come from some scare-mongering media report. They are from the handbook of the Recommended Dietary Allowances published in November, 1989 by the US National Academy of Sciences. They are the official word on American nutrition.

There are numerous other authoritative sources indicating the degradation of our food. Dr Robert Harris, Professor Emeritus of Biochemistry at MIT, documents enormous destruction of nutrients in vegetables in modern cold storage.[3] Every time you eat an apple and see the flesh turn brown within a few minutes, remember that is a sign that the apple has oxidized in storage, and has lost most of its vitamins.[4] Dr Theodore Labuza, Professor of Food Technology at the University of Minnesota, reports up to 90% losses of thiamin in the drying of meats.[3] Professor Darryl Lund of the Department of Food Science of the University of Wisconsin, shows that blanching of vegetables and fish, can destroy one-third to one-half of their thiamin, riboflavin, niacin, pyridoxine, and vitamin C.[3] Similar large losses of B-vitamins and vitamin C occur in the pasteurization and ultrafiltration of milk.[5] Dr Henry Schroeder, foremost American authority on nutrient content of foods, reports that freezing of meats can destroy up to 50% of the thiamin and riboflavin, and 70% of the pantothenic acid.[6]

If you add up the nutrient losses that have accrued to our food since the late 1940s, there is not a great deal left. First came degradation of the soils by use of nitrogen/phosphorus/potassium fertilizers, that do not contain the minerals essential to human health. Then came development of modern food processing that has stripped our food of many of its vitamins.

Now we have also irradiated foods that do not rot, and may be years old and devoid of vitamins by the time you eat them. And 1992 is the first year of the bioengineered foods, the genetic alteration of which changes their nutrient content in yet unknown ways. Tomatoes that don't freeze and die in a sudden frost because they contain genes from the arctic flounder may be great for farmers, but they leave human bodies out in the cold. No athlete can develop top performance from such poor raw materials.

The only way to obtain decent vegetables and fruits is, avoid all processed produce and buy fresh, outside the mainstream of the produce industry:

1. Buy your produce close to the ground that it came from.
2. Buy only organic vegetables and fruits, if possible, straight from the farm.

3. Buy at local farm outlets.
4. Buy only certified organic produce, preferably from
   health food stores and local markets.

Fatty Fatty Fatty

You can't help but notice the ad campaigns by the meat industry, claiming that beef, veal, and pork are both healthy and low in fat. Both claims are essentially false. This bogus image is being desperately paraded to save a failing market. Beef consumption has dropped steadily, from a peak of nearly 95 lbs per person per year in 1976, to less than 70 lbs. [7]

For some years, the Colgan Institute has published articles in numerous magazines, decrying the woeful state of American meat. Wide publicity for our articles in the last two years prompted the National Livestock and Meat Board, and various state meat councils to write us letters of complaint. In reply we quoted government and university sources for fat and drug content of meats, and challenged the meat industry to prove its figures.

Since we sent them our data, the National Livestock and Meat Board have been strangely silent. We requested that they contribute a statement to this book, but they have not deigned to reply. They had their chance: now I'll give you the facts.

It's true that the meat industry is now breeding leaner meat, but it is still not nearly lean enough. Let's do the numbers. According to USDA figures one of the leanest beef cuts is doublebone sirloin steak.[8] A 12 oz. sirloin, dry-broiled and trimmed, yields 6.6 oz. of meat, including 1.8 oz. of fat. When you exclude the 107 grams of water content (57%) which has zero calories, the lean meat left is 61 grams. The fat left is 19 grams including 9 grams of saturated fat. Lean meat (protein) is 4 calories per gram, fat is 9 calories per gram. So the juicy sirloin steak works out as:

Fat   19 grams x 9 calories = 171 calories = 41%
          (including 81 calories of saturated fat)

Protein   61 grams x 4 calories = 244 calories = 59%

Total   415 calories

So, being as generous as possible to the meat industry, one of the best lean cuts is still 41% total fat, 19.5% saturated fat. That's way above the government health recommendations of 30% total fat, 10% saturated fat. Almost all other cuts of beef are even fattier.

Pork is worse. Now touted as "the other white meat" clever advertisements by the National Pork Production Council try to dupe consumers into believing that pork is as healthy as poultry. On March 23, 1990 the Center for Science in the Public Interest filed a petition with the Federal Trade Commission to stop the pork industry's misleading ads. By USDA figures, fat calories in average trimmed cuts of pork run a whopping 53%![9] Compare the photos of decent, organic, free-range pork we bought from the farm, with the cut we bought from the supermarket. No

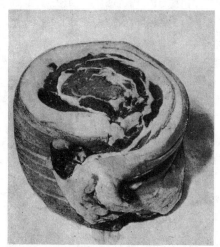

Figure 3. Pork from a factory farm, confined lifelong and given steroid hormones, antibiotics and other drugs.

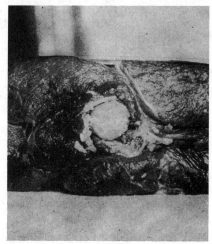

Figure 4. Free-range pork bred without drugs.

athlete should put the supermarket version into his body. The fat in an average pork chop would grease two sumo wrestlers.

Meat Pollution

If you value your health, fat content alone is enough to turn you off meats. But that's only the beginning. Most meats in America are seriously contaminated with antiobiotics, hormones, pesticides, and other chemical residues.

In 1991, the Centers for Disease Control (CDC) in Atlanta released figures showing that approximately half of the 15 million pounds of antibiotics made annually in America, are used on livestock and poultry. Over 90% of pigs and veal calves, 60% of cattle, and 95% of all poultry have antibiotics routinely added to their feed.

This routine use of penicillin and tetracycline derivatives in animal feed has caused the breeding of drug-resistant strains of bacteria, which now remain in the meat until you eat it. This problem was first confirmed in 1986 when CDC tracked a drug-resistant strain of salmonella from an infected herd of cattle, to diners who ended up in hospital with salmonella poisoning. Since then, following numerous outbreaks, CDC has issued public warnings that chickens and eggs may carry drug-resistant salmonella and campylobacter. These food-poisoning bacteria *kill* 2,000 Americans every year and make another six million people sicker than hell. At least *half* of all raw chicken (and eggs) sold in America is contaminated.[10]

And the only way to make it safe is to cook it to death. The official advice for eggs is to fry both sides for *seven minutes* each. Thanks CDC, I tasted those leather eggs once in Las Vegas, and offered to eat the menu instead.

Literally hundreds of other drugs are used on livestock, and there are huge stocks of banned drugs still in use. In 1989, the pesticide heptachlor, banned as a carcinogen since 1978, turned up in 400,000 Arkansas chickens. The antibacterial drug sulfamethazine, another known carcinogen, is a further example.

Beyond a certain minimum level that will not contaminate dairy products, it is illegal for use on dairy cattle. The FDA reported in 1988 that one-quarter of all milk samples tested were contaminated with sulfamethazine. Sounds so bad you may think I am exaggerating. Don't take my word for it. You can confirm all these horror stories and more by calling the US Department of Agriculture (USDA) Meat and Poultry Hotline, (800) 535-4555.

But don't expect government agencies to do anything great to protect you. Testing of meat and poultry is done by the USDA itself. Their own internal audit investigations show they do it very badly. The 1988 report shows inspection errors, lost samples, incomplete testing, and allowing meats to proceed to market that should have been impounded. Overall, 78% of the meat inspection reports examined were deemed inadequate.[11] You have to protect yourself.

Healthy Meat

The free-range organically grown meat that made America great, the meat that everyone used to eat, is now a hard-to-find luxury. With all the publicity given to organic farming and clean food, you would think the market is booming. No way. The going is tough to convert to chemical-free, low-fat livestock. **Health Foods Business** reports that, of 59 companies who attempted to "go natural" up to 1987, less than a dozen were still in business in 1990.[7]

The big reason is cost. It is impossible to produce low-fat livestock that are free of antibiotics, hormones, and pesticides that are also cost-competitive with mass produced livestock. First, they need space, preferably free range. To stay lean, cattle like people have to exercise. They exercise by foraging. But the land they forage on has to be clean, free of pesticides. So you have a double-whammy cost of more land per animal, and clean land too. With over 90% of America's agricultural land, pesticide contaminated, you pay an arm and a leg for any bit that isn't.

Then you need feed that is chemical free. Mary Lou Bradley, owner of B3R Country Meats, one of the best sources of clean meat, has a grain bill 10% higher than the average cattle rancher. Then you send them to slaughter earlier and leaner. Bill Dunkelberger of Lean & Free Meats, has his beef slaughtered at 1,000 lbs, compared with 1,300 lbs for mass produced beef. That's 300 lbs of meat per animal that he doesn't get paid for. So his prices have to be higher. But in return, you get beef that is naturally 25% leaner. For those athletes who want top

Table 2. Natural Meats Suppliers*

Beef/Veal
B3R Country Meats Inc., 2100 West Highway 287, Childress, Texas 79201 (817) 937-8870
Clean and Lean, Peach Valley Ranch, Honeywood, Ontario, Canada (519) 925-6628
Coleman Natural Beef Inc., 5140 Race Ct., #4, Denver, Colorado 80216 (303) 297-9393
Lean & Free Products, Inc., 5265 Rockwell Dr., NE, Cedar Rapids, IA 52402 (800) 383-BEEF

Poultry
Health is Wealth, Sykes Lane, Williamstown, NJ, 08094 (609) 728-1998
Rocky the Chicken, PO Box 1817, Sebastopol, CA 95473 (707) 829-5432
Shelton's Poultry, 204 Loranne, Pomona, CA 91767 (714) 623-0634
Zacky Farms, 200 N. Tyler Avenue, SO El Monte, CA 91733 (800) 858-0235

*Source: The Colgan Institute, San Diego, CA.

performance, some of the best sources of clean, lean meats are given in Table 2. Eat them hearty.

Fishy Business

With all the bad reports about the fats, hormones, and pesticide residues on meats, and the salmonella contamination of poultry and eggs, fish has fast become the popular alternative source of protein. American fish consumption increased 25% since 1980.

Then, disaster! In 1992, Consumers Union published results of a six-month investigation of the fish industry. They bought fish from the same places you buy it, supermarkets, grocery stores, and speciality fish shops. They sampled seven popular varieties, salmon, flounder, sole, catfish, swordfish, lake whitefish, and clams. It all smelled!

Almost 40% of the fish samples were beginning to spoil at the time of purchase. Ninety percent of the swordfish were contaminated with mercury. Half the whitefish and 40% of the salmon contained polychlorinated biphenyls (PCBs). The clams were laced with arsenic and lead. And this is the one that really got me: almost half of all the fish samples were contaminated with bacteria from *animal or human feces.*[12]

Microbiology experts reported to Consumers Union that sewage outflows were not the source of fecal contamination of the fin fish, only the clams. The fin fish became contaminated **after** being caught. The report cites a litany of appalling sanitary practices during handling, processing, and distribution. Fecal coliform counts above 10 per gram is the standard for contamination. One in five of the Consumers Union samples had counts *exceeding 100 per gram*. Vomit city!

The Centers for Disease Control report that fish and shellfish cause about 10% of all outbreaks of food poisoning in America. But, as Dr Sanford Miller of the University of Texas Health Science Center points out, fish poisoning is greatly under-reported. Often an upset gut and general malaise is attributed to 'flu or stomach bug rather than the tuna sandwich you ate yester-day. No athlete can afford these drains on health and training.

The American fish industry is a stinking mess. Preliminary results of the Food and Drug Administration's review of 3,852 fish-processing plants released in February 1992, were so bad that, as I write, they are hastily staffing their new Office of Seafood to try to regain control. They would not put a number on it, but they did tell me that the problems would take years to solve.[13] If you are going to use fish as a low-fat source of protein, you have to protect yourself.

Finding Good Fish

If fish smells fishy, it's kaput. Fresh fish has virtually no smell. As soon as it starts to go bad, fish produces a chemical called **tri-methylamine** which gives the fishy odor. It's a definite sign of spoilage.

The next trick is to avoid certain fish altogether. Avoid swordfish (mercury and PCB contamination), lake whitefish (PCB contamination), oysters, mussels and clams (lead con-tamination), the large tuna species, yellowfin and bigeye (mer-cury contamination). Don't buy from stores that display cooked and raw fish on the same layer of ice, even if they are separated. Don't buy from stores that pile the fish up so high that the top fillets get heated by the case lights. And never buy a whole fish unless it is completely embedded in ice, has bright bulging eyes, and vivid color.

Many ocean and lake areas are so badly contaminated that the fish from them are deliberately mislabelled so you don't know where they come from. But, if you can find out, don't buy Great Lakes fish, fish from the Los Angeles Basin, the San Francisco Basin, the New Jersey coast, Puget Sound, and the Boston Harbor area. The Environmental Protection Agency, and numerous other studies, [14] report that all are heavily contaminated.

Buy the fish from Alaska, Australia, and New Zealand, whose waters are low in pollutants. Unfortunately, even some

Alaskan fish are now threatened by leaking radioactive wastes from defunct Soviet testing sites on the islands of Novaya Zemlya and from widespread radioactivity in runoff of the Ob and Yenisey rivers in Siberia.[23] So if that Alaska or Artic salmon glows in the dark - bury it.

I didn't include Scandinavian fish because trade restrictions have made most of it history. So that "fresh Norwegian salmon" isn't. For poor man's salmon, buy only the small species of tuna, skipjack, and albacore. Being lower on the food chain, they are only lightly polluted. Buy flounder and sole, the least polluted fish in the Consumer Union Study. Buy Australasian orange roughy: extremely low-fat and virtually contamination free.

As a staple of athletes and the most eaten fish in America, canned tuna deserves the last word. There is no bacteria problem because the canning involves high heat that kills everything. But tests by Consumers Union showed that 50% of the cans they bought contained filth from insects, rodents, and birds. In the early '70s there was a similar stink over canned fish. With a massive clean-up effort, tuna was cleaned of virtually all filth by 1979.[12] But since then, almost all canning has moved outside the US, to countries that have low-low standards of hygiene. So it will be a hard problem to fix.

Overall best tuna in the Consumers Union study was canned albacore (white tuna). Best water-packed brands of albacore for taste and cost are Bumble Bee, Lady Lee, and Empress Fancy. At less than one gram of fat per 100 grams (31/2 oz.), and 24 grams of first-class protein, tuna is still one of your best choices.

Food for Athletes

This book spends a lot of chapters on vitamins, minerals, and other nutrient supplements. But make no mistake, for top performance **food is first.** After 18 years of research on thousands of athletes with every diet known or dreamed of, we have a handle on the food that works. **The basis of the optimum sports diet is whole grains and vegetables.**

Every kind of domestic vegetable you can think of forms a good source of carbohydrate. Many fruits do also, although they should be kept as a minor food resource because of their high content of simple sugars. Go very easy on fruit juices. Most of them contain higher levels of sugar than sodas. Orange juice causes more insulin bursts in America than Coke and Pepsi combined.

The top 20 grains and legumes for athletes are given in Table 3. Why legumes? Because beans combined with grains form complete proteins, although not as good as proteins from animal sources. Incidentally, you don't have to eat them at the same time as some dopey books on food combining suggest. The body is much cleverer than that. It will take the amino acids from morning beans on toast and combine them with the amino acids from evening rice to provide all the essential amino acids.

Table 3. Top Twenty Grains and Legumes for Athletes*

Best Protein Sources Over 20% Protein Under 20% Fat	Best Carbohydrate Sources Under 5% Fat Over 70% Carbohydrate
Soybeans	Brown Rice
Split Peas	Whole Barley
Kidney Beans	Whole Buckwheat
Dried Whole Peas	Whole Rye
Wheatgerm	Foxtail Millet
Lima Beans	Wild Rice
Black-eyed Peas	Whole Corn
Lentils	Pearl Millet
Black Beans	Whole Wheat
Navy Beans	Rolled Oats

*Source: The Colgan Institute, San Diego, CA.

The other common query about vegetable proteins, is whether the quality is as high as proteins from meats and dairy foods. Using the old method of protein equivalency ratios (PER), vegetable proteins do not score as high.

But scientist have known for decades that the PER standard bears little relation to human needs for amino acids or to the bioavailability of proteins.[15] PERs were derived in Victorian times, and the only reason for survival of such an archaic method is the fierce lobbying and powerful influence of the meat and dairy industries over the last fifty years.

Finally, it seemed that nutrition science had prevailed. In 1992, the FDA decreed that protein quality be evaluated by a new method that takes into account all the recent advances in determining human needs for amino acids.[15] Evidence reviewed by an expert committee of the Food and Agriculture Organization of the United Nations, and independently by protein expert Dr Vernon Young and his colleagues at the Massachusetts Institute of Technology, shows that, in the past, animal proteins have been over-valued, and vegetable proteins, especially soy protein, have been under-valued.[15,16]

The tongue-twister name of the new method is **Protein Digestibility Corrected Amino Acid Score**, or **PDCAAS** for short. Trust the FDA to make it as complicated as possible. I wrote to them suggesting the simple name **Protein Score** or **PS**, but they would have none of it.

By the PDCAAS, the quality of a food protein is assessed by its content of essential amino acids, the ratios of these amino acids to each other, and their bioavailability. Best quality soy protein is given a PDCAAS of 1.0.[17] That means it provides high quality protein, complete in all essential amino acids.

So it does, but it isn't the best. The new method of protein analysis is fine, but in complete contradiction to PCDAAS scores achieved by other proteins, such as whey protein and egg protein, the FDA has decreed that 1.0 is the maximum score to be permitted on food labels.[18] That may be OK for couch potatoes, but when you read the research in Chapters 12, 13 and 32, you will see how nonsensical it is for athletes.

Another big problem with a lot of bean and soy products is taste. I have yet to find a good vegieburger, and bland to tasteless is the best you can say for soydogs. But by the time this book comes out, the problem should be solved. Dr Arthur Spanier of the USDA has just reported to the American Chemical Society, that USDA scientists have isolated the natural compound that gives beef it's meaty flavor. The 8-amino-acid compound, termed BMP, can be added directly to foods such as tofu, to make them taste almost exactly like the best cuts of beef. That may cure an errant physician friend of mine who wanders along the soy aisle at food trade show,s peering into sizzling pans of soy dogs and soy bacon, loudly proclaiming "Hmm, fried prophylactics."

Many people can't stomach beans and soybean products however they taste, because the undigested sugars, **raffinose** and **stachyose**, ferment in their gut with explosive results. If you are an unrepentant athlete who is determined to remain vegetarian, a new product, Beano, in the cooking eliminates the problem. Made by Akfarma of Pleasantville, New Jersey, Beano contains an enzyme, **alpha-galactosidase,** which digests the errant sugars for you. It also works for sufferers from the effects of raw broccoli, cabbage, falafel, oat bran, whole wheat, and other whole grains that contain gas-producing sugars. A boon for anyone making gut-wrenching efforts in their training.

Eat A High-Fiber Diet

If you base your diet on grains and vegetables, you will naturally get large dollops of fiber. It does a lot more than the popular claims of keeping you regular, holding down cholesterol, and preventing colon cancer.[19] For athletes, fiber is essential to reduce bodyfat and to stabilize blood sugar.

The bodyfat effect is covered in Chapter 13. The blood sugar effect is equally important. Studies of diabetes show conclusively, that a high daily intake of dietary fiber stabilizes glucose so effectively, that many pre-diabetic patients never have to succumb to the use of insulin, and many diabetics can reduce or even eliminate their insulin.[20,21]

The Colgan Institute recommends that athletes get 40 grams of fiber daily. But it isn't quite that simple. Loosely defined, fiber is not a food for humans. It is that part of plant foods that the human system cannot digest. There are hundreds of different fibers, each with different physiological effects. Science is still trying to sort out which one does what. The six basic categories are: **celluloses, hemicelluloses, gums, mucilages, pectins** and **lignins**.

To ensure the best results, you should eat some of each, from the soluble fibers like pectins in apples and carrots, and the gummy fiber in oat bran, to the insoluble celluloses in wheat bran and other grains. As with all foods, one key to optimal sports nutrition is variety.

Table 4. Fiber 10. The best common sources of fiber.*

Each food choice contains about 10 grams of dietary fiber		
Grains	**Vegetables**	**Fruits**
½ cup All Bran	½ cup mixed beans	2 cups raisins
1 cup Rolled Oats	½ cup peas	3 pears
½ cup Fiber One	½ cup lentils	3 bananas
½ cup Bran Buds	1 cup peanuts	4 peaches
1 cup Grapenuts	2 cups soybeans	4 nectarines
3 cups Puffed Wheat	3 cups steamed vegies	4 oz. blackberries
4 Shredded Wheat	3 cups pumpkin seeds	4 oz. raspberries
2 cups sweet corn	4 servings mixed salad	5 apples
3 slices rye bread	4 large carrots	6 oranges
4 slices wheat bread	5 cups cauliflower	10 dried figs
4 oz. bag popcorn	5 cups broccoli	20 prunes

*Source: The Colgan institute, San Diego, CA.

Never use psyllium or other medical fiber preparations to get your fiber. Use food. For the best variety of fiber, see Table 4. When buying cereal, get the plain kind, and buy **unsulfered**, **unsugared**, dried fruits separately to mix with it. The fruits mixed into most of the muesili-type cereals we have tested are abysmal.

Avoid New Wave Junkfood

Used to be that junkfood meant a double-bacon-cheeseburger with all the trimmings. But today, it is dressed in shiny "health-food" packaging and lurks on every supermarket shelf. Modern packaged processed foods can contain any number of 2,000 preservatives, emulsifiers, conditioners, thickeners, synthetic dyes and other chemicals that have no place in an athlete's body.

A loaf of "wheat" bread I picked up at the supermarket yesterday contained 53 ingredients. In contrast, a loaf of excellent local whole-wheat bread contains five ingredients including the water. You are eating the bread for the grains. Make sure you get what you pay for.

Become a skilled label reader. Ignore the bread and baked goods that scream "WHOLE WHEAT." Most contain only a sprinkle thrown at the dough vat from a great distance. Turn to the "Ingredient List" that legally cannot lie. It may be hidden with the tiniest permissible print, but the first and therefore largest ingredient will usually read "enriched flour." That means white flour with all the nutrients removed and only a few added back again.[19] Leave it on the shelf.

Don't rely on the "Nutritional Information" list either. I can get excellent nutrition information scores by grinding up cockroaches. But anyone who reads the ingredients wouldn't buy them. The Ingredients List is the key. Any time you see a lot of chemicals, or even a lot of ingredients in a simple food like bread or baked goods, leave it for people who have no care for a healthy body.

Here's a good example of the Madison Avenue wordscams that now bedeck our food. A new squad of athletes I was training were all chewing in the gym. "Granola bars, Doc. Healthy stuff," said one worthy. I looked at the label. Ingredients included peanut butter, chocolate coating, and chocolate chips: 170 calories, with 100 of them from fat. That's 58% fat, worse than most candy bars. The relation between those bars and real granola is non-existent.

How about turkey roll labelled "90% fat-free." Not bad you might think: only 10% fat. Pul-e-e-e-e-ze! Ingredients are given by weight. The real numbers for a 100 gram (3 1/2 oz.) serving are:

Water weight	70 grams	0 calories
Fat weight	10 grams	90 calories
Protein weight	20 grams	80 calories
	Total	170 calories

The actual fat content of this supposed low-fat food beloved of athletes is 90/170 calories, a whopping 53%. That's higher fat than regular ice-cream.

God Dwells In The Details

To sum up, aim to eat only certified organic vegetables, fruits and grains. Avoid all imported produce. Avoid all hormone and drug-infested meats and dairy foods. Eat only certified drug-free organic meats and poultry. Avoid all American fish, except flounders, sole, and albacore. Eat Australasian fish freely. Avoid all processed junk food.Use your eyes and nose to test for freshness, and read the ingredients not the advertising.

Some folk may think I go overboard in this chapter. After all, say my critics, millions of ordinary people eat the Standard American Diet (SAD) of processed and contaminated food every day, and come to no apparent harm.The key words are *apparent* and *ordinary*. Most people are sedentary and overweight and subject to spiralling incidence of all sorts of diseases including cancer.[22] Their bodies are capable of very little. No successful athlete can be that way. Athletes are not ordinary. You are reading this book because you are extraordinary: you want to excel. Excellence grows only from attention to detail.

Before Bela Karoli came to America, US gymnastics was in the doldrums. He brought with him his unique focus on detail, a half-inch placement of the hand here, a hairs breadth turn of the foot there, even the way a gymnast moves her eyes. The result: multiple Olympic golds. Bela is one of those rare masters of movement, who know above all that God dwells in the details.

I want to instill into you the same precision, the same attention to detail about your nutrition. The biochemistry of nutrition is exact. Only the best will build you a premium body. If you make this book your bible of sports nutrition, I want it to be able to make you a champion.

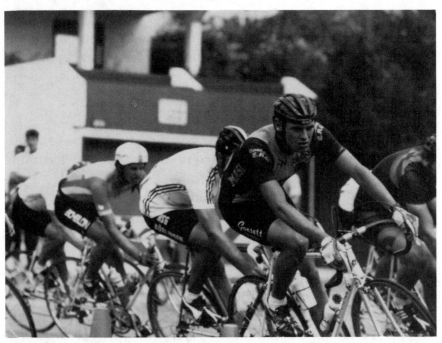

Champion cyclist Howard Dorfling leading the pack. Howard used the Colgan Institute program in his development from club cyclist status to membership of the U.S. Cycling Team.

Chapter 5

Give
Me Air

A recent headline in **USA Today** ran, "101.8 Million People Are Breathing Unsafe Air." That came from a congressional report on data dragged from a reluctant Environmental Protection Agency by Rep. Henry Waxman (D-Cal). Waxman concluded, "The magnitude of this problem far exceeds our worst fears."

Waxman is right. Air pollution is a massive health problem. Let's look at Los Angeles, one of the worst areas in the nation. Dr Bart Ostro, an epidemiologist with the California Department of Health Services, examined 320 apparently healthy, non-smoking men and women in north-central Los Angeles, who had kept daily logs of respiratory symptoms for six months. Onset of symptoms correlated with smog and the day following a smoggy day.[1]

But that was only coughs and colds and shortness of breath. Dr Russell Sherwin and colleagues at the University of Southern California found a lot more serious evidence. They examined the lungs of 85 Los Angeles residents aged 14-25 who had died in homicides or traffic accidents. Evidence of smog damage was severe, including chronic bronchitis, inflamed bronchial glands, and tiny holes "burned" in the lung tissue. Ozone was definitely involved, because chimpanzees exposed to ozone develop identical holes in lung tissue.[2]

The immune system is also weakened. Acting on

thousands of reports by physicians of increases in immune-related diseases, in April 1992 the US National Research Council asked immunologists all across America to redouble efforts to identify environmental pollutants that are causing immune damage.[3] Air pollutants are especially suspect. Incidence of asthma, for example, has risen 58% since 1970.[4]

To sum up the evidence of many studies, in February 1992, Dr Jane Hall and colleagues at California State University and the University of California, reported that the air quality of the Los Angeles Basin "remains the worst in the nation," and that 12 million residents experience respiratory disorders and an increased risk of death as a direct result of air pollution.[5]

Don't think you can overcome air pollution because of your healthy athletic lungs. Your muscles, bones, organs, even the enamel of your teeth are all rebuilt continuously out of what you eat, drink, and breathe. Over 98% of the you that is reading this page is entirely reconstructed from the substances that entered your body during the last 12 months, including all the man-made chemicals, particulate matter, and toxic gases in your air.[6] The quality of your body structure and its performance is dependent on the quality of what you put into it. To the degree that the air you breathed was polluted in the last year, so is your flesh today.

Don't think that I'm overstating the case and that air pollution is a minor problem for healthy athletes. One promising British runner protested my ban on athletes training in Griffith Park, one of the worst polluted areas in Los Angeles. He went right on and ended up in the hospital still protesting, "But Doc, it's only a wee bit of bronchitis." I remember a sweet young lass who once told me she was only a wee bit pregnant...

Smog Poisoning

The dirty yellow-brown pall blanketing the San Bernardino Freeway as I race this morning towards the Sierra Mountains, is mute evidence of the continuing release of our primary industrial pollutant, nitric oxide, throughout Los Angeles. Nitric oxide reacts with sunlight to form the brownish toxic gas nitrogen dioxide. Despite the shiny new Clean Air Act, levels are not declining.

The other main contributor to the haze and the smell is ozone from car exhausts and from the action of sunlight on nitrogen dioxide and certain man-made hydrocarbons. But the worst is the unseen danger of carbon monoxide from the burning of gasoline, oil, and coal. Carbon monoxide (CO) is tasteless, odorless, colorless, and deadly.

However good the diet and the training, unless you also combat these pollutants in your air, you cannot develop top potential. Unfortunately, although there are thousands of air pollutants, science knows next to nothing about the detrimental effects of most of them. Here we will examine only two, ozone and carbon monoxide, because at least with these we have some decent data on athletes.

Ozone

Some folk are confused about ozone. After all, the ozone layer protects us from solar ultra-violet and it is man-made chlorofluorocarbons that are making holes in it. And ozone is used in biochemistry to kill bacteria. So it must be good. Right? Wrong! The ozone layer 12 miles straight up does protect us. The same concentration at ground level would kill you in a minute.

It is ozone's capacity to kill bacteria that also damages people. Until man-made pollution raised the ozone levels in our ground level air, there was very little of it around, just enough to give you that stimulating whiff of "sea air" as you came to the coast. Now in our urban areas ozone is present in toxic concentrations everywhere.

At a level of only 0.3 parts per million (ppm) in air, ozone inflames human lungs, even while resting in a chair. Athletes in heavy training breathe up to 20 times the air of sedentary folk and breathe deeper, sucking the ozone in each breath into the deepest reaches of your lungs. Studies show that the threshold level of ozone for lung damage in athletes is less than 0.2 ppm.[7,8] To put that in perspective, 0.2 ppm is an EPA Stage 1 Pollution Alert. The federal ozone limit for clean air is 0.12 ppm. Los Angeles has about 170 days per year when ozone exceeds 0.2 ppm, running up to 0.9 ppm. New York has about 100 days, Phoenix - 80, San Diego - 70, and Houston - 60. No athlete can maintain an optimum body with such exposure.

The first problem that ozone creates is inflammation of the bronchioles, much like the inflammation that occurs in asthma. Breathing is inhibited and the energy cost of each breath increases. Consequently, the maximum amount of oxygen the athlete can take in (VO2max) is reduced. Numerous studies have shown that athletes breathing air with ozone levels at peak daily levels of our major cities, suffer up to 10% reduction in maximum performance.[9-12] That's the difference between winning and last in many sports.

But acute effects of ozone on performance are the minor problems. The real guts is the continuing damage done to your body that will prevent you achieving top potential. Ozone damages tissue by generating **free radical chain reactions**, damaging bronchioles of the lungs by attacking polyunsaturated lipids in cell membranes, and damaging and killing red blood cells by generating **hydrogen peroxide** in the blood.[13] These are long-term effects that can hurt performance for weeks following even a few days of ozone exposure.

Studies of rats exposed to low levels of ozone give us an idea of the damage many athletes are doing to themselves while training in our major cities. In one study, rats were fed a diet adequate in all nutrients, equivalent to the human levels of the Recommended Dietary Allowances. They were then exposed to levels of ozone of 0.1 ppm, the low end of current daily levels in New York and the Los Angeles Basin. Almost all the rats developed lung lesions.[14]

Coming up to the 1984 Olympics, I lambasted the US Olympic Committee in print and on television for holding events such as the marathon in highly polluted areas, just to suit the mighty TV sponsors.[15] The USOC replied by getting some tame scientists (dependent for their livelihood on university grants from Olympic sponsors) to claim that athletes could adapt to the air pollution by training in it. Thankfully, the best coaches agreed with me. Legendary running coach Bill Dellinger had already experienced the disaster of trying to train in smog when he was a 5,000 meter Olympic runner himself, training for the Tokyo Olympics. In 1964, his squad came and trained in Los Angeles. "All we got out of that was a bad cold," says Dellinger.[12] He failed to medal.

Bob Sevene, coach of Joan Benoit Samuelson, who won the womens Olympic marathon gold medal in 1984, also took the smart approach to protecting his athletes from smog. "We'll arrive in Los Angeles on Friday, rest on Saturday, run on Sunday, and leave."[16]

Carbon Monoxide

The human body had very little exposure to carbon monoxide during evolution. Consequently, in developing its system to extract oxygen from the air, it could not also develop a system to exclude carbon monoxide.

As your blood cells circulate through the bronchioles of the lungs, hemoglobin in the cells absorbs oxygen from the air, and disposes of carbon dioxide waste. The newly oxygenated blood then flows to muscles and organs. That's the way your body should work. But hemoglobin, the red, oxygen-carrying pigment in your blood, has a 210 times greater affinity for carbon monoxide than for oxygen. When a molecule of carbon monoxide and a molecule of oxygen compete for attachment to hemoglobin, the carbon monoxide wins every time. In air polluted with carbon monoxide, the blood will pick up every molecule of this toxic gas in preference to oxygen.

For every molecule of carbon monoxide that enters the blood, less oxygen is available to muscles and brain. It is like an

immediate loss of conditioning. Maximal oxygen uptake
(VO2max) is reduced and performance declines.[17] In the
blood, carbon monoxide forms a toxic compound called
carboxyhemoglobin (COHb) that is carried to the muscles and
damages every cell it touches. The body doesn't even notice. It
didn't experience carbon monoxide during evolution and has
developed no defense. That's why suicide by car exhaust is so
popular.

Studies show that the VO2max of sedentary healthy men
is reduced in direct proportion to the level of carboxyhemoglobin
in the blood. This reduction begins at 2.6%, a very common blood
level of carboxyhemoglobin in non-smoking, urban dwellers.[18]
With their much greater use of air, athletes are found to be in
double jeopardy.[19,20]

In an excellent study, Dr John Nicholson, a physician and
athlete in New York City, recruited 16 runners and 10 other
volunteers to act as controls. All were young, healthy non-
smokers and not overweight. Blood levels of carboxyhemoglobin
were measured at the Cardiovascular Center of New York City
Hospital. At 5:15 p.m., on three separate weekdays (in the midst
of rush hour), half the runners were taken to Central Park where
they ran for 30 minutes. The other half ran on FDR Drive for 30
minutes. The non-runner controls stood beside FDR Drive the
for the same period.

In both Central Park and along FDR Drive, blood levels
of carbon monoxide (measured as COHb) increased three-fold
above the levels at rest. Levels rose also in the standing controls,
but to less than half the level found in runners. So even with
moderate exercise, athletes are exposed to at least double the
toxic effects of carbon monoxide.[21,22]

Combating Air Pollution

We are less than two years into the twenty-year
compliance schedule of the new Clean Air Act and there are
already political moves to gut it. Vice President Dan Quayle

(Gawd help us!) chairs the President's Council on Competitiveness. In April, 1991 the Council persuaded the EPA to change the rules to allow factories, utilities, smelters, and all the worst industrial sources of pollution, to rewrite their own permits on emissions without public notice. So don't expect the government to protect you: you have to protect yourself.

The first and obvious strategy if you are serious about your athletic career is, don't live or train in major cities. Unlike contaminated food and water, there is no way to avoid contaminated air if you live in it. You can't run and you can't hide.

The latest study on the Los Angeles Basin indicates that residents are receiving toxic doses of air pollutants even while they sleep.[5] All these unfortunate folk are growing toxic bodies. Their health, their performance, even their life expectancy is permanently reduced.

Don't be one of them. Top athletic performance is one of the greatest thrills, the greatest challenges, and the greatest satisfactions in life. You have one body and one shot. It's worth relocating your job, house, even changing your lover or spouse to give yourself the best shot. Do not get to an age when it is all over and accuse yourself in the mirror, "You never even let me try."

If life demands that you live and train in a city, there are a few helpful precautions:
  1. Never exercise during smog alerts unless in a building with purified air.
  2. Never exercise in rush hours.
  3. Avoid smokers and tobacco smoke environments.
  4. Exercise in parks or traffic-free areas.
  5. Exercise *early* in the morning before pollution counts rise.
  6. Avoid underpasses, tunnels, areas of trees, areas of close, tall buildings. These trap and concentrate pollutants.

The other major defense against air pollution is nutrient antioxidants. Most pollutants cause their damage by oxidation.

Mechanisms of oxidation damage are explained in Chapter 20. There are yet no studies of antioxidant use to combat air pollution in athletes, but animal studies give us some idea of the extent of protection you can achieve.

In one report, two groups of rats were exposed to 0.1 ppm of ozone in air, the level exceeded every day in New York and Los Angeles. One group was supplemented with high doses of vitamin E. The other was given vitamin E in the diet equivalent of the RDA for humans. Most of the RDA group developed lung lesions within two weeks. Over 80% of the high-dose vitamin E group remained healthy throughout the study.[14]

In another report, rats were given either 100 IU or 1,000 IU of vitamin E per kilogram of food, and exposed to 0.8 ppm of ozone (the high end of current levels in Los Angeles). The rats given the high-dose vitamin E were far better protected.[23]

Rats have tougher and more adaptive lungs than men. It is clear that RDA level intakes of vitamin E are insufficient to protect you from even low levels of ozone. It is equally clear that high levels of vitamin E, taken for its antioxidant action, afford a considerable measure of protection.

It is understandably difficult to get volunteer athletes to expose themselves to toxic gases to test antioxidant protection. So scientists have to try and do it sideways. In one of the few human studies, Dr E. Calabrese gave 12 healthy volunteers 600 IU of vitamin E daily for four weeks. He then exposed their blood cells *in vitro* (in the test tube) to hydrogen peroxide, an oxidation product of ozone. By the second week of supplementation, the vitamin E afforded considerable protection against oxidation damage to red blood cells.[13]

Because of the principle of synergy we covered in Chapter 1, vitamin E alone is unlikely to provide optimum antioxidant protection. So I recommend that all athletes exposed to air pollution use multiple antioxidants. Some scientists may object that the evidence is yet insufficient to justify such a recommendation. Fortunately, there are other sound reasons for athletes to use antioxidant supplements with plenty of evidence to back them.

All is made clear in Chapter 20. That chapter also specifies how you can develop your personal antioxidant program by applying the principles of biochemical individuality and lifestyle dynamics. And you get some protection from air pollution thrown into the bargain.

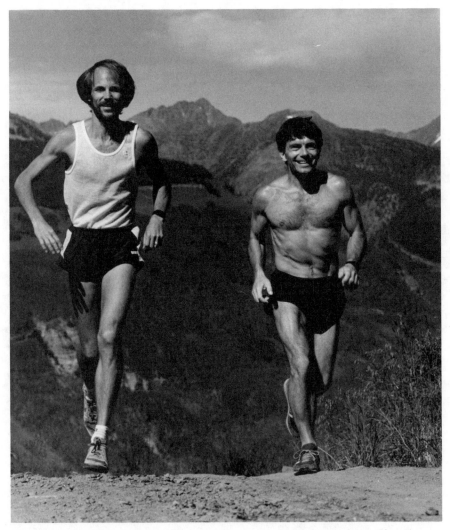

Dr Colgan at 10,000 feet up Vail Mountain running with Olympian Jeff Galloway.

Chapter 6

Body Pollutants

Toxic chemicals in our water (Chapter 2) and toxic gases in outside air (Chapter 5) are not the only pollutants to affect athletes. Most Americans today are exposed to toxic chemicals in the home and at work. To reduce insurance costs and to avoid liability, many companies do not publicize the possible damage to health caused by their products and procedures. You have to learn to protect yourself.

Most urban pollutants do not make you sick right away. They build into your body over long periods, progressively disrupting its function. Usually they remain undiscovered until they cause full-blown disease.

The Augusta Chemical Company, for example, was aware that a compound they used, **betanaphthylamine (BNA)** causes bladder cancer. In 1984, they cooperated with the National Institute of Occupational Safety and Health (NIOSH) to notify their workers about BNA, and screen them for bladder cancer. In 586 workers screened, 13 were found to have already developed bladder cancer, and 26 others showed precancerous changes in the bladder. This notification and screening saved a good many lives.

But the tragedy of it was, nearly one worker in every two had never heard of BNA, and almost three-quarters of the workforce were unaware that it is toxic. Of those workers that did know BNA is harmful, most had only learned about it *after* developing bladder symptoms.[1]

In the early 1980s, NIOSH studies identified 253 actual workplaces, distributed over 43 states, with a total of 245,480 workers, who were exposed to toxic chemicals without being properly informed of the dangers. In 1985, Public Citizen, the consumer arm of the Ralph Nader organization, obtained these studies under the Freedom of Information Act. Many of these workers remain unprotected today. The studies give company names, the toxic chemicals involved, and the diseases they cause. If you have any suspicions about your workplace, it's worthwhile checking to see if it is on the list.[2]

But that's only the measured tip of the toxic iceberg. In 1989, looking at only one harmful chemical, **cadmium**, NIOSH estimated that 1,500,000 workers may be exposed. Cadmium is a proven cause of lung and prostate cancers.[3] Many workers are aware it is dangerous, but recent studies show cancer, kidney, and lung diseases in workers exposed to *legal* levels of cadmium. The International Chemical Workers Union is currently pressing the Occupational Safety and Health Administration (OSHA) to lower exposure standards to a safe average level of 1 mcg per cubic meter, that is 100 times *less* than current legal levels. Meanwhile, you have to protect yourself. If you work in or near cadmium-using industries, such as electroplating, battery makers, plastics manufacturers, metal alloy plants, and car manufacturers, then you are likely to be exposed.

Formaldehyde, another known poison, is a similar problem. In 1982, Anne Gorsuch, then Administrator of the Environmental Protection Agency (EPA), said that the problem of wide industrial use of formaldehyde was "trivial." Assistant Administrator John Todhunter agreed, and nothing was done. Industry lobbyists were happy to avoid the costs of making formaldehyde safe. Then Gorsuch and Todhunter were ousted in the big EPA scandal. The Colgan Institute was among the many scientific organizations that protested to the new administration about formaldehyde. In 1984, the EPA began a new survey of this chemical. Its report finally appeared in April 1987, indicting formaldehyde as "a probable human carcinogen." If it can cause cancer, realize how it can inhibit your quest for a premium body.[4]

There are over 780,000 workers in the garment industry exposed to formaldehyde, plus many hundreds of thousands in and around the plywood and particle board industries. In addition, formaldehyde is used in the manufacture of adhesives, detergents, dyes, fertilizers, insecticides, leathers, paints, paper, and plastics. If you work in any of these occupations, you may be at risk.

Even with chemicals that are well controlled, the occupational risk is not eliminated. Rubber compounds and vinyl chloride emissions have been tightly regulated since the 1970s. Yet rubber vulcanization workers still have *10 times* the average risk of oesophageal cancer.[5] And workers in vinyl plastics industries have double the risk of lung cancer, and *200 times* greater risk of liver cancer, than the general population.[6]

The Colgan Institute recommends all athletes to adopt the strict rule we have in our laboratory. **If you can't eat it, don't touch it or sniff it.**

Avoid The Mercury

I watched a champion bodybuilder suddenly fall over sideways after a couple of reps of lunges with two-and-a-quarter (225 lbs). Later he told me, "I've been getting these dizzy spells, Doc. And I'm not using any juice." He had been to his physician who could find nothing wrong. All the usual blood tests were normal. But a change in his work gave me the clue. Four months earlier, he had taken a job making latex paint.

I asked some critical questions: How did he feel when driving? Pete said he got shaky and irritable for no reason, especially on freeways, like he was scared of driving. He also said he got embarrassed and mad when people looked at him, and was embarrassed to come to the gym. His sleep was disturbed, he had no appetite, he ached all over, and muscle was dropping off. For a guy who used to be Mr. Easygoing, these were big personality changes. I told him it might be mercury.

We all get a little mercury from our food and air, but a specific urine test for mercury showed he was excreting 25 times the normal level. At the paint factory where he worked, they did wear protective masks and gloves, at least some of the time. But some latex paints exude such high levels of mercury vapor, that it pervades the whole area. NIOSH estimates that at least 67,000 Americans are exposed to toxic levels of mercury at work, in jobs ranging from mining to medicine.[7] Our case illustrates how easy it is for toxins in the workplace to silently wreck your training.

The most insidious symptom was his loss of confidence, something you would think was entirely mental. No way. Mercury poisoning attacks the brain, to cause a condition marked by shyness, fearfulness, and timidity. Left untreated, it produces the Mad Hatter Syndrome, satirized in **Alice In Wonderland**, so-called because hatters used to suffer a high incidence of insanity from the mercury used to make animal fur into felt for hats. If you are concerned to be an elite athlete, then avoid mercury like the plague. It can reduce the strongest athlete to a frightened mouse.

Mercury poisoning can be cured if caught early. With our bodybuilder, we used the proven mercury detoxifiers, vitamin E and selenium.[8] He also changed his job. Last week he was back up to full sets of lunges with two-and-a-quarter, smiling the while.

Get The Lead Out

Lead is another toxic metal that man has used with gay abandon to poison the environment. We got at least some of it out of the gasoline, so there is now less in the urban air. But, worse sources of lead pollution are still with us. Except for occupations that expose workers to lead, most of the toxic lead burden in American bodies comes from our food.

For a test, Dr D.G. Mitchell bought 122 canned foods and drinks in the usual lead-seamed cans. Average lead content was 80 mcg per pound of food. Some canned baby foods showed over

100 mcg of lead.[9] In another test, **Consumer Reports** found that one 4 oz. serving of canned beans, can also serve you with 60 mcg of lead.[10]

Because of the lead pollution of air and food, the bodies of Americans today carry a toxic lead burden over *50 times* greater than in the past.[11] It makes us pretty sick. The medical text, **Subclinical Lead Poisoning**, shows how even small amounts of lead can cause fatigue, depression, and memory loss.[12]

Over the last 20 years, the Food and Drug Administration has progressively lowered the allowable limit for lead in foods. Now they consider there may be *no safe level of lead*. In work going on at the University of Cincinnati Medical School, researchers have shown that inner-city children have problems with motor coordination and balance caused by lead. The average blood level of lead in these children is 18 mg/dl, well within the allowable limit of 25 mg/dl set by the Centers for Disease Control. If you are an athlete, motor coordination and balance are crucial. Avoid leaded gasoline, canned foods, leaded paints, pewter ware, and some cosmetics, and get the lead out of your life.

You can't avoid all lead, so the second line of defense is good nutrition. Adequate intakes of zinc, iron, calcium, and phosphorus reduce absorption of lead, [13] and vitamin E works well to detoxify the lead that is already weighing down your body.[13] But remember the principle of synergy. Complete nutrition every day is the best strategy.

Can The Aluminum

If you phone the FDA they will tell you that aluminum is not toxic in the amounts found in American food and water. This is the same government agency that told you that the lead in your drinking water was "harmless", until the Clean Drinking Water Act Amendment in 1986, which outlawed all new lead pipes and lead contaminated substances in the water supply. All recognized authorities on lead toxicity had been calling for removal of lead water pipes since the 1960s because of the clear evidence that even small amounts of lead cause irreversible brain degeneration.[14] But it took until 1986 and a new law before the FDA changed its tune.

Now we are in the same position with aluminum that we were with lead 20 years ago. The silver metal is well entrenched in and around our food and water. Meanwhile, scientists who have measured the toxic effects of aluminum on brains and bones, are campaigning for its total removal from the food chain.

Evidence that aluminum can cause brain degeneration began to surface in the late '70s. At the University of Toronto, Dr D.B. Crapper and colleagues, showed that aluminum given to cats turned them into idiots. Examination of the cats' brains after death found destroyed areas filled with what are called **neurofibrillary tangles.** These areas showed high concentrations of aluminum (12 mcg/gram), the same level of aluminum found in destroyed areas of the brains of some victims of Alzheimers disease.[15]

Also in the '70s, other evidence began to accumulate showing that even small amounts of aluminum interfere with the metabolism of the essential minerals fluoride and phosphorus. Over a long period this toxic effect results in loss of minerals from the bones and osteomalacia (soft bone disease) and osteoporosis (fragile bone disease).[16] Crunch time for aluminum came in 1979. Groups of dialysis patients given aluminum salts to reduce high phosphate levels, all went raving mad and lost so much essential minerals that their bones snapped like toothpicks.[17] No athlete can afford weak bones.

Aluminum was hastily and quietly removed from dialysis fluids. But the problems persisted, because aluminum continued to be given by mouth in antacids and other medications. Until the early '80s, it was still widely believed that oral aluminum could not be absorbed and was harmlessly excreted. Only after hundreds more patients had been turned into permanent lunatics, did the medical profession finally accept that oral aluminum is readily absorbed. And when kidney function is reduced, as in dialysis patients, the body can't get rid of it. So in a very short time, the brain retires to la-la land.

So what, you say? My kidneys are fine. Doubt if it will save you. Any big jolt of aluminum will overwhelm the kidneys' capacity to excrete it, and start depositing permanently in your brain and bones. In the **New England Journal of Medicine** on 21 February 1991, a study by Dr I.B. Salusky and colleagues of UCLA Medical School, shouts a warning. After one year of treatment with low levels of aluminum previously thought to be safe, dialysis patients doubled their aluminum levels, and showed evidence of rapid bone disease.[18] Another recent study in the British medical journal **Lancet**, shows brain dysfunction in patients with similar levels of aluminum previously thought to be completely safe.[19]

These diseases happen pretty quick and obvious in patients with reduced kidney function. In athletes like you, the accumulation of aluminum is likely to be much slower and unnoticed, insidiously eating away at your bones and brain.

I have cited only a fraction of the studies. The evidence against aluminum is now so strong that it is criminal neglect to continue to permit addition of the metal to our food and water, and allow its use in contact with food. But then, US health authorities were criminally negligent for 20 years over the lead problem. So don't expect the government to protect you. You have to protect yourself.

As a still accepted food additive, aluminum is added to food everywhere. Aluminum salts are used routinely in water treatment. In summer they are added to public water supplies in massive amounts. Historians of the future might wonder whether the deliberate addition of aluminum to drinking water, like the deliberate use of lead water pipes, might have been ways to eliminate large numbers of the population before they got too old and burdensome to keep.

To eliminate aluminum, first, don't drink the water, unless you first distill it. Distill is the right word. Water filters don't remove aluminum. Second, avoid aluminum containing or citrate containing antacids (citrate makes aluminum more easily absorbed). Third, read labels for the words alum, alumina, aluminum, aluminate. Ditch any product that contains them. Likely candidates, salt (sodium silico aluminate), bread and baked goods (potassium alum), processed cheese (sodium aluminum phosphate), flour, pancake mix, pickled vegetables, almost all antacids, aluminum canned beverages, buffered aspirin, douches, underarm deodorants, and toothpaste. Don't use them.

Aluminum pots and pans are not a huge worry, unless you stew everything for hours. They give you only 2-3 mg aluminum per day. You get more than that from raw vegetables, and one antacid tablet gives you up to 50 mg. Healthy kidneys can excrete several hundred milligrams of aluminum per day.

Toxic Medicines

Sounds like a contradiction: medicine is supposed to ease illness not cause it. But if you read the **Physicians Desk Reference**, you will see the sad truth that most medicines are toxic, and have no place in a healthy body.[20] Famous physician Dr Peter Latham said it right, "Poisons and medicines are oftentimes the same substance given with different intents."[21]

The bottom line for athletes is not to take any form of drug, even aspirin, unless absolutely unavoidable. If presently you swallow prescribed or OTC drugs by the handful, you are not to blame. Pharmaceutical conglomerates spend billions of dollars indoctrinating us that every sniffle or twinge spells health disaster without their nostrums. Prescription drugs are sometimes necessary for the really sick. But for any of the minor ills, to which the hard-trained body is prey, drugs simply add a further toxic burden.

In eighteen years of work with athletes, we have found that prescribing drugs for minor ills in otherwise healthy people, is mostly a placebo medical strategy to maintain the athletes' humor while waiting for Nature to do the healing. Avoid it every way you can.

Chapter 7

Rest
And Sleep

Some respected recent texts on sports nutrition don't even mention rest and sleep.[1,2] So it may seem unwarranted to include a chapter here on the subject. It's not only warranted, it's vital. Bodily growth and repair occur *only* during rest or sleep, never during training. Successful development of an athlete is always a delicate balancing act between three variables: a training program of progressive overload, the correct raw materials (nutrients) to maintain and repair tissue and build new tissue, and sufficient rest and sleep to permit the repair and new growth to take place.

Numerous texts discuss only the nutrition you need before, during, and after athletic performance. But that's only half the picture. The main business of nutrition is to build a better body. That work takes place only during rest. Even if your training and nutrition program came straight from the mouth of God Almighty, without adequate rest your body will fail to adapt.

Some athletes tell me they need only six hours of sleep a night. My reply is, "Maybe you can get by, but you will never reach full potential." After 18 years in the business, I have seen it many times. The short sleep athletes are the first to succumb to that big killer of sports careers - **overtraining.** Many recent studies document that the overtraining syndrome occurs primarily because of insufficient rest.[3,4]

The great coaches have always known. Swimming great

Jim Councilman of Indiana University, for example, makes his athletes sleep nine hours a night, plus a nap in the afternoons. With a tip of my hat to Jim, the Colgan Institute gives similar advice. You have to allow your nutrition the space it needs to work.

There's no way you can gut it out by will power. Just the opposite. Athletes who are falling into the overtraining syndrome often start to train harder to "break the plateau." Instead of improving they get worse faster.[5] You can't beat overtraining with more work because, by the time it becomes noticeable, your body is already shot.

Studies show that the neuroendocrine system becomes exhausted, altering hormone levels so that optimal performance is impossible.[6] Some severely overtrained athletes have developed Addison's Disease, characterized by the permanently reduced function of the adrenal glands, so that they no longer maintain proper hormone levels. That's the finish of any elite sports career.

The other big problem is suppression of immune function. Overtrained athletes become progressively more susceptible to infection.[8] They also get more injuries, especially muscle and tendon injuries, the type that can cut training for months.[4] My friend, Olympian Jeff Galloway, who has taught thousands of athletes how to run, put it best. **"The single greatest cause of improvement is remaining injury-free to train."**[9]

Compelling evidence of depressed immunity also comes from athletes with poor training advice, who increase their training intensity without increasing their rest. They almost all get sick or injured, which promptly cancels any benefit of the extra work.[10] In contrast, carefully balanced training and rest can *enhance* immunity.[11] So if you want optimum performance, you better get it right.

The general rule for rest is to get 71/2-91/2 hours sleep a night. For athletes who train twice a day, and you should if you want the maximum training effect, a 30-60 minute nap after your first training session, is invaluable. It may be a hard habit to get into, but persevere. You'll thank me.

How to Recognize Overtraining

The basic conundrum an athlete faces is, how intense should training be? There is a wide range of biochemical individuality in responses to exercise stress. And this genetic component is further modified by past training and by nutrient intake as well as rest. The trick is to have an individual monitoring system for signs of overtraining that tells you to back off and increase your rest. The system we use is very simple yet very effective.

Waking Heart Rate: The first sign is waking heart rate. After monitoring the heart rates of athletes for more than a decade, the Colgan Institute has developed this simple rule of thumb. Get into the habit of taking your pulse immediately on waking and recording it. Do it before you get out of bed. It is less accurate at other times because emotions, activity, having just eaten, type of food, caffeine, and alcohol, all affect heart rate. The rule is, **if your waking pulse on any day is elevated by more than eight beats per minute above its average level for the preceding week, you are falling into overtraining.**

Waking Bodyweight: The second sign is waking bodyweight. Your weekly average weight should not vary by more than 2 lbs, even if you are frantically working to gain muscle. Most athletes working hard at the weights gain less than 10 lbs of muscle per year. The rule is, **if your weight drops by more than 3 lbs on any day from a previously stable bodyweight, you are falling into overtraining.**

Insomnia: The third sign is insomnia. Running guru Dr George Sheehan first turned me onto this one.[12] One complication is training late at night. The Colgan Institute advises against training at night because the adrenocorticotrophic hormones (e.g. adrenalin and noradrenalin) generated by the exercise, interfere with normal sleep. The rule is, **if you don't train at night yet start to suffer from restlessness, inability to fall asleep, or too early awakening, you are falling into overtraining.** You may also experience abnormal mood swings during the day, and a loss of motivation. Cut back!

Immunity: An optional measure, but invaluable if you have access to it, is immune function as measured by the complete blood count (CBC) part of a usual SMAC blood screen. Our rule is, if you show elevated counts of **segmented neutrophils** (segs), **lymphocytes** (lymphs) **monocytes**, (monos) or **eosinophils** (eos), or a combination of elevated counts of these immune cells, **and no infection or illness can be found,** then you are falling into overtraining. More detailed explantions of immunity are given in Chapter 22.

Curing The Overtraining Syndrome

You cannot resolve overtraining by simply increasing your sleep. From long experience our one-week-cure rules of thumb for all athletes are:

1. Stop training entirely for one week. Running athletes can jog *lightly* for a mile or two each day. Strength athletes can stretch for 30 minutes each day.
2. Reduce protein intake to 15% of total calories..
3. Increase carbohydrate intake to 70% of total calories. Use predominantly complex carbohydrates of low glycemic index.
4. Increase antioxidants to 200% of usual intake. How to determine you individual antioxidant intake is detailed in Chapter 20.
5. Increase sleep to 9 hours solid per night.

Better still, avoid overtraining. Monitor the signs and back off training and increase your sleep at the first inkling. Even if you follow every detail of this book to design a brilliant individual nutrition program, it will not help unless you also have sufficient rest and sleep to enable the nutrition to do its work.

Part II

Fuel

Nothing tastes as good as lean and mean feels.

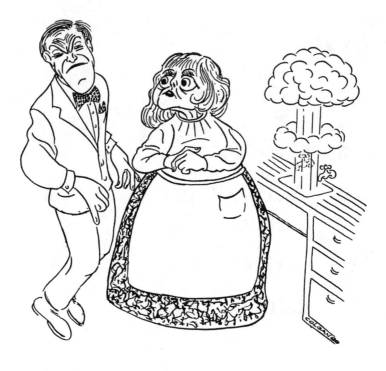

"It's not the water pollution we mind: It's the god-awful smell"

Chapter 8

Smart Fats

In March, 1990 major US health authorities finally agreed that everyone over age two should reduce their total intake of fats to 30% of daily calories, with saturated fats less than 10% of calories. These figures were first proposed as a health standard more than 20 years ago. It has taken that long for the sluggish committees of the American Heart Association, the National Heart, Lung, and Blood Institute, and the National Cancer Institute to come to agreement.

Meanwhile, nutrition science has advanced rapidly. The recommendations now in effect are far too high and way, way behind science. They present a completely false picture of the health effects of fats. Athletes who follow the current US health recommendations on fats,[1] are unlikely to achieve optimum performance.

At the other end of the scale some folk, such as devotees of Nathan Pritikin, think that all fats are bad, and the less we eat the better. This simplistic viewpoint had led a lot of people into dietary error. There are good fats and there are bad fats, and those who want premium bodies should make a clear distinction between the two.

The body can use all types of fat as its largest source of energy. They provide about nine calories of energy per gram. An athlete who is 15% bodyfat, carries 12% of his fat as energy reserve. The other 3% is essential bodyfat that acts as insulation and cushioning for vital organs. You see media reports of athletes claiming them to be less than 3% bodyfat. They are probably hype or instrument error. In 18 years, we have never found an athlete less than 4.5%. Below that, you are on the edge of illness.

The 12% energy reserve in a 175 lb athlete of 15% bodyfat is worth 75,000 calories, enough to run 150 miles. That is much more than he will ever need for sports. Compare this with sugar in the form of glycogen, the body's other main energy source. In the same athlete, his 450 grams of glycogen reserve at four calories per gram, are worth only 1,800 calories. Because of the body's cycle of glycogen use with exercise, and because of an obligatory minimum level of glycogen for muscle to function, that is only enough to run about 20 miles. So the limiting energy source for exercise is always sugar, never fat. Most of the energy reserve of fat is simply dead weight that inhibits performance. Athletes gain no benefit from carrying it, nor from eating the fats that put it on.

Essential Fats

To understand what fats an athlete needs we have to dip into a smidgen of biochemistry. Bear with me, it's worth it. Food fats and oils are all composed of fatty acids. As the name implies, a fatty acid consists of a fat bit and an acid bit. Its chemical make-up is a carbon chain made of carbon and hydrogen atoms. Different fatty acids have different length chains. Short-chain fatty acids, such as butyric acid from butter, have four carbons. Fish oils and the long-chain fats that comprise most of the human brain have 20 to 24 carbons.

Saturated fats, as the name implies, have all their carbon atoms "saturated" with hydrogen atoms, that is, they will not hold any more hydrogen. Unsaturated fats have empty spaces where hydrogen atoms are missing. These spaces link up with molecules of other substances in the body, so they make unsaturated fats much more biologically active. In contrast, saturated fats have no empty links and are virtually inert. Their only biological role is as calories, to be burned for energy. Because almost all athletes carry more energy reserve of fat than they will ever use, they have no need for saturated fats at all. They are difficult to avoid in our fat-laden food supply, and you will not avoid them entirely. But to achieve optimum sports nutrition, you should make every effort to **eliminate saturated fats from your diet.**

Athletes do require special fats, as the major components of cell membranes, around every cell of the body. These fatty acids are also used in exclusive ways in the brain, inner ear, eyes, adrenal glands, and sex organs. In these very active tissues, special fats are essential for the high level of oxygen use and energy transformation required for optimum performance.[2] Without these special fats you would quickly sicken and die. With a deficient supply, optimum performance is impossible.

Your body has the ability to change the long-chain fats of more than 16 carbons into unsaturated forms, and to lengthen already unsaturated fats, by inserting empty spaces called double bonds. Through this ability, it can make almost all the myriad of different fats it needs. But there are two essential fatty acids that you cannot make, **linoleic acid** and **alpha-linolenic acid**, both of which are long-chain (18 carbons). They have to be provided by your diet. Linoleic acid and alpha-linolenic acid are all the dietary fats an athlete needs.

Fish Oils and Olive Oil

Throughout this book I recommend the qualities of the fish oils, eicosapentanoic acid (EPA) and docosahexanoic acid (DHA). The body itself also produces EPA and DHA, in brain cells, the inner ear, the adrenals, the sex glands, and other highly active tissues. EPA and DHA are made in the body from alpha-linolenic acid in the diet. But if you don't get sufficient alpha-linolenic acid, which is highly likely with our degraded food supply, then the body can use exogenous EPA and DHA from fish.

Not any old fish will do. The best sources of EPA and DHA are the high-fat cold-water fish: salmon, sardines, mackerel, and trout. Low-fat fish like haddock, sole, and flounder contain insignificant amounts. Clams, oysters, and scallops contain high *proportions* of EPA and DHA in their fats, but only small total amounts. Also, as we saw in Chapter 4, American supplies of these shellfish are contaminated. So, despite what you may read in popular health books, shellfish are a poor source.

To understand how essential fatty acids work and how fish oils fit into the nutritional picture, Figure 5 shows the main conversions that take place in your body. You can see how dietary fish oils can substitute for alpha-linolenic acid. In fact, because of an age-related decline in the conversion enzymes that enable the body to make EPA and DHA, fish oils may be preferable for athletes over 30.

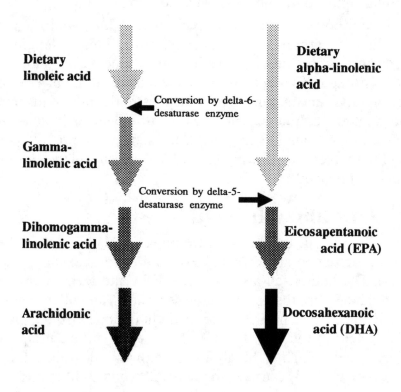

Figure 5. How the human body uses and converts the two essential fats.

If you use fish oils to obtain your EPA and DHA, then there is no need to seek alpha-linolenic acid in vegetable oils. Consequently, you can use extra virgin olive oil in cooking and in salads. It is a good source of linoleic acid, the first essential fatty acid, but contains no alpha-linolenic acid.

Extra virgin olive oil, recommended for athletes for more than a decade by the Colgan Institute, contains high levels of a monounsaturated fatty acid, called **cis-oleic acid**. Although not essential, repeated studies have shown that dietary oleic acid lowers serum cholesterol, and has other beneficial effects on blood lipids.[3,4]

Also, extra virgin oil is the most palatable and easy to use of the good vegetable oils. Make sure it is **extra virgin**, which by law describes unprocessed olive oil. Preferably ensure the brand you use is also organic. The Flora company noted below is one reliable source.

One other aspect of Figure 5 deserves note. An age-related decline of the conversion enzyme, **delta-6-desaturase**, inhibits conversion of linoleic to gamma-linolenic acid. Without this step, your body cannot use linoleic acid. So we recommend that all older athletes take some preformed **gamma-linolenic acid** in their diets. Two good sources are evening primrose oil and borage seed oil supplements. One good, though expensive source is the widely available Efamol brand of evening primrose oil. A better, more economical source is Borage Power from Nature's Herbs.

Vegetable Essential Oils

The best vegetable source of linoleic and linolenic acids is flax or linseed oil. This oil was available freely for food use in America for hundreds of years. At the Colgan Institute, we have used it for eighteen years in nutrition programs. For a few years, however, it was under a senseless restraining order, because of wild claims of its use to cure disease made by some irresponsible nutrient supplement companies. Now thankfully, it is back on the market again. Two excellent brands of certified, organic, cold-pressed flax oil are Flora, Box 950, Lynden, Washington 98264, phone (800) 446-2110, and Omega Nutrition, 1720 La Bounty Road, Ferndale, Washington 98248, phone (604) 322-8862. They are also available in health food stores.

Other sources of the two essential fatty acids are pumpkin seeds, walnuts, and soybeans. The dark green leaves of leaf vegetables also contain small amounts.[5] The fat content of common seed oils is shown in Table 5. This table applies only to cold-pressed unprocessed oils. As we see below, when even the best oils are processed into margarine and refined cooking oils, they lose their healthful attributes.

The only other common seed oils that contain significant quantities of linoleic and linolenic acids are hempseed and rapeseed oils. The healthy hempseed oil was widely used until a century ago. Then the hallucinogenic effect of smoking the leaves was rediscovered. I say rediscovered because the Chinese knew about marijuana over 4,000 years ago, and discarded it as an inferior drug. Now marijuana is the largest cash crop in some states of America. But if you buy or grow hemp plants for oil, men with large feet and shiny badges will visit you and cause you considerable mischief.

In contrast, rapeseed oil *was* illegal until the mid-1980s, but is now FDA approved. As the table shows, rapeseed oil has very healthy levels of linoleic and linolenic acids. It was illegal until recently because it contains a toxic fatty acid called erucic acid. Erucic acid still found in European rapeseed oil is linked to heart disease in reports in reputable medical journals.[6]

Approval came from development of low erucic acid rapeseed plants by Canadian growers. They dubbed the oil from these plants "canola," I guess an abbreviation of "Canadian oil." Tests of the harvested canola seeds by the Canadian Grain Commission show erucic acid levels of about 0.6%.[7] This level does not pose a threat to health. So if the canola oil is pure, and guaranteed not to be blended with toxic European rapeseed oil,

Table 5. The percentage of fats in vegetable oils: The good, the bad, and the ugly.*

	Polyunsaturated Fats		Mono-unsaturated Fats	Saturated Fats
	Linoleic Acid	Linolenic Acid		
The Good Oils				
Flaxseed (linseed)	15	54	22	9
Pumpkin seed	45	15	32	8
Soybean	42	11	32	15
Walnut	50	5	29	16
Canola	26	8	57	9
Second Best				
Almond	17	--	68	15
Virgin Olive	12	--	72	16
Safflower	70	--	18	12
Sunflower	66	--	22	12
Corn	59	--	25	16
Sesame	45	--	45	13
Rice Bran	35	--	48	17
The Bad Oils				
Peanut	29	--	56	15
(Contains Carcinogenic Fungus Aflatoxin)				
Cottonseed	48	--	28	24
(May Contain Toxins)				
The Ugly Oils				
Palm	9	--	44	48
Palm Kernel	2	--	18	80
Coconut	4	--	8	88

*These percentages hold only for fresh unprocessed, cold-pressed oils that have not been hydrogenated.

Source: The Colgan Institute, San Diego, CA

go for it.

Processed Oils Are Bad Fats

Type of oil is not the only problem in trying to find healthy essential fats. In fact, the worst problem is what industry does to the oil. All the oils in Table 5 remain healthy, *only* if they are unprocessed. US health authorities will not tell you this yet, because they lag far behind the research. And there is also a powerful food oils lobby that works to stop this information becoming public.

Modern processing changes the chemical character of fatty acids in oils so that the human body can no longer use them. To understand this problem requires a smidgen more biochemistry. All nutritionally important fats are in what is called a **cis** chemical configuration. That is, the hydrogen atoms on the carbons are all on the same side of the molecule. Because of their slight electrical charge, the hydrogen atoms repel each other and put bends in the carbon chain. These bends are the essential shape of the molecule that make it possible for all the special biological functions of fats to take place.

This essential **cis** configuration is destroyed by modern processing procedures, including heating, hydrogenation, bleaching, and deodorizing. These procedures are applied to almost all mass-produced fats and oils today. They change the healthy **cis** configuration into an unhealthy **trans** configuration. Processing rotates the hydrogen atoms, so that they lie on opposite sides of the fat molecule. The molecule then straightens out, loses its essential shape, and loses its ability to perform the biological functions required by the body.

Hardly any trans fatty acids occur in Nature, so the human body has never developed the mechanisms necessary to use them. Today, almost all processed fat and oil products, cooking oils, margarines, and fats used in breads, cookies, candies, chocolate, frozen dinners, pies, and processed meats, contain high levels of nutritionally damaging trans fatty acids.[2,8,9] If you want a premium body, **eliminate all processed oils from your diet.**

How Much Fat

Total fat needs for athletes are a lot lower than the 30% of calories recommended by US health authorities.[1] In trying to estimate the best intake, some researchers point to highly athletic groups such as the Tarahumara Indians. Even in their 50s, both men and women of this Mexican tribe perform fantastic running feats of 100 miles or more on diets that get only 9-12% of their calories from fat.[10]

Other researchers point to low rates of degenerative disease in countries such as Japan, where calories from fats are about 15% of the diet. There is no longer any doubt that such diets lower serum cholesterol and reduce the amount of fats you have to carry in your blood.[11]

But virtually no controlled studies have been done on the amount of fat that produces optimum performance in sports. From 18 years of work directly with athletes, the Colgan Institute has found that the strongest predictor of performance related to fats is bodyfat level. The lower the better.

As detailed in Chapter 11, bodyfat is deposited mainly from the fat an athlete eats. Every ounce of extra bodyfat increases the energy required to move your body. Therefore, for a given energy capacity, it reduces the maximum possible speed. Also, every ounce of extra bodyfat increases body temperature during exercise, not only because of the extra weight and insulation, but also because you have less water for cooling. Bodyfat is only 50% water, whereas muscle is 75% water. Except for the essential fatty acids, the only fat you should eat is that which you can't avoid. **Aim to keep total fat intake below 15% of daily calories.**

In a 3,000 calorie diet, 15% is only 450 calories. That is 50 grams of fat. About 20 grams will be unavoidable saturated fats. That leaves you two tablespoons each of olive oil and flax oil, and maybe a knob of butter on your toast. Add two meals of cold-water fish per week, plus a daily capsule of gamma-linolenic acid, and you are doing all that we know about fats to improve your performance.

Lower That Fat!

A great deal of the fat in our food is hidden, either by false advertising or by not being mentioned at all. So keeping your fat intake below 15% of calories is a tough job. Milk, for instance, is heavily touted for athletes. An 8 oz. glass of regular milk contains 87.6% water (0 calories), 3.8% fat (69 calories), and 8% carbs and protein (64 calories). That makes it more than 50% fat. Don't drink it. Even "low-fat" 2% milk is over 25% fat. Don't drink that either.

The milk example is a good indication how you have to become an avid label reader for all packaged and processed foods. Refuse to buy any food that does not give the fat content. Fat content is given by weight, so add a zero to get the approximate calories of fat. Then find the total calories per serving of the food, always given on the label. If the fat calories are more than a fifth of total calories, leave it on the supermarket shelf.

Take regular vanilla ice-cream, for example. Fat content is 8 grams per serving. Add a zero to get 80 fat calories. Total calories per serving is 160. Fat content is 80/160, that is 50%. Not an acceptable food. Contrast ice-cream with low-fat frozen yogurt, which today can be made to taste just as good. Fat content is 2 grams per serving. Add a zero to get 20 fat calories. Total calories per serving is 110. Fat content is 20/110, that is 18%. Low-fat frozen yogurt is a good, low-fat food.

Many foods have no fat labelling, especially protein foods such as meat, fish, eggs, and cheese. A rule of thumb to avoid the high-fat varieties is - fish first. If you just can't stomach a high-fish diet, then Table 6 gives a Top Ten and an O.K. Ten of common protein foods. It also gives a Worst Ten, foods all athletes should avoid.

Table 6. Ranking of Fats and Cholesterol in 30 High Protein Foods**

Top Ten Less than 5% Fat	O.K. Ten 5% to 20% Fat	Worst Ten 30% to 60% Fat
Eat These		**Avoid These**
Cod	Shrimp*	Beefburger*
Sole	Tuna*	Pork Roast
Halibut	Chicken Breast	Bologna
Flounder	Buffalo Steak	Frankfurters
Lobster	Sardines	Beef Roast*
Crab	Herrings*	Bacon
Mussels	Salmon	Steak, T-Bone
Scallops	Lamb or Veal	Pork Sausage*
1% Cottage Cheese	Riccota Cheese	Cheddar Cheese*
Turkey Breast	Eggs*	Cream Cheese*

** Fat Content by weight
* Over 100 mg cholesterol per 100 gm serving: Eggs have over 500 mg per 100 gms.

Source: Colgan Institute, San Diego, CA

Some of the new prepared meats are also very low in fat. Hormel has a 97% fat-free frank (by weight), that is only 20% fat calories. Healthy Choice, Butterball, and other brands all make 98% fat-free (by weight) sliced turkey and sliced chicken. By calories they are only 15% fat. And Turkey Tree has 99% fat-free ground turkey meat that makes excellent turkeyburgers that are only 7% fat calories.

Many athletes coming to the Colgan Institute complain that you can avoid fat only by eating foods that taste like sawdust, that you cannot get equivalents to normal food. Not so. Table 7 shows a typical shopping basket of cereal, bread, yogurt, crackers, snacks, cheeses, meat, dressing, candy, and ice-cream. On the smart side, a day's fat intake from all these foods is only 16 grams. On the dumb side it is 104 grams. The choice is yours.

Table 7. Smart and dumb choices in shopping for fat.*

Item	Smart Choice	Fat (gms)	Dumb Choice	Fat (gms)
Cereal	Quaker Puffed Wheat	0	Quaker 100% Natural	5
Yogurt	Yoplait Light	0.5	Yoplait Custard Style	5
Bread	Wholewheat Breadsticks	1	Bran Muffins	8
Crackers	Ak Mak Crackers	2	Keebler Wheatables	6
Cheese	Lifetime Cheddar	3	Kraft Casino Cheddar	9
Cottage Cheese	Weight Watchers 1%	1	Skaggs Regular	5
Meat	Zacky Farms Turkey Roll	1	Oscar Meyer Bologna	8
Butter	Butter Buds	0	Regular Butter	11
Dressing	Tasti Italian	0	Lawry's Italian	9
Snacks	Mini Ricecakes	0	Butter Thins	6
Candy	Fibar Raspberry	3.5	Kudos Granola Bar	12
Ice-Cream	Dreyers Grand Light-Mocha	4	Hagen-Daz Mocha	20
Total Grams Fat	**Smart**	**16**	**Dumb**	**104**

*Source: Colgan Institute, San Diego, CA

Cut The Chips and Dips

Potato chips, corn chips, crackers, puffs, rinds, stix, and bits all appear to be dry foods, therefore not high in fat. Wrong! Most dry crackers are so high in fat that major brands, such as Nabisco, don't dare put the fat content on the label, for fear of losing customers.

Companies that produce lower fat types of crackers do include a fat analysis, but even these are way above our cut-off of 20% fat calories. Hains Stoneground Wheat Cheese Crackers, for example, are about 130 calories per serving with 3 grams protein, 17 grams carbohydrates, and 6 grams fat. Our simple rule of thumb is to add a zero to the fat and compare it with total calories, that is 60/130. The crackers are over 40% fat, twice the healthy limit.

Puffs and chips, stix and bits are much worse. Ruffles plain potato chips, for example, 90 calories of fat in 154 total calories. That is 58% fat. For crackers, Ak Mak Original are only 18% fat. And you can substitute pretzels for chips. Most brands of pretzels are under 20% fat. The best snack of this kind is rice cakes. Many brands use whole grain rice, and fat content is a fat zero. Lean enough for you?

Fake Fats

Three fake fats have appeared on the market. First was **Olestra** by Proctor & Gamble, made out of sugar and vegetable oil. It tastes like vegetable oil, but by chemical wizardry, the Olestra molecule is too big and dense to be digested.[12] Studies of Olestra show that it can be used anywhere that regular fats are used without changing the taste or texture of the food. It contributes zero calories.

Because Olestra has no calories, there are also high hopes for its use in weight reduction. The problem is that it encourages people to eat foods that taste fatty, which may promote a fat-eating habit for all food. Also, it has zero nutritional value. On both counts, Olestra has no place in an athlete's body.

Better than Olestra is **Simplesse**, from the Nutrasweet Company. Simplesse is a fat substitute made from egg white or milk protein. The protein is specially granulated in microfine granules, which gives it the taste and texture of fat. One gram of the Simplesse (4 calories) can replace up to three grams of regular fat (27 calories) in foods.

Because it is a protein, Simplesse cannot be used in cooking. But, it is already an ingredient in ice-cream, yogurt, butter, mayonnaise, cream cheese, and chocolate. Protein expert Professor Vernon Young of M.I.T. told me, "Before Simplesse, Americans concerned with fat consumption were often forced to deprive themselves of their favorite rich foods, or to eat less tasty and less satisfying products instead of the real thing. Now everyone can reduce fat intake with pleasure, not penalty." If you have to have an ice-cream or chocolate fix, Simplesse could be a boon. Just don't make it a habit.

Finally there is **Caprenin** from Proctor & Gamble. It is not really a fake fat but rather a reduced-calorie fat, yielding only 5-6 calories per gram instead of the usual nine calories of most fats.[13] Not much of an advantage. Caprenin is already being used to reduce the fat content of candy and chocolate. It might help a bit if you are a chocaholic. But it has no value for athletes.

Medium Chain Triglycerides

A lot of sports supplements now include **medium-chain triglycerides** (MCTs) in the mix, with the idea that these fats actually cause the body to lose fat. Some supplements sold for cutting up and fat loss make specific claims such as "will help you lose that last pound of fat to achieve the raw shredded look."

This belief that one special kind of fat can help you lose bodyfat arose from the use of MCTs in medicine with patients who have trouble absorbing fats.[14] MCTs have the unique property of bypassing the usual mechanisms by which the body stores fat.[15,16] So they are more available than most fats for use as energy. Also, although MCTs are readily used for energy, they are not deposited as bodyfat no matter how much of them you eat.

The studies that triggered the use of MCTs in sports were done with diabetics and weight-loss patients, who were given MCTs in place of the usual long-chain fats. On low-calorie diets, these patients lost more weight than patients given ordinary fats.[17,18] But muscle loss was substantial, making it difficult to determine whether MCTs actually aid fat loss or not. Also, the total diet was over 50% MCTs, that is over 50% fat, a very unhealthy arrangement.

More recently, MCTs have been tested with healthy non-obese men and women *not* on low-calorie diets, with an entirely different result. Dr Valerian Dias and colleagues at the University of Calgary reported that with MCTs as 51% of calories, fat oxidation is increased and protein oxidation is reduced.[19] The subjects didn't lose weight, but the MCTs were burned for energy preferentially, thereby sparing muscle.

MCTs may therefore have a place in sports nutrition as a short-term aid in sports such as bodybuilding, gymnastics, and ballet. In the week or so before competition, when it is critical to maintain muscle while keeping bodyfat as low as possible, MCTs could form a fuel source that maintains energy for training and spares muscle, but cannot be deposited as fat.

To achieve this effect, a high proportion of the diet (about 50%) must be MCTs. So most of the pills sold for this purpose contain far too little. You need a liquid source such as the TwinLab brand, providing at least 100 grams of MCTs a day for an 1,800 calorie diet. Use this strategy only briefly, however, because a 50% fat diet cannot maintain a premium body.

Conclusion: The Fat Rules

As we discussed, the athlete's need for fats is minimal. You need only the essential fatty acids, linoleic acid, and alpha-linolenic acid. Other fats should be avoided. You can achieve this goal by following these rules:

1. Eliminate saturated fats from your diet.
2. Use extra virgin olive oil as your main source
   of fat.
3. Eat two meals weekly of cold-water fish; salmon,
   trout, mackeral, and sardines.
4. Athletes over 30 take a daily capsule of gamma
   linolenic acid.
5. Keep fat intake down to 15% of total calories.

Fake fats and MCTs may also have some special uses, but they do not form part of the nutrition you need to build a premium body. And the going is tough to keep other unwanted fats at bay. But it's worth the effort. Stick with it and you will be amazed how your body remodels itself into a leaner, meaner framework.

Chapter 9

Carbohydrates: Premium Fuel

Make a clear distinction between nutrients that are building materials, and nutrients that are fuel. Proteins, vitamins, minerals, and essential fats are predominantly building materials. They are used long-term to grow a better body, like putting new tires on your car or installing a new carburetor. All carbohydrates, are predominately fuel. They are used short-term, like gas in the tank. So the types and amounts of carbohydrates to provide the right fuel mix, and the timing of their intake to provide an optimum supply, are critical for any particular performance to succeed.

Chapter 8 showed you how **carbohydrate is always the limiting fuel,** because no matter how lean athletes are, they have fat calories to spare. The body uses variable amounts of fat during extended exercise, depending on biochemical individuality, blood oxygen levels, blood free fatty acid levels, and conditioning.[1] But you never have to worry about running out. With carbs, however, you can run out in a heartbeat.

That's simple stuff, well known to athletes. But there are basic misconceptions about fat that make it even more important to get your carb intake right. A while ago I went to breakfast with some of the San Diego Padres. A couple of chunky lads were yaffling fried eggs, and fatback bacon like there was no tomorrow. "Why are you eating all that fat?" I asked. "High energy, Doc, 9 calories a gram," said both of them, sing-song as if they learned it from a book. They are dead wrong.

If you throw fat on the fire, it yields at least 9 calories per gram -- fast. But it doesn't work that way in the human body. Despite its high caloric *content,* in muscles, fat burns very slowly for energy. The biochemistry works like this. Primary fuel for exercise is **adenosine triphosphate (ATP)**. It's a lot easier for the body to break down muscle glycogen and blood glucose into ATP than to break down fat. Consequently, ATP is formed *a lot faster* from carbs than from fat. The rate of ATP synthesis from carbs is about 1.0 mol/min: from fats the rate is only 0.5 mol/min.[4] So carbs yield approximately **twice** as much energy as fats. During anaerobic exercise which uses only carbs as fuel, energy formation jumps to 2.4 mol/min, almost five times the energy that can be derived from fat.[4] **Carbs are the highest energy fuel.**

Some researchers have made big news of the discovery that the higher the level of an athlete's conditioning, the more fat he can use for fuel.[3] True, but feed him properly on carbs, and he will beat his fat-burning performance every time.[4]

The effect of forcing the body to use fats for fuel is well documented. If athletes are exercised until muscle glycogen and blood glucose are at low levels, then the body burns predominately fats. Performance declines dramatically.[5] Consequently, athletes should design their carbohydrate nutrition so that they burn as little fat as possible.

You may think that this advice does not apply to short events such as the shot-put or high jump. But, to excel in sport, *all* events require long training sessions. During training, *all* athletes will achieve the best levels of performance by designing their nutrition so that the body derives as much energy as possible from glycogen or glucose.

The Training High

Besides carbs being the limiting fuel and the highest energy production fuel, there is a third reason that makes them critical for optimum performance. **Training should always end**

on a physiological and psychological high. You cannot achieve this goal without the proper carbs.

The physiological effect of carbs is easy to understand: the psychological effect is more subtle. But it's there. Studies show that perception of fatigue during exercise, with all its damaging effects on motivation and self-worth, directly parallels the decline in muscle glycogen stores.[6] Those findings make carbs the king of foods for athletes.

Say you are a 5,000 meter runner doing repeat 400s. Given that you have a decent coach who has you on the right training progression, the last repeat should always be the best. If it isn't; then likely your carbs are wrong. Say you are a weight-lifter training on repeat snatches. The last snatch should always be the best. If you can handle only a lower weight on the last rep, then likely you are running on empty. You are setting yourself up for mediocrity.

The point is, your training and your carbohydrate nutrition must be designed to fit your body exactly, so that you finish every training session with the best performance of that session. To do so is critical because **your muscles and brain always register and remember the last rep**. If you are slower and weaker and out of energy towards the end of training, then you will be slower and weaker and out of energy in the final, crucial minutes of competition. To grow faster and stronger and a whole lot happier, you have to arrange your carbs so that you finish exercise with fuel to spare.

Timing of Carbohydrate Intake

The easiest way to achieve correct carb nutrition is to divide carbohydrates into three categories: carbs before exercise, carbs during exercise, and carbs after exercise.

There are now 25 controlled studies showing that taking carbohydrates during exercise enables the athlete to postpone fatigue and perform at a higher level.[7] Many popular articles and ads for carbohydrate drinks and bars have stressed these findings, as if guzzling carbs on the run is the most important way for athletes to use them. But most of the studies have been roundly and rightly criticized, because many of the subjects did not have optimal levels of muscle glycogen at the *start* of exercise.[7] So the additional carbohydrates taken during exercise were merely boosting an already deficient supply.

Would these athletes have performed even better if they had no carbs during exercise, but began with a higher level of muscle glycogen? You betcha! Basic biochemistry tells us right away that carbs taken *between* exercise sessions have to be more important than those taken *during* exercise. It works like this. Glucose in the blood from carbohydrates just digested cannot be used by the muscles nearly as effectively as muscle glycogen formed from carbohydrates taken some hours previously. Unlike muscle glycogen, which can be used directly for energy, blood glucose first has to go through a chemical conversion called **phosphorylation**. Sounds complicated but, as the name implies, it is only a simple conversion of the glucose by adding phosphate. This conversion is done by an enzyme called **hexokinase**. Hexokinase is the limiting step in the body's use of glucose.

Unfortunately, the hexokinase in human muscle has only a low level of activity. This biochemical limitation keeps the maximum use of blood glucose for energy much lower than the maximum use of muscle glycogen for energy.[8] Studies with athletes have confirmed that the level of glycogen in the muscles *before you start exercise,* is the most important fuel determinant of performance.[9]

Carbs Between Exercise

So in designing your carbohydrate nutrition, the primary goal should be to achieve the highest levels of muscle glycogen between the finish of one session of exercise and the start of the next. To do this you have to begin eating carbohydrates immediately after you finish a session. In a series of excellent studies, Dr John Ivy and colleagues at the Exercise Physiology and Metabolism Laboratory of the University of Texas at Austin, have shown that muscle glycogen synthesis after exercise, occurs in two phases, a very rapid rate of synthesis for about 4-6 hours (most rapid in the first 2 hours), then a much slower rate for the next 24 hours.[10,11]

The most rapid rate of glycogen synthesis occurs immediately after exercise because the low level of glycogen remaining in the muscles, stimulates activity of an enzyme called **glycogen synthase** that controls glycogen storage.[12] You have to hit the carbs when glycogen synthase is really dancing.

The amount and type of carbs are also important. Ivy and colleagues have found, that the maximum rate of synthesis in the first 4 hours after exercise occurs by feeding athletes 225 grams of glucose polymers in liquid form.[11] Above that there is no further effect.

Glucose polymers are complex carbohydrates made by extending glucose molecules so that they are more slowly digested than simple sugars. Ads for sports drinks and bars have made big play of the term "glucose polymer" as if it is some new scientific wonder. In fact it is old news. Many of the new drinks use variants of the starch, maltodextrin. Maltodextrin has been in wide use in foods for at least 50 years. Nevertheless, we have found that modern liquid carbohydrate repletion drinks, such as TwinLab's Ultrafuel, are more easily digested and cause fewer problems of gastric distress, than the old standby complex carbs such as bananas and fig bars.

Complex carbs are not the whole story. Immediately after intense exercise you need sugar quickly, to take advantage of the high levels of activity of the glycogen storage enzyme, glycogen synthase. So take a little in addition to glucose polymers. Athletes often avoid glucose because they think simple sugars cause a detrimental insulin burst. They do if you have not just exercised.[13] But when your muscles have a high demand for glycogen replacement, the glucose is shunted into muscle so fast that no insulin instability can occur. A little fructose also helps.

Fructose preferentially replaces hepatic (liver) glycogen.[14] As we see in chapter 32, this combination is also crucial to anabolism. Rule 1 for optimum carbohydrate nutrition is: **Take 225 grams (8 oz.) of liquid complex carbohydrates, glucose and fructose immediately after exercise.**

How Much Carbs?

For the whole period of glycogen repletion before the next bout of exercise, Dr David Costill and colleagues at Ball State University have reported that muscle glycogen levels plateau at an intake of 650 grams of carbohydrates per day.[15] The actual amount different athletes need, however, varies widely depending on biochemical individuality, training intensity, and training duration.

In ultra-endurance sports such as ultra-running and Ironman distance triathlons, where training can be up to 6 hours per day, the amount of carbohydrates required to maintain muscle glycogen stores can be much higher than 650 grams. James Bond (the real one), while training on a program from me to run the Western States 100-mile race, could eat 900 grams of carbohydrates a day and not put on an ounce. James won the coveted Western States silver buckle at age 53.

Another example is Julie Moss who trained with me for years as she climbed the ladder of triathlon success to become world champion. Julie would ride 2-3 hours in the early morning, then arrive at my office. We would run together for 8-15 miles, then go straight to the pool and swim for an hour or so. After that 5-6 hour exercise bout, and a break for lunch, Julie would hit the weights in the afternoon. Depending on the training schedule, she would be exercising 7-9 hours per day, 6 days a week. Carbohydrate intake required to maintain muscle glycogen was up to 1,200 grams per day. Her bodyfat was always under 10%, and she got leaner as the season progressed.

Controlled studies on cyclists report similar findings. In simulations of the Tour de France, researchers gave the cyclists high-intensity training on successive days for 5 hours per day. Subjects burned over 900 grams of carbohydrates per day.[16] And that was with cycling which uses only 40% of an athlete's total muscle mass.[17] Running, which uses about 60% of total muscle mass, has a higher energy cost. Cross-country skiing, which uses up to 80% of total muscle mass, has at least double the energy cost of cycling.

Because of these differences, the Colgan Institute has developed a system shown in Table 8 that can help you devise your own program. I have kept the table as simple as possible. If your training hours or bodyweight are between the categories listed, then interpolate for the amount you need. Say you are a long jumper of 165 lbs training 3 hours a day. Your weight is midway between 154 and 176. Go to the 3-hour column and take the midway figure between 600 and 700, that is 650 grams of carbohydrates per day.

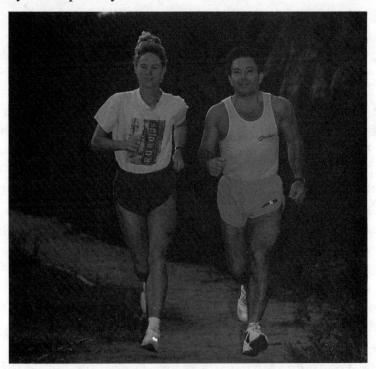

Dr Michael Colgan training with Julie Moss.

Table 8. Estimate of daily carbohydrate requirements (grams) for different bodyweights and training durations.

| Bodyweight | | Daily Training (hours) | | | | | |
kg	lbs	2	3	4	5	6	7
40	88	200	300	400	500	600	700
50	110	300	400	500	600	700	800
60	132	400	500	600	700	800	900
70	154	500	600	700	800	900	1,000
80	176	600	700	800	900	1,000	1,100
90	198	700	800	900	1,000	1,100	1,200
100	220	800	900	1,000	1,100	1,200	1,300
110	242	900	1,000	1,100	1,200	1,300	1,400
120	264	1,000	1,100	1,200	1,300	1,400	1,500

Say you are a gymnast of 90 lbs, training 5½ hours a day. On the 88 lbs row, 5½ is midway between 5 and 6 hours, that is 550 grams of carbohydrates per day. Rule 2 for optimum carbohydrate nutrition is: **Use Table 8 to select the daily amount of carbs you need in terms of bodyweight and hours of training.**

Because of biochemical individuality in carbohydrate use, the overall guide should always be your bodyfat level. Provided you follow the fat rules in Chapter 8, Table 8 is designed to allow a little overfeeding of carbohydrates for most athletes. So if you find yourself putting on more than a pound a week, cut back. At the other end of the scale, if you do a very strenuous sport like cross-country skiing, you may need to eat a little more carbs than the level in the table in order to maintain bodyweight.

The slight bias towards overfeeding is deliberate for two

reasons. First, a small daily insufficiency of carbohydrates is not noticed by healthy athletes. But over weeks of training, it leads inevitably to progressive exhaustion of glycogen stores,[18] setting the athlete up for the overtraining syndrome detailed in Chapter 7. Second, and very important, slight overfeeding of carbs reduces the use of muscle protein for fuel, and therefore spares that vital muscle tissue.[19]

We have covered the importance of taking 225 grams of carbs immediately after training. But that's not the end of it. The timing of eating carbs the rest of the day and the type of carbs you eat are also critical for optimum glycogen repletion. First, to maintain glycogen synthesis, you have to maintain a steady flow of carbohydrates across the intestinal wall. If that flow is interrupted for even a couple of hours in the 24 hours after heavy exercise, then glycogen storage is reduced.[20] This reduction occurs because the activity of the storage enzyme, glycogen synthase, is dependent on a steady flow of insulin.[21] Anything that causes insulin levels to fall is detrimental to glycogen repletion. Rule 3 for optimum carbohydrate nutrition is: **Eat carbohydrates in small meals throughout the day.**

As we saw above, except during and immediately after exercise, simple sugars cause insulin fluctuations that inhibit glycogen synthase activity, and reduce glycogen storage. Slowly digested carbohydrates, that is those with a low glycemic index, cause much smaller rises and falls in blood glucose and insulin levels than sugars.[22] At the Colgan Institute, we have found that these carbohydrates, especially the starches from whole grains and legumes (beans), are much more effective in glycogen repletion than sugars such as glucose or sucrose, or highly processed starches. In controlled studies, Dr David Costill at the Human Performance Laboratory of Ball State University has made similar findings.[23,24]

The basic problem athletes face is to identify the slowly digested carbs amongst the huge array of everyday foods. The Glycemic Index developed by Dr David Jenkins to assist diabetics provides the best approach.[22] A section of the glycemic index pertinent to athletes is shown in Table 9. Eat less of the foods on the left and more of the foods on the right. Rule 4 for optimum carbohydrate nutrition is: **Ditch the sugar. Eat mainly carbs with a low glycemic index.**

As you can see from the table, the sugar fructose is an anomaly. It has a low glycemic index and does not cause sharp fluctuations in blood glucose or insulin. These findings have persuaded some athletes to eat fructose by the spoonful and to seek out high-fructose foods. Not a good idea. Fructose is only

Table 9. A section of the glycemic index. Comparison of common foods with equivalent substitutes that have a lower glycemic index.

Eat Less		Eat More	
Food	**Glycemic Index**	**Food**	**Glycemic Index**
Sugars		**Sugars**	
Glucose	100	Fructose	20
Honey	87		
Vegetables		**Vegetables**	
Parsnips	98	Soybeans	15
Carrots	90	Kidney Beans	30
White potatoes	70	Lentils	25
		Sweet Potatoes	48
Fruit		**Fruit**	
Bananas	65	Apples	36
Raisins	68	Oranges	40
Grains		**Grains**	
White flour spaghetti	56	Whole wheat spaghetti	40
Cornflakes	85	Oats	48
White rice	70	Brown rice	60
White flour pancakes	66	Buckwheat pancakes	45
White bread	76	Whole wheat bread	64

half as effective as complex carbs for repletion of muscle glycogen.[25] High fructose diets also cause a rise in blood fats,[26] and a rise in blood uric acid levels.[27] Both are degenerative conditions that wise athletes avoid.

Nevertheless, a little fructose can be helpful. After digestion, complex carbohydrates are converted to glucose to enter the bloodstream. Most of the glucose bypasses the liver.[28] Fructose, however, is mostly metabolized in the liver, and yields greater repletion of liver glycogen than glucose.[29]

The small amount of fructose added to glycogen repletion drinks such as TwinLab's Ultra Fuel is sufficient, without seeking additional fructose in other foods. At the Colgan Institute, we restrict the fructose content of the diet to 10% of total carbohydrates. That permits 2-4 of these glycogen repletion drinks per day.

Use of such drinks, that are predominantly glucose polymers, may also be essential for optimal repletion of muscle glycogen, especially in athletes who train more than four hours per day. Recent simulations of the Tour de France in which athletes rode 5 hours daily, show that cyclists cannot fully replete without them.[16,30,31] Rule 5 for optimum carbohydrate nutrition is: **Use glycogen repletion drinks that are predominantly glucose polymers, but also contain a little fructose.**

Carbohydrate During Exercise

During exercise, the glycogen content of muscles *always* decreases. And, as we have seen, muscle glycogen is the highest energy fuel, better than liver glycogen, much better than blood glucose, and far and away better than fats. Also, as the level of muscle glycogen declines, the maximum level of performance declines. So, having your muscles full of glycogen at the *start* of exercise is the ideal state. There is no way that you can fully compensate for sub-optimal levels of muscle glycogen by taking carbohydrates on the run.

Many athletes, however, eat a diet that provides

insufficient carbohydrates *all the time*. Numerous studies show that the carbohydrate intake of endurance athletes range between 40% and 55% of total daily calories.[32,33,34]

The brilliant research of Dr David Costill who first alerted me to the importance of carbs in 1974, has shown conclusively that this range of intake by athletes in heavy training, progressively depletes the muscles of glycogen.[24] These studies indicate that many athletes may *never* achieve full levels of muscle glycogen. For them, taking carbohydrates during exercise may be the only way to maintain performance. But it will never be their best performance, because bodies cannot use blood glucose as effeciently as muscle glycogen. So if you want the best, study the rules given above and keep your muscles full.

That's not the end of it. Recent studies show that even with high levels of muscle glycogen, eating carbohydrates during exercise can give you an edge. And very long events (over 3 hours), may require carbs on the run to compensate for declining levels of muscle glycogen. In the final stages of long events, such as the Ironman Triathon, liver glucose and blood glucose from the digestion of carbs taken during the race, can provide 90% of the carbohydrate energy.[35]

Non-athletes typically have resting muscle glycogen levels in the range of 100-120 mmol/kg.[36] Elite athletes eating sufficient carbohydrates have much higher levels. They range from 170-200 mmol/kg. But for long events it is still not enough. One recent study showed that subjects with starting levels of glycogen of 180 mmol/kg, when made to cycle at 70% VO2max without taking any carbohydrates during exercise, showed fatigue and insufficient muscle glycogen after two hours.[37]

These findings bear on all athletes, even those in short event sports, for two reasons. First, as we saw above, many athletes habitually eat insufficient carbs. Taking carbs during exercise will help compensate. Second, in order to excel all athletes have to do long training sessions that inevitably deplete muscle glycogen. Taking carbs during training will help achieve that important goal of the **Training High**, always finishing training with your best rep.

Timing Carbs For Competition

The next question is, when do you take the carbs? Because of the time they need to digest, it is essential to take in the first carbohydrates 3 hours prior to exercise. Costill has shown that complex carbs taken 3-4 hours before exercise raise blood glucose and improve performance.[38]

Some athletes suffer intestinal distress if they eat on the day of competition. The best way to overcome this problem is to habitually take carbs 3 hours before training. Start with 10-20 grams, and gradually increase the amount over several months up to 100-150 grams. Using this method at the Colgan Institute, we have taught marathon runners with sensitive guts to safely take up to 200 grams of carbs before races in the form of carbohydrate replacement drinks. Rule 6 for optimal carbohydrate nutrition is: **Habitually take 100 grams of a carbohydrate replacement drink 3 hours before exercise.**

Don't use candy, honey or sucrose, as some books advise. Many studies show that taking these sugars, *before* exercise results in reduced performance.[13,39]

Once the exercise begins, the minimum level of carb intake required to improve performance is 40 grams per hour.[17,40] Some books suggest that carbohydrate during exercise is beneficial only during the last stages of long exercise, when muscle glycogen stores are depleted. Don't believe them!

At the Colgan Institute we have measured respiratory exchange ratios which provide a good measure of carbohydrate use for fuel. We found that if you begin sipping carbs right after you start exercise, respiratory exchange ratios typically increase. Other researchers have similar findings.[40] Although the definitive studies are not yet done, this evidence suggests that the increased blood glucose levels that result from taking complex carbohydrates throughout exercise, permit a higher overall rate of carbohydrate use throughout, and an increase in performance throughout.

After analyzing all the research to date, the Colgan Institute recommends 70-90 grams per hour as optimum. Above 90 grams, many athletes run into gastric distress. To achieve that level you need to drink a bit over a quart of carbohydrate rehydration beverage per hour. Note the rehydration part. Don't use solid foods. They deplete your water. As we saw in Chapter 2, hydration is always your first priority.

Research up to the mid-1980s indicated that a 7% solution permitted the best supply of both water and carbs. The latest research shows that carbs in the beverage can range from 5% to 10% and still provide about the same absorption. Above 10%, gastric emptying is inhibited, and you get less water and less carbs per hour.[41]

The best fluid replacement drinks contain predominantly glucose polymers or glucose plus a little fructose. There are plenty of exotic carb sources hyped by the makers of drinks. Inulin, for example, a starch extracted from flowers, has a glycemic index of only 11, the lowest of any available starch. Some supplement manufacturers have praised inulin to the skies as a miracle carb. But there is not a stick of evidence. No controlled studies at all. Stick to mostly maltodextrin or glucose. Much cheaper and we know it works.

Drinks that fulfill the criteria for supplying hydration and carbs include several commercial drinks designed for companies by the Colgan Institute from their experimental drink, Crux. It was developed to supply carbs and hydration at high altitudes, where the need for water and energy is always competing with nausea and intestinal upset. Crux has been used on four Everest Expeditions and numerous other mountain projects. It has also become popular with runners and triathletes in ultra-distance events, where upset gut is a persistant problem.

Crux is not distributed commercially but an equivalent drink that is widely available is TwinLab's Hydra Fuel. Along with

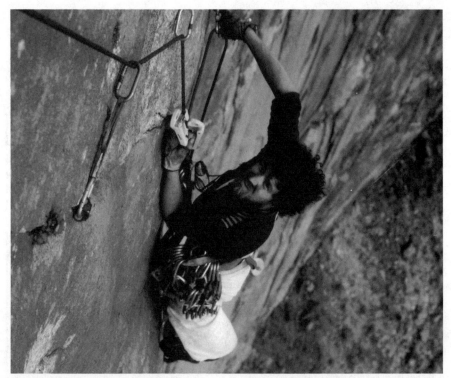

Famed climber Craig Calonica has used the carbohydrate drink Crux on numerous climbing expeditions, including two to Mt. Everest.

glucose polymers, and glucose this drink provides a little fructose, to help replenish liver glycogen.[29]

To maintain carb intake of 70-90 grams per hour during exercise, you need to drink a lot, about one 8 oz. glass every 15 minutes. Carrying a dispenser bottle and sipping repeatedly is definitely the best way. Elite long-distance runners and cyclists often carry two or three bottles and change them frequently at aid stations. Rule 7 for optimum carbohydrate nutrition is: **Sip a 5%-10% carbohydrate rehydration beverage at a rate of 1 quart (35 oz.) per hour during exercise.**

Carbs Are King

As with all the chapters in this book, I have space to cover only a tiny fraction of the research. It is my job to give you the right fraction, the studies that represent the state of the art of sports nutrition worldwide. I believe these rules for carbs make the grade:

Table 10. Rules for carbohydrate intake.

Seven Rules for Carbohydrate Nutrition
1. Take a carbohydrate replacement drink containing 225 grams (8 oz.) of glucose polymers with a little glucose and fructose immediately *after* exercise.
2. Use Table 8 to select the daily amount of carbs you need in terms of bodyweight and hours of training.
3. Eat carbohydrates in small meals throughout the day.
4. Eat mainly carbs with a low glycemic index.
5. Use glycogen repletion drinks that are predominantly glucose polymers, but also contain a little fructose.
6. Habitually take 100 grams of complex carbs 3 hours before exercise.
7. Sip a 5%-10% carbohydrate rehydration beverage during exercise, at a rate of 1 quart (35 oz.) per hour.

If you don't have a personal coach -- get one. And accept only the best. That way you will get the right progression of training. Then, if you ever run out of gas, you know that the fault is not a training program too arduous for you, but very likely your carbs. Don't go it alone. If a water pipe bursts in your house, you send for the plumber, the guy who knows how to fix it fast. Yet plumbing is a simple skill compared with training an athlete. Plain dumb to think you can do it yourself. Put your talent in my hands for nutrition, and in the hands of the best coach you can find for training. Give yourself the best of chances to reach your true potential.

Chapter 10

Carbo Loading

The last chapter showed you that the greater your muscle glycogen stores at the start of long, hard exercise, the better your performance. Carbo loading is a complex strategy, used only before competition, that enables you to super-load your muscles with glycogen. Done well it is highly effective. The problem is, few athletes know how.

Scandinavian researchers Bergstrom and Hultman first reported carbo loading in 1967.[1] They and other research teams used a three-part technique often called the Astrand method after the famous sports physician. It begins 6-7 days out from competition. The athlete does a session of exhaustive exercise then does light exercise for 1-2 days, then does another session of exhaustive exercise so as to severely deplete glycogen levels. Over this depletion exercise period, the athlete eats a very low-carb diet (less than 10% of calories), so that no glycogen repletion can take place. Then, for the next three days, the athlete eats a very high-carb diet (over 80% of calories), and exercises very lightly, hardly at all on the last day.

In elite athletes, during the depletion phase, muscle glycogen levels typically fall from 150 mmol/kg ww to 25 mmol/kg ww. During the super-compensation phase, glycogen levels typically rise to 225 mmol/kg ww, giving the athlete 50% more muscle glycogen than normal at the start of competition. Some athletes achieve more than double their normal levels. [1,2,3]

Sounds simple, but don't you believe it. The Astrand method has a big problem. When your muscles are severely depleted of glycogen by exhaustive exercise, and you eat very little carbohydrate to replace the glycogen, the body burns its fat and muscle protein for energy. This predominant use of fats puts you into a condition called **metabolic acidosis** or **ketosis**. Ketosis is accompanied by muscular weakness, fatigue, nausea, headache, dizziness, confusion, irritability, anxiety, and a marked decline in performance. Not a state to be in a few days before competition. Except for the special case of bodybuilders dealt with below, athletes should do everything to avoid ketosis during carbo loading.

Fortunately, brilliant studies by Dr David Costill and colleagues at the Human Performance Laboratory of Ball State University, Indiana, show that it is unnecessary to deplete glycogen to the degree that promotes ketosis in order to achieve carbo loading. In fact, their method is only a mild deviation from your normal carbohydrate nutrition, coupled with the usual tapering of training before competition. During days 6-4, carbohydrate intake of 50-60% of daily calories is coupled with a normal training taper of say 80%, 60%, and 40% of normal training, depending on the event. During days 3-1, carbohydrate intake is increased to 70% of daily calories and training is tapered to zero on the last day before competition.[4,5]

This Costill method does not achieve quite as high levels of glycogen as the Astrand method. Costill readily agrees that glycogen synthesis is correlated with the degree of depletion.[6] But it keeps the athlete in much better condition, so it achieves at least the same increment in performance.[4,7]

Carbo Loading Problems

But there are more pitfalls. Simply switching to a high-carbohydrate diet as you taper before competition, will not produce much glycogen loading. That only works if your previous training has been severe enough to keep you in chronic partial glycogen depletion. The secret is that depletion has to be sufficient to stimulate the activity of the glycogen storage enzyme, **glycogen synthase**.[8] Without that, the excess carbs turn into bodyfat - just more dead weight to carry. We have tested a lot of athletes at the Colgan Institute who put on fat when they thought they were loading glycogen.

Another problem is that glycogen depletion, and therefore loading, occurs *only in the muscles exercised.* Clever studies have shown that if you exercise one leg to exhaustion, for example, then sit around and eat carbs for three days, the glycogen content of that leg will increase two-fold above its pre-exercise level. But the glycogen content of the other leg will remain unchanged throughout.[9,10]

This discovery is virtually unknown among athletes. But it is vital to performance. Typically, athletes are advised to do long, slow aerobic exercise such as jogging or walking the Stairmaster to exhaustion for the depletion phase of a carbo loading cycle. *This advice is completely wrong.* A marathon runner, for example, will deplete and subsequently load his leg muscles by exhaustive jogging. But arms and shoulders are hardly used in slow running. In the marathon race, where he is running as fast as he can aerobically, it is often exhaustion of glycogen stores in the arms, shoulders, neck, and back that let him down. Those muscles will not load with glycogen above habitual levels with a bout of jogging that primarily depletes the legs.

Another example is bodybuilders who need to load glycogen throughout the body to achieve maximum muscle size, hardness, and definition. Typically you will see them riding a stationery bike or walking the Stairmaster in order to deplete. Wrong way! What they need to do is very high repetitions with light weights in the widest variety of exercises they can think of. Only then will the muscle fibers throughout the body deplete. And only then will the muscles subsequently load glycogen above habitual levels.

Another frequent error is to use intense exercise for

depletion. It is true that the more intense the exercise, the faster you use up muscle glycogen.[11] The problem is that intense exercise also causes muscle soreness that can last 5-8 days, and interfere with performance during competition. Heavy exercise also exposes you to risk of injury.

How to Load

The next problem is the loading itself. As we saw in Chapter 9, to maintain activity of the storage enzyme, glycogen synthase, you have to maintain a steady flow of insulin with as little fluctuation as possible in blood levels of insulin. To do this, carbohydrate intake should be as even as possible.[12] You should start the loading with a 200 gram drink of glucose polymer solution, such as TwinLab's Ultra Fuel, immediately after the second session of exhaustive exercise. Immediacy, and glucose polymers are both important variables, because studies show that delaying the start of carbo loading even two hours after the finish of depleting exercise reduces the loading response.[13] So does the initial use of solid carbohydrate foods.

After the first hour, you should eat 100 grams (3 1/2 oz.) of carbohydrate foods or drinks every 1-2 hours, up to 1,200 grams in the first 24 hours. Except for very big men (225 lbs +), loading more than this amount is detrimental, because the maximum range of carbohydrate absorption in us normal size folk is 50-100 grams per hour.[13,14]

After the first 24 hours, the loading response diminishes. So taper off your carbohydrate intake so that you are eating your normal total dietary calories of food, but with 80% of the calories from carbs. Anything above your normal dietary calories will likely end up as bodyfat.

Keep your liquid intake high throughout loading, because every gram of glycogen requires 2.7 grams of water to store it.[11] Even slight dehydration will reduce the loading response and put heavy stress on blood and kidneys.

Many athletes break all these rules and then wonder why

they never seem to get the benefits of loading. Sports medicine expert Dr Gabe Mirkin told me of a comical case where the athlete ate almost two loaves of bread at each sitting, then was surprised when he got chest pains and heart irregularities. I'm surprised his gut didn't explode. Another case occurred at the Colgan Institute where a "myopic" triathlete inadvertently followed the carbo loading schedule for bodybuilders. He drank very little and ended up sick and dehydrated, unable to compete.

Probably the silliest errors are beliefs that carbo loading increases your power or maximum aerobic output. The amount of glycogen in your muscles does nothing for strength, power, or VO2max. It simply enables you to continue longer at your maximum aerobic pace. So if you are a marathon runner who can cover 20 miles at a 6:45 per mile pace, but can never break 3 hours because you fade in the last 6 miles, then carbo loading is a dream come true. Keep your usual 6:45 pace and it will sail you through the finish in 2 hours and 57 minutes. But if you set off at a 6:30 pace because you think the extra glycogen can make you faster, you will die around Mile 15.

Far from increasing power, for short events (less than 2 hours), glycogen loading is a definite liability. First, there is insufficient exercise to use the extra glycogen. Second, and more important, doubling your glycogen store will increase your water and glycogen weight by 4-5 lbs. If you don't believe that reduces your performance, try competing with a five-pound bodybelt. One try will convince you. In fact, the extra glycogen is worse than a bodybelt. It also creates tightness and stiffness of muscles. In long events, the benefits far outweigh these disadvantages, but in quickies they are deadly.

The Colgan Institute carbo loading program is detailed in Table 11. Developed from practical use of the technique with hundreds of athletes, it lies between the Astrand and Costill methods, incorporating the best features of both. It permits you to achieve the highest levels of pre-contest glycogen, while maintaining the health and well-being essential to successful competition. But don't wait until an important competition to try it. Make regular carbo loading cycles part of your training program. That way you make the errors when there is no gold medal or folding green at stake.

Table 11: Colgan Institute carbo loading program for endurance athletes.

Days Away From Competition	Complex Carbs (% daily calories)	Fluids (% usual intake)	Exercise
5	40%	100%	Light intensity to near exhaustion
4	40%	100%	Light 30-60 minutes max.
3	80% (after exercise)	150%	Light intensity to near exhaustion. Include resistance excercise session
2	75%	150%	Light intensity 30 minute max.
1	75%	150%	Light intensity 15-30 minute max.
Day of Competition	200-250 grams between 3 and 1 hours before competition	Drink up to 30 minutes before competition.	

Source: Colgan Institute, San Diego CA.

Some tips in using the table. Except for your essential fatty acids, avoid all fats throughout the cycle. In the second session of depletion exercise (Day 3), include light, high-repetition resistance exercise with weights and machines. Use as wide a variety of movements as possible to deplete muscle fibers throughout the body. Immediately you finish this second session, which should be by noon on Day 3, take 200 grams of complex carbs in the form of a glucose polymer drink such as TwinLab's Ultra Fuel. Continue to eat carbs in small snacks at a rate of 75 grams per hour until bedtime. The greatest amount of glycogen loading occurs in the first 10 hours. If you do it right you will wake on Day 2 feeling great.

Continue eating carbs in small meals evenly spaced throughout Day 2. They should constitute 75% of your total calories. But, and this is vital, do not eat much more carbs than your normal daily amount calculated from Chapter 9. Keep water intake high (see Chapter 2). You should be urinating every 3 hours.

On Days 2 and 1, do only very light exercise, but do some. Don't lay around as various books suggests. My friend and mentor Arthur Lydiard the New Zealand Olympic coach with more gold medalists to his credit than anyone else I know, stipulates "Move the legs every day."

Day 1 is a repeat of Day 2. On Day 0, competition day, take 200-250 grams of complex carbs, as a glucose polymer drink, between 3 hours and 1 hour before performance. Drink water up to 30 minutes before performance. If you have followed the rules, you are now ready to roll with more than double your usual level of muscle glycogen. Go for it!

Carbo Loading for Bodybuilders

Bodybuilders are a special case who use carbo loading not to boost their energy supply, but rather to increase their muscle size and density. Demands on the body are smaller during bodybuilding competition than during other sports. Consequently, bodybuilders can push themselves to greater physical extremes before competition. Neither ketosis nor dehydration limit their posing ability, so they can carry carbo loading to the limit.

In addition, elite bodybuilders add another wrinkle called **sodium depletion/potassium loading**. This procedure dehydrates the body even further. It also redistributes some of the remaining body water from the body cavity into the muscles, giving the physique a leaner, harder look.

The bodybuilding carbo loading procedure developed by the Colgan Institute, detailed in Tables 12 and 13, has proved very effective with champion bodybuilders such as Jeff Smullen shown here. It begins 6 days out from competition with a reduction of carbohydrate intake to 20% of calories. Protein makes up most of the rest of the diet. Don't eat more than normal. Fluid intake is 150% of normal. Sodium, which is usually low in the diet of bodybuilders, is increased to 150% of normal. If you don't usually watch your sodium intake, then don't increase it. Keep your training at its normal duration and intensity.

Keep your potassium intake very low. Fresh vegetables and fruits are high in potassium. So is meat, poultry, and fresh fish. Avoid them. See Chapter 12 for the best sources of protein.

Day 6 begins **ketone** measurement. As the body begins to burn more fat because of the low carbs in the diet, the kidneys produce substances called ketones that are excreted in the urine. You can measure the level of ketones by catching some mid-stream urine in a cup and dipping it with Ketostix, available from most drug stores. The chemically coated stick changes to different colors depending on the level of ketones. The first day should show zero.

Day 5 is a repeat of Day 6, except for training which should be of light intensity but long duration, high repetitions to exhaustion. Ketone measurement should show 5-15 on the Ketostix, and you also feel fatigued, irritable, and uncomfortable.

Day 4 is a complete repeat of Day 5. Now you feel really bad! You are irritable, very tired, confused, aching, and convinced that the whole thing is a crock of bovine scatology. Persevere. Workout somehow with high reps, long duration to exhaustion. If you just can't manage it, take 25-50 grams of medium chain triglycerides to boost your energy.

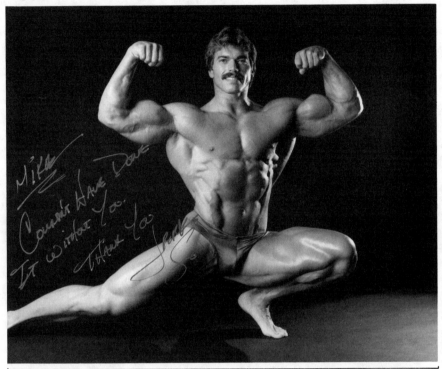

Bodybuilder Jeff Smullen used a program from the Colgan Institute, including a carbo loading regine to help him win the Tournament of Champions.

One good tip. During ketosis, the body also loses some of its acid buffering capacity. You can boost this capacity and feel a lot more comfortable by taking a teaspoon of bicarbonate of soda in 12 oz. of water. Better still, use a commercial buffering supplement such as TwinLab's Phosfuel. But augment your buffer store in this way only towards the end of Day 4. Ketones should now read in the range 15-40.

Table 12: Pre-competition carbo loading for bodybuilders.

Days Away From Competition	% daily calories Complex Carbs	% daily calories Protein	Training	Fluids
6	20%	60-70%	Normal	150%
5	20%	60-70%	High repetition to exhaustion with as wide a range of movements as possible	150%
4	20%	60-70%	High repetition to exhaustion	150%
3	80%	10%	High repetition to exhaustion	Medium
2	70%	10%	Light 30-60 minutes	Low
1	70%	10%	Light 30-6- minutes	Low
Day of Competition	Low	0	Pose &pump	Low

Source: Colgan Institute, San Diego, CA.

On Day 3, work out with high repetitions, light exercise, and posing practice for two hours in the morning. Use medium chain triglycerides only if absolutely essential. Immediately after training, take 200-250 grams of carbs as a glucose polymer glycogen repletion drink. Continue to take 100 grams of complex carbs every two hours for the rest of the day.

On Day 3, you also eliminate all the sodium from your diet. Reduce protein intake to 10% of total calories. Increase potassium intake to normal levels. Reduce water intake to normal levels. By evening, ketones should read 0-5.

On Days 2 and 1, weigh yourself carefully in the mornings. On Day 2, you should be up by 2-3 lbs. On Day 1, you should be up by 4-5 lbs. On both Days 2 and 1, drink only 50% of your normal water intake. Keep sodium intake at zero from now to competition. Increase potassium intake to 150% of normal. Keep carb intake moderately high, enough to load but not enough to bloat. Keep exercise very light, posing only. Ketones should read zero from now through competition.

One good tip. Don't use diuretics. If you do the loading right, your body will drop water fast. You can always drop a half-pound more in the sauna on competition day. To combat the cotton mouth caused by dehydration, use sugarless gum.

On contest day you should be 5-6 lbs heavier, all in the muscles. Keep all food and fluid intake low. A little simple sugar or candy right before going on stage will carry you through. A little pumping will help, but posing practice is probably better. Follow the game plan exactly, and you should come in hard and shredded.

Big caution. Carbo loading for bodybuilders as described here is a highly unnatural and potentially dangerous state in which you temporarily manipulate body water, sodium, and glycogen. The only reason I am including it in this book is to prevent some of the bad messes that people get into when they attempt to do it the wrong way. Consult your physician before ever trying it. If you do so, it is at your own choice and risk.

The procedure has worked well for bodybuilders on

programs from the Colgan Institute, but there is a great range of biochemical individuality in responses. In a book, I can't give you the personal eyeballing that enables us to adjust the procedure to suit individuals. So, if you do try it, then do it in practice and with caution.

One common problem is retention of sodium which makes you retain water and blow up like the Pillsbury Doughboy. If that happens, you have to put your feet up (to avoid edema) and wait it out. Thereafter, skip the sodium/potassium bit. Your biochemistry may not be built for it.

Table 13: Pre-competition sodium depletion/potassium loading for bodybuilders.

Days Away From Competition	Sodium	Potassium	Ketostix*
6	Medium	Low	0 - 5
5	Medium	Low	5 -15
4	Medium	Low	15 - 40
3	0	Medium	0 - 5
2	0	High	0
1	0	High	0
Day of Competition	0	0	0

*Ketostix are used to measure ketones in your urine. The appearance of ketones at the levels shown on Days 5 and 4, indicate near exhaustion of body glycogen stores which prepares the muscles to supercompensate by loading glycogen on Days 3, 2, and 1. If ketones fail to appear (Ketostix, negative) it usually means you have done insufficient depletion training.

Source: Colgan Institute, San Diego, CA.

Chapter 11

Battling The Bulge

After reviewing more than one hundred studies on body composition of athletes, sports medicine specialist Jack Wilmore of the University of Arizona concluded, "there is a high negative correlation between percentage of bodyfat and performance..."[1] Fat is just dead weight. From baseball, boxing, bodybuilding, cycling, football, gymnastics, karate, running, skiing, track and field, weightlifting, and wrestling, it is the low-fat body that wins. To be a champion, you have to lose the pudge. The good news is, given the correct nutritional help, we have **never** found a single athlete that couldn't do it.

But some coaches, usually sporting fair spare tires of their own, still encourage athletes to eat like hogs, with the notion that a bit of extra padding never hurt anyone. Mainly it's because they have little idea how to get their boys (or themselves) lean and mean, while preserving power and speed. Consequently, many athletes who come to me for nutrition programs, are skeptical that a few extra pounds can reduce their performance. I get them to run 400 meters flat out. Then after recovery, I give them a 10 lb well-padded bodybelt to wear, and get them to run another one. They never doubt the detrimental effects of bodyfat again.

Most athletes we see at the Colgan Institute are initially overfat for optimum performance. Wilmore's analysis shows that bodyfat of elite male athletes runs from 4.0% in wrestlers, to 8-12% in runners, to 16% in shot, discus, and football. The elite male average is below 12%. For elite female athletes, bodyfat runs from 8% in bodybuilders, through 10-15% in gymnastics and running, to 25% in discus and shot. The elite female average is about 15%. The bottom line is, the more fat you can pare off your body while preserving muscle and health, the better your performance.

When Ivan Lendl's career was slipping in 1985, I got a call. Though he was already less than 10% bodyfat, I advised his people that if he lost another 5 lbs of fat, while carefully maintaining his muscle, he would be faster, and his game would improve. He did and the result is tennis history.

Detrimental Dieting

Sadly, many, many athletes do not have access to the nutritional programs that would enable them to lose bodyfat safely. Often they use methods that decimate both their performance and their health. Boxers, wrestlers, and martial artists, for example, are notorious for starving and dehydrating themselves to the point of illness in order to "make weight" in a lower weight class.

When Professor Charles Tipton at the University of Arizona examined the diets of high school wrestlers, he found that they used two main methods of reducing weight. The first method was to crash diet by reducing calories to dangerously low levels, sometimes below 500 calories a day. The second method was to dehydrate the body severely for a week to reduce water weight.[2] Other studies have found numerous cases of kidney malfunction in wrestlers who dehydrate to make weight.[3,4]

In another study of college wrestlers, Suzanne Steen and Dr Shortie McKinney analyzed their nutrition over a whole wrestling season. Many of the wrestlers were below the RDA levels in protein, vitamins A, B_1, B_6, and minerals, iron, zinc, and magnesium - **all the time**.[5]

Dancers and gymnasts are worse. In one recent study, Connie Evers of the University of Iowa examined the diet of students enrolled for dance. Seven out of every ten were under-nourished.[6] To keep bodyfat down, they dieted severely, with the consequence that their food supplied insufficient vitamins and minerals, even at the conservative levels of the RDA. Some of the students took vitamin supplements, but generally not enough of them to bring their nutrition up to par.

The same goes for gymnasts. Dr Robert Moffat of Western Washington University made an extensive analysis of the diets of female high school gymnasts.[7] He found that they were deficient in vitamin B6, folic acid, calcium, zinc, and magnesium. And nearly half their food was garbage, consisting of cakes, candy, and sodas.

Endurance runners fare little better. The energy expenditure of their sport allows them to eat more yet, remain slim. In that extra food, they also get increased amounts of vitamins and minerals automatically. Nevertheless, studies abound showing that runners do restrict their food and often have poor nutrition. For example, Dr Patricia Deuster and colleagues at the Uniformed Services University in Bethseda, MD, found that highly trained women runners, who had qualified for the women's Olympic Marathon Trials, had marginal iron and zinc status, and an average food intake of only 2,400 calories per day, too low for their level of training (up to 100 miles running per week). Many of them also had low dietary intakes of calcium, magnesium, iron, copper, and zinc, despite regular vitamin supplementation.[8]

In a study we did on 12 male and 11 female marathon runners at the Colgan Institute, every one was concerned to keep bodyfat as low as possible and used a weird assortment of diets to achieve this goal. When they first came to us, almost all of them had deficient iron stores and low bodily levels of zinc, vitamin B6, vitamin B12, and vitamin C.[9]

Even field athletes use detrimental diets in attempts to maximize muscle and minimize bodyfat. Drs M. Faber and J. Spinnler Benade of the South African Medical Research Council measured the diets of elite male and female discus, hammer, and javelin throwers and shotputters. Of the males, many had calcium and magnesium intakes below the conservative levels of the RDA. Of the females, 90% were below the RDA for calcium, 70% were below the RDA for iron or magnesium, and 40% were below the RDA for zinc.[10] Over 100 other studies report dietary deficiencies as bad or worse than the examples given here.[11] Clearly, many athletes are not getting the right nutritional advice to maintain low bodyfat levels in a way that provides the nutrition essential for top performance. Don't be one of them.

Pathological Diets

The main reason that athletes have so much trouble losing bodyfat is the wholesale misinformation on dieting that pervades the weight-loss industry in America. Most popular diet books and weight loss programs appear to be designed to distort people's nutrition and disrupt their metabolism so as to make them fatter and sicker.

Most of the methods used are so opposed to what is known in nutrition science, that a cynic might conclude they are designed to keep people repeatedly coming back to highly profitable and terribly unsuccessful diet programs for the rest of their lives. In 1992, Americans are slated to spend $36 billion on weight-loss, and there are a lot of rich companies who want to keep it that way.[12]

That's putting the truth hot and heavy so I better review some heavy evidence to support it. Studies by Dr Paul La Chance and Michelle Fisher at the Department of Food Science at Rutgers University, analyzed a slew of the best of the diet books. They found that popular diets, including the Atkins, the Beverly Hills, the Carbohydrate Cravers, the California, the F-Plan, the I Love America, the Pritikin, the Richard Simmons, the Scarsdale, and the Stillman, were all seriously deficient in vitamins, minerals, and fiber.[13] Combined with the food and caloric restrictions that these diets impose, such deficiencies are an invitation to illness.

The popular weight-loss programs hyped on television are little better. Although many of them do include vitamin supplements to make up for their deficiencies, the most they achieve is quick, nasty, and very temporary weight-loss. According to Marketdata Enterprises, the smart market-tracking company in Valley Stream, NY, more than eight million Americans sign-up for weight-loss programs every year. Almost all of them fail miserably.

In April, 1992 the National Institutes of Health convened a panel of thirteen of the country's leading medical specialists on weight-loss headed by Dr Suzanne Fletcher, editor of the **Annals of Internal Medicine.** Dr Walter Glinsman and colleagues from the Food and Drug Administration analyzed 75 lbs of documents provided by weight-loss centers (ironic that the panel cited the documents by weight). The report concluded, there is no good evidence that any popular weight-loss program has much chance for long-term success. The public is being presented with anecdotal reports of individual successes and not being told that most who try the various programs either drop out before completing them or regain most or all of the weight lost.[14]

One of the scientific studies presented at the conference from Dr Thomas Wadden of Syracuse University, is typical of the results of diet programs. In 1983, three groups of overweight women were put on the best form of weight-loss programs used by commercial diet centers. One group was put on an 800 calorie diet. The second and third groups were put on 800 or 1,200 calorie diets and also given the much touted behavior therapy, the popular counselling support, and other razz-ma-tazz used by centers such as Weightwatchers.

All groups rapidly lost weight. The second group, on 800 calories plus behavior therapy, was the best. Over 90% of them lost more than 20 lbs. Within a year, however, almost half of the women in all three groups had gained it all back. Within five years, 81% had gained it all back - and more. Incidentally, the behavior therapy groups were **less** successful at keeping off the pudge than the simple calorie restriction group.[14]

If that's not enough to convince you that dieting doesn't work, then look at the record of the prestigious and expensive, medically supervised programs such as Optifast and Medifast, often run through hospitals and medical clinics. The Colgan Institute tracked 13 people who rapidly lost weight on these programs. Eight of them regained most of it within 12-18 months. Today, four years later, only three have remained slim and two of those have been on continuing programs from us.

A larger study confirms our findings. In 1988, San Diego State University reported on 200 people who lost an average of 84% of their excess weight on these medically supervised diets. Incidentally, the diets cost at least $1,500 and include an extended course of behavior therapy sessions on how to keep weight off. Didn't work! Within three years, they regained 60-80% of the pudge.[15] Recently, the Federal Trade Commission commanded these companies to stop using the cloak of medical legitimacy to make overblown claims.

Why Diets Don't Work

There are three main problems with popular diet programs, all of which occur because they do not follow the findings of nutrition science:

1. They are concerned with reducing *weight* rather than the correct approach of reducing bodyfat.
2. They strip off vital muscle which is the major body component that burns the fat in the first place.
3. They take off weight far too fast, thereby throwing the body into a defensive, fat-preserving condition.

The true purpose of weight reduction is to dispose only of excess bodyfat while retaining your muscle and body water. Yet virtually none of the current commercial programs make any attempt to differentiate between these three weight components.

Some programs are even designed to partially dehydrate participants so as to show quick success. Any high school wrestler can tell you how to lose 5 lbs of water in two days, by stopping drinking, sitting in the sauna, or taking diuretic drugs or diuretic foods, such as melon and black coffee. But such tactics only stimulate the body to produce more anti-diuretic hormone, which causes it to grab back every drop of water and more, as soon as you take a hearty drink. Meanwhile, as we saw in Chapter 2, the dehydration decimates health and performance.

Muscle loss is even worse. Nutrition scientists have known for decades that, on low-calorie diets of 800 - 1,200 calories per day, up to 45% of the weight lost comes from the body cannibalizing its own muscle tissue.[16] Since the mid '80s, we have had a lot of models coming to the Colgan Institute for programs, because the new look is toned muscles rather than the sockfuls of pudding that passed for arms and legs in the Marilyn Monroe era. In vain attempts to look toned and thin without doing the necessary resistance exercise, many of these women exist on 500 - 800 calories a day, and have lost most of their muscle. They look slim, but measure up to 30% bodyfat. Technically, they are obese! Muscle is hard won and easily lost. No athlete can afford to waste an ounce of it.

Retaining muscle is also essential to losing fat. Bodyfat itself has very low metabolic activity. It burns few calories.[17] Muscle is the furnace in which bodyfat is burned. The less muscle you have, the lower your basal metabolic rate, and the harder it is to lose fat.[18] Any diet program that reduces muscle is a recipe for failure.

The next big problem with commercial diets is that they stimulate the body to accumulate the fat again once you stop. It happens like this. Because of public preference and patronage for programs claiming quick results, in order to compete in the marketplace, companies set calorie levels far too low (800 - 1,200 calories). Undereating to this extent causes rapid fat loss (and muscle loss). The body recognizes the fat loss as an attack on its energy reserve and immediately takes all sorts of defensive action. Two of these defenses combine to decimate your efforts to keep the fat off. First, your body increases the quantity and activity of an enzyme called **lipoprotein lipase,** the main enzyme it uses to collect and store fat.[19] Second, it slows your basal metabolic rate, further reducing your ability to burn fat.[20]

The lipoprotein lipase activity and the reduced metabolic rate continue for weeks after you stop the diet, because the body has a memory for exactly how much fat it had and wants it back. So it grabs and stores every molecule of fat you eat, even at the expense of bodily need for energy. The net result is the familiar post-diet fatigue and ravenous appetite that quickly returns every ounce of the flab, plus a little bit more for "insurance." Please don't follow commercial diets or popular diet books. If you do, your athletic career is likely to be nasty, debilitating, and short.

Fat Calories Are Fatter

It's still a common myth that a calorie is a calorie, whether it comes from carbohydrate, fat, or protein. Not so. Fat calories are fatter. That is, numerous recent studies show that you put on more bodyfat by eating fat than by eating the *same number of calories* from carbohydrate or protein. [21,22,23]

Dr Wayne Miller and colleagues at the University of Illinois did a convincing series of studies with rats. They gave one group of rats a diet containing 42% fats not too different from the standard American diet, or SAD (so aptly initialled). They gave a second group a low-fat diet of Ralston Purina animal chow. Both groups ate as much as desired.

Over 60 weeks, both groups ate almost exactly the same number of calories (36,000 per rat). Common beliefs in the weight-loss industry about calorie intake and bodyfat, would predict that both groups of rats would be equally fat. No way Jose! The high-fat group were very plump with an average bodyfat of 51%. The low-fat group were lean (for a rat) with an average bodyfat of 30%.[24] There is no longer any doubt that fat calories pack on the bodyfat.

Two reasons fat calories are fatter. First, evolution programmed mankind to store fat against times of food shortage that were frequent in earlier centuries. Consequently, fat oxidation (use of bodyfat for fuel) is not related to fat intake.[25] We are designed to be able to store far more fat than we use. Second, although the body can convert excess carbohydrate and protein to fat, it takes more than two grams of either to make one gram of fat. Add to that the metabolic cost of the conversion, which uses about a quarter of the calories contained in the excess,[26] and it becomes obvious that you have to stuff yourself with carbs or protein before you grow much fat.

One last wrinkle. How much fat you gain also depends on the type of fat you eat. Recent studies show that unsaturated fats are oxidized for fuel by the body more easily than saturated fats. That is, much of the saturated fat eaten is directly stored.[27] So avoid animal fats like the plague.

Calorie Counting Hogwash

Few people realize that the calorie counts on food labels and calorie charts have little to do with the caloric value of foods to any particular human being. Calorie counts for foods are obtained by burning the food in a bomb calorimeter and measuring the heat produced. A bomb calorimeter is not a human body. The values of four calories per gram for carbohydrates and proteins, and nine calories per gram for fats, are rough approximations made up almost a hundred years ago. They have become an entrenched and prevailing myth of the diet industry.

The caloric values of carbohydrates, proteins, and fats vary not only with particular foods that contain them and your dietary composition. They vary also with each person's biochemical individuality which affects the digestibility and efficiency of the use of food by the body. Just the example of dietary composition should be enough to convince you of the nonsense of calorie charts. Table sugar mixed with water, for example, provides more energy and puts on much more bodyfat than table sugar eaten by the spoonful.[28] One very good reason for avoiding sugared sodas.

We did one study at the Colgan Institute with four men and two women aged 23-40 whose weight and bodyfat were stable, that is, did not vary week to week by more than 2%. For six weeks, they reduced their usual lunch by 250 to 400 calories every day, and kept all other meals strictly at their usual levels. According to the American diet industry, that's a sure fire prescription for losing weight.

Over the six weeks, subjects reduced their so-called "caloric intake" by a total of 8,400 to 18,900 calories. According to the calories in - calories out myth that dominates American dieting, they should have lost substantial weight. At approximately 3,600 calories per pound, they should have lost between 2.25 and 5.25 pounds. In fact, only one man and one woman lost any weight, the man 1.5 lbs and the woman 0.75 lbs. The other four lost nothing at all.[29] Counting calories just doesn't add up.

Lotions, Potions, and Drugs

The prevalence of cottage cheese thighs in America is a boon to the cosmetics industry. Anti-cellulite creams abound made by such prestigious houses as Elizabeth Arden, La Prairie, Clarins, Chanel, Lancome, and hundreds of lesser companies.

The advertising is a plethora of hyperbole and mendacity. Some brochures claim that the creams help break down cellulite to release the toxins it contains. Others claim to increase circulation to carry the toxins away, "that are the main cause of cellulite," or to release water trapped in unsightly ripples under the skin. The worst blatantly state that their creams or lotion will remove cellulite wholesale.

None of these work a jot. As Dr Peter Foder, president of the Lipoplasty Society emphasizes, there are no toxins, and there is no trapped water. Cellulite is just ordinary bodyfat sitting under the skin in tiny pockets separated by connective tissue. You cannot remove a molecule with creams or lotions unless they contain a beta-adrenergic agonist drug that can penetrate the skin and enter the fat beneath.[30] All such drugs are still experimental. It will be years before the FDA approves one. Then it will be strictly prescription, and therefore v-e-e-e-ery expensive. Meanwhile, all the cellulite creams and lotions are a useless snake oil scam.

Over-the-counter weight-loss remedies are no better. Recently the FDA banned, as ineffective or unhealthy, more than one hundred substances sold for weight control. These include:

> Fiber pills (the amount of fiber is negligible)
> Herbal teas (contain diuretics, cause only
>   temporarywater loss)
> Artificial sweeteners (no evidence that users lose
>   weight)
> Guar gum (has fatally blocked throat or intestines)
> Glucomannan, Spirulena (bulking agents that don't)
> Gymnema silvestre (taste blocking herb)
> Starch blockers (putrify intestines)
> Intestinal peptides (not active orally)
> Grapefruit pills, Lactate (hype and dreams).

The only two substances now permitted to be sold freely for weight-loss are benzocaine and phenylpropanolamine (PPA). Benzocaine is just a local anaesthetic aimed at numbing the taste responses of the mouth and throat to food. PPA is a stimulant that does appear to suppress appetite a bit. But is also tends to raise blood pressure and cause nausea even in healthy young people.[31] And even the makers of over-the-counter weight-loss drugs containing PPA do not recommend them for long-term weight control. Athletes we have measured while they were using these drugs show no additional fat loss at all.

There are drugs that will strip off bodyfat. We discuss the most effective in Part VII of this book. But the side-effects are horrendous. Don't use them. The following program will enable you to take off all the bodyfat you want -- and keep it off for life.

Permanent Fat Loss

As part of biochemical individuality, people differ widely in their **inherited** tendencies to accumulate bodyfat. That's obvious. But some theories have extrapolated the obvious to claim that each person is designed to be comfortable and healthy only at a certain level of fat, and that the body will always revert to that level.[32] They are dead wrong!

The habitual amount of fat that you carry is not ordained by your genes. It is caused by what you eat and what you do. We know now that neither the number of fat cells nor their size is genetically fixed.[33] Fatness is much more dependent on your lifestyle.

From the principle of physiological dynamics, your body has no internal reference system for a fixed level of fat, only for an habitual level. When you remain at a particular level of fat for a year or two, the body develops all the adipose cells, capillaries, enzyme counts, peripheral nerves, hormone levels, and connective tissue to support it. It comes to recognize that level of fat as self and will defend it vigorously. That is your **fatpoint.**

The body constantly monitors its fatpoint with hormonal messengers, such as glycerol, which warn the brain to take defensive action if even a single ounce is suddenly used for fuel. So the usual forms of dieting (one popular program claims "10 pounds in 6 weeks,") can't possibly work. As we have seen earlier in this chapter, by slowing metabolism, increasing fat storage, and increasing appetite, your body's fatpoint defenses will defeat you every time.

But it's far from hopeless to change your bodyfat level. In fact, it's easy. Reliable studies show that it takes years of overeating to grow fat.[34] In other words, the body shifts its fatpoint *up* very slowly. To shift it *down*, you have to operate the same way, very slowly. Rule 1 for permanent fat loss: **Lose no more than half-a-pound of fat per week.**

Studying athletes for the last 18 years, we have found that the **most** you can reduce your food intake to reset the fatpoint is 10% per day. Any weight loss of more than half-a-pound per week is a warning that you are reducing too much. You will see little change for the first two months, but over a year, your fatpoint will edge downward by 3-6%. Meanwhile, your body is remodelling its adipose cells, hormones, enzymes, capillaries and other tissues to suit. In a year to eighteen months, you have reset the fatpoint without arousing a single bodily defense.

To ensure that you are losing fat and not muscle, it is essential to get your body composition measured each two months. After testing dozens of systems, the Colgan Institute recommends only two, underwater weighing and near infra-red inductance using the Futrex 5000 device. Go to the same facility each time, because systems are all calibrated differently. Rule 2 for permanent fat loss: **Get your fat measured every two months.**

The only type of food you need to cut from your diet is saturated fats. As we saw earlier, this food puts on more bodyfat than any other. When excess carbohydrate or protein is eaten, the body makes complex metabolic adjustments to promote glycogen storage in muscle, and increase the use of protein or sugar for fuel.[35] Hence you have to eat a big excess of these foods before they are converted to bodyfat. But when excess saturated fats are eaten, metabolism remains unchanged. Virtually, all the excess is promptly layered onto belly, hips, and thighs.[36] Rule 3 for permanent fat loss: **Avoid all saturated fats.**

These include the fats in all meats and most dairy foods and the high levels of saturated fats in some vegetable oils detailed in Chapter 8. If you focus on eliminating all saturated fats, then given our fat-loaded food supply, you might be able to keep intake down to 10% of total calories.

Don't use popular diets or weight-loss centers to help you. As we saw most of the programs are deficient in vitamins and minerals. It is no use to athletes to reduce bodyfat if they also deplete the body of essential nutrients. Rule 4 for permanent fat loss: **Avoid all commercial diets.**

The same goes for lotions, potions, and over-the-counter drugs touted for weight control. The lotions and potions don't work at all. The drugs are temporary at best, and saddled with side-effects that crucify performance.[31] Rule 5 for permanent fat loss: **No drugs or witches' brews.**

There are a few nutrients that can help. The first is l-carnitine. Fats are burned for energy inside muscle cells at structures called **mitochondria**. But the fats are stored in adipose cells and cannot pass through the mitochondria membranes unless they are transported by l-carnitine.

The amount of fat burned depends a lot on the level of l-carnitine in the muscle. The higher the level, the greater the amount of bodyfat used for fuel. Although the body makes l-carnitine, it may not make an optimum amount for athletes, because muscle carnitine levels are rapidly depleted even during moderate exercise.[37] There is reasonable evidence that oral supplements of this amino acid raise muscle carnitine levels.[38] And a recent study with athletes shows that supplementation with two grams per day of l-carnitine significantly increased their use of fat during exercise.[39] Rule 6 for permanent fat loss: **Maintain l-carnitine status.**

The second nutrient that helps with fat loss is the essential element chromium. In the 1970s, Dr Walter Mertz of the US Department of Agriculture established that chromium is essential for normal insulin metabolism. As such, it is important for growth of muscle and control of bodyfat.[40] The RDA handbook recommends 50-200 mcg chromium per day.[41] Other studies show that some sedentary subjects require 290 mcg per day, to remain in chromium balance.[42] From these figures, the range of daily chromium needs for sedentary people is at least 50-290 mcg. The most recent study by the US Department of Agriculture indicates that 90% of US diets contain less than 50 mcg chromium per day.[40] So chromium deficiency is widespread.

Athletes use about twice as much chromium as sedentary

people, even on moderate exercise days.[43] So they are likely to be doubly deficient, with all its detrimental effects on maintenance of muscle and use of bodyfat for fuel. To overcome these problems, at the Colgan Institute, we supplement athletes with 200 - 600 mcg of chromium picolinate daily. Rule 7 for permanent fat loss: **Maintain chromium status.**

There is more to controlling insulin than chromium. Except for during and immediately after intense exercise, every time you eat simple sugars, especially sugared drinks, blood sugar rises precipitously and causes an insulin burst. The liver then balances the insulin see-saw by turning the excess into triglycerides (fats) which are promptly deposited as bodyfat.[44]

So you should do everything possible to keep insulin production stable. An obvious strategy is to avoid most simple sugars. Athletes need to base their diets on complex carbohydrates that are slowly absorbed and do not disturb insulin metabolism. The right carbohydrates are detailed in Chapter 9. Rule 8 for permanent fat loss: **Cut the sugar: eat mainly complex carbs.**

Another nutrient, or rather non-nutrient that helps regulate insulin metabolism is fiber. It retards the digestion of sugars and fats so that less quick sugar and less high calorie fat bombard the system.[45] High fiber diets (30-50 grams per day) create a slow, even energy uptake that favors use of food for energy rather than for deposition as bodyfat.[46] And insulin also remains stable. The right fiber to use is detailed in Chapter 4. Rule 9 for permanent fat loss: **Eat a high fiber diet.**

In a just published report, Gilbert Kaats of Health and Medical Services of San Antonio, Texas and his colleagues at the University of Texas, combined my Rules 5, 6, and 8 in a study that emphasizes their effectiveness.[47] First, they gave groups of five overweight men and women simply low-calorie, low-fat, diets of 1,250 calories per day for women and 1,650 calories for men. Over eight weeks, subjects lost very little weight. Then for another eight weeks, they supplemented the diets daily with:

Chromium picolinate:	400 mcg
L-carnitine	200 mg
Fiber	20 gm

At the end of the second period, subjects showed an average weight loss of 15.1 lbs, including an average fat loss of 11.8 lbs. Spectacular! The bodyfat reduction was far too fast to last, but it does underline the importance of chromium, carnitine, and fiber status if you want to achieve permanent fat loss.

Two other nutrients that help regulate insulin metabolism are omega-3 fatty acids, the eiosapentanoic acid (EPA) and docosahexanoic acid (DHA) found in fish oils. Dr Leonard Storlien and colleagues at Garvin Institute of Medical Research in New South Wales, Australia have shown that animals supplemented with fish oils do not develop disorders of insulin metabolism, even when given a diet that normally causes diabetes.[48] That's the sort of protection an athlete needs. Rule 10 for permanent fat loss: **Maintain omega-3 fatty acid status.**

Two more strategies for losing bodyfat concern exercise. The usual advice is aerobic exercise and more aerobic exercise, and the more intense the better. It is dead wrong! Except at low intensity such as brisk walking or slow jogging, aerobic exercise, including running, rowing, cycling, swimming, and aerobics all strip off muscle almost as much as they strip off fat. That's why most long distance runners and cyclists are skinny and weak. They have a great endurance but no power. Running guru Dr George Sheehan once admitted to me that he couldn't do a single sit-up. A dozen chins or 30 push-ups are beyond many of the elite runners that we test.

Remember what we said earlier about muscle. It's the engine in which bodyfat is burned. Do everything to preserve it. The correct exercise for fat loss is low intensity, high repetition, high variety resistance exercise training. The minimum is four sessions of 30 minutes weekly. We have used our Bodyshape

Program now with hundreds of cases, and compared them to aerobic exercise. The resistance training is definitely superior. The secret is that, while burning fat, weight training preserves or even increases the engine of muscle mass, making it progressively easier every week for the body to burn more fat. Rule 11 for permanent fat loss: **Weight train to maintain lean mass.** Rule 12 for permanent fat loss: **Do low intensity, high duration aerobic exercise daily.**

Also, train in the mornings. Numerous studies show that exercise raises the resting metabolic rate (RMR), not only while you are doing it, but for up to 18 hours afterwards. You burn more calories per hour **all day.**[49,50] But if you work out in the evening and then go to sleep, RMR drops like a stone, and you lose the major fat-loss effect. Rule 13 for permanent fat loss: **Train in the mornings to boost RMR.**

The final rule is so important, not only for losing fat, but also for gaining muscle, that I gave it a separate chapter. Probably the single greatest influence on bodyfat is your **anabolic drive.** This complex of hormonal influences is fully described in Chapter 32. Rule 14 for permanent fat loss: **Maintain your anabolic drive.**

If you apply these simple rules honestly and don't lose bodyfat and keep it off, I'll quit sports medicine and blimp up to 300 lbs on Haagen-Daz. Then I can join Oprah Winfrey on TV and complain how all weight-loss programs are a scam. When she wheeled that cart on stage with 60 lbs of fat to show what she had lost, I bet $100 she would regain it in a year. I won. Even the rich and famous fall victim to the frauds of commercial weight loss.

Table 14. Fourteen Rules for Permanent Fat Loss.

Rules For Permanent Fat Loss
1. Lose no more than 1/2 lb of fat per week.   2. Get your fat measured every two months.   3. Avoid all saturated fats.   4. Avoid all commercial diets.   5. No drugs or witches' brews.   6. Maintain l-carnitine status.   7. Maintain chromium status.   8. Cut the sugar: eat complex carbs.   9. Eat a high fiber diet.   10. Maintain omega-3 fatty acid status.   11. Weight train to maintain lean mass.   12. Do low intensity, high duration aerobic exercise daily.   13. Train in the mornings to boost RMR.   14. Maintain your anabolic drive.

Part III

Building Materials

The FDA interpretations of the Nutrition Labelling and Education Act completely satisfy the statutory requirement for public confusion.

Michael Colgan, Nutrition Certification Course, 1992

Chapter 12

Protein For Growth

Confused about protein and amino acid requirements? No wonder. At one extreme we have the Recommended Dietary Allowances (RDA) of 0.75 grams of protein per kilogram bodyweight for sedentary folk. No additional protein is specified for athletes, no matter how intense their training.[1] Uninformed physicians, nutritionists, and dietitians (often funded by the meat or dairy industries), parrot the RDA as right for everyone. And (with paychecks in mind) they usually specify that your protein should come from animal sources like beef, eggs, or cheese - all high-fat, high-cholesterol foods that have been losing their market share like crazy.

At the other extreme, we have the wild claims of some supplement suppliers. Their tubs of "protein" powder are now so big they make great garbage bins once you empty them. Take a few handfuls of these "wonder" amino pills or this "ultimate" protein shake, say the ads, and Bingo! You'll grow bigger than God.

Like Tweedledum and Tweedledee the tame commercial scientists and the supplement hustlers snipe at each other with very little science and even less common sense. To clear up this mess, I will spell out the science of protein nutrition in as non-technical a way as possible. I will explain what types of protein you need and how much, what amino acids you need and when, in order to achieve the premium athletic body.

This stuff is leading edge. It is therefore a ready target for criticism by researchers whose thinking is biased by obsolete theories, or the source of their next research grant. If you quote this chapter and someone tells you different, then read the research references given. You will see that I have kept the scientific faith. As you pursue your quest for excellence, remember the words of Maeterlinck, "Each progressive spirit is opposed by a thousand mediocre minds appointed to guard the past."

Building Blocks for Bodies

Suck all the water out of a lean athletic body and what is left? Mostly protein. Over 50% of the dry weight of your body is protein. Even the hemoglobin that carries the oxygen in your blood is protein. The structure of your genes and your brain cells is totally protein. All bodily functions, from the blink of an eye to the creation of new muscle, are controlled by thousands of different enzymes -- and all enzymes are proteins. So you better get your protein nutrition right if you have aspirations to become a champion.

And you have to get it right *all the time*. You can make big mistakes with fats and carbs and correct them easily. But your mistakes with protein build right into your structure, and hamper performance for months. Whenever I lecture on this topic, at least one student will object that I am overstating the case. "Aw, come on Doc, you have your genes at birth. They may be made of protein but they can't be affected by nutrition." Dead wrong. Many athletes don't appreciate the dynamics of body structure. Body proteins are not there forever. They die.

Experiments using radioisotope techniques show that over 98% of the molecules of the human body are completely replaced each year.[2] Bits and pieces of all your structures are constantly being replaced with new proteins. In six months your biceps, your blood, your enzymes, even the structures of your genes are all completely replaced. The body you have today is built almost entirely from what you have eaten over the last six months.

If the proteins you eat are poor quality, then all the structures of your body, muscles, bones, blood, teeth, and pinkies will be poor quality. Oh, the human system is super ingenious at making do with inadequate building materials, patching, stitching, and pinch-hitting, but it can't build premium tissue from garbage. A Twinkies and coffee diet produces a Twinkies and coffee body. For optimum performance you have to eat optimum protein to build optimum structure -- period.

That Pesky RDA

In attempting to assess the RDA for protein, successive committees of the US National Academy of Sciences, Food and Nutrition Board have repeated a basic error for the last 50 years. They have studied only sedentary individuals. They have relied on data from protein put in and protein excreted from the body in feces and urine of subjects confined to metabolic wards. Other losses in skin, sweat, and hemolysis (blood loss) are usually estimated. No allowances are made for exercise or muscle growth.[1]

These studies have little relevance for athletes. Losses of protein in sweat, for example, increase substantially when you exercise.[3] So do losses by hemolysis (death of red blood cells).[4] Use of protein for energy also increases dramatically, providing 5-10% of the total energy supply.[5] If you push exercise so that muscle glycogen becomes depleted, then the body literally eats its own muscle tissue for fuel.[3]

How then can the RDA committee and numerous media pronouncements on nutrition still come to the conclusion that exercise does not increase protein requirements? Simple, they have not kept up with new research over the last decade that demonstrates the increased protein needs of athletes. The 1989 handbook of the RDAs (the latest issue), quotes as its reference sources studies done from 1964 to 1977 (1, p. 71). If you want to be a champion, get this handbook, study it carefully to confirm what I say, then see how it makes like a discus, over a large, deep body of water.

How Much Protein?

Evidence for the protein needs of athletes has been accumulating since 1974. Dr I. Gontzea and colleagues at the Institute of Medicine in Bucharest were the first to show that exercise causes the body to use protein at a much faster rate. Like the RDA studies, they also measured nitrogen balance, but added the essential variable of exercise. A positive nitrogen balance means that the body is obtaining sufficient protein from the diet. A negative nitrogen balance means that the body has insufficient input of protein, and is therefore cannibalizing muscle and other protein structures to provide its daily needs.

First, the athletes were instructed to stop exercising and

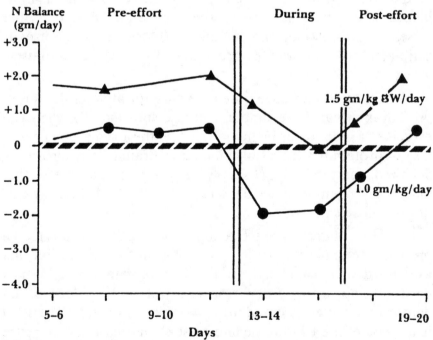

Figure 6: Effects of exercise on nitrogen balance at different levels of protein intake. Redrawn from Gontzea, References 6 and 7.

remain sedentary for two weeks. They were given a daily ration of 1.0 grams of protein per kilogram bodyweight (33% above the RDA). As long as they remained sedentary, this level of protein intake maintained a positive nitrogen balance. Then they were given workouts of 2 hours a day. As Figure 8 shows, nitrogen balance dropped to negative within two days. Protein intake one-third above the RDA was insufficient to meet the increase in protein needs caused by the exercise.[6,7]

Gontzea fed another group of athletes a higher level of protein at 1.5 grams per kilogram bodyweight (twice the RDA). As Figure 8 shows, as long as they remained sedentary, nitrogen balance was positive. But when they were given the same 2-hour a day workouts as the first group, nitrogen balance dropped to negative within four days. So even 1.5 grams per kilogram bodyweight was insufficient to meet the increased protein demand caused by the exercise.[6,7]

The studies of Gontzea were published in a reputable international nutrition journal but were not acceptable to some American scientists, because they originated in a foreign medical school. Now, however, there are new studies in the U.S. that are not so easy to ignore. At conservative Tufts University, Dr William Evans and colleagues, at the USDA Human Nutrition Research Center, have shown that men who regularly exercise with the endurance sports of running, cycling, or swimming require more protein than the RDA. Their findings show that regular, moderate endurance exercise increases protein needs to about 1.4 g/kg/day.[8]

Other new studies of endurance exercise support this figure. Dr CN Meredith and colleagues reported in the **Journal of Applied Physiology** that active endurance athletes aged 23 to 59, required an average protein intake of 1.26 g/kg/day.[9] Dr Peter Lemon and colleagues at Kent State University, Ohio, leading lights in the area of protein needs, repeated the experiments of Gontzea and found that endurance athletes in regular training require 1.14 - 1.39 g/kg/day.[10]

These researchers all examined athletes doing moderate levels of training. Excellent studies that simulated the Tour de France show that, if you increase the intensity and duration of endurance exercise, protein needs increase even further. The "Tour de France" cyclists, doing five hours of intense riding per day, required up to 1.8 g/kg/day to remain in protein balance.[11,12,13] That's almost 2½ times the RDA.

Growing Muscle

What about strength and short-event athletes, who are especially concerned not only to maintain protein status, but also to increase muscle growth. There is no doubt that very high protein intake, 3.0 g/kg/day, maintains a highly positive nitrogen balance.[14] But the use of nitrogen for building muscle is not controlled by the protein you eat. It is controlled by processes in the liver that hold the available store at precisely the level required to meet bodily demand. All excess protein is simply broken down into carbohydrates and urea wastes.

Despite what the supplement ads imply, it is not protein *intake* that controls muscle growth, but rather the demand for growth caused by the trauma of intense exercise. No one ever grew an ounce of muscle from simply gulping protein. Muscles grow from pushing poundage - period.

So the trick is to match your individual protein intake to your training program. If, and only if, you are doing intense strength or speed workouts (over 3 hours per day), then there is evidence that very high protein intake does yield greater muscle growth. Dr Frank Consolazio and colleagues at the Letterman Army Institute of Research in San Francisco, gave healthy men either 1.4 g/kg/day or 2.8 g/kg/day of protein in a 3,600 calorie diet. Then they trained the hell out of them to near exhaustion for 40 days. Subjects on the lower protein intake, which we have seen is sufficient for most endurance athletes, gained 1.21 kg of lean mass. Subjects on the higher protein intake gained a massive 3.28 kg (7.2 lbs) of lean mass.[15] When you train hard for muscle you need a lot of protein to keep pace.

Other studies support these findings, including one on Romanian weightlifters, the strongest athletes in the world. Over three months of training the weightlifters increased their protein intake from 2.2 g/kg/day to 3.5 g/kg/day. Even though these men were already near the top of their potential, they made huge, further gains of 6% in muscle mass and 5% in strength.[16]

They were eating protein at a level of about 450% of the RDA. But before you grab that protein bar, remember they were also training up to *five* times a day. If you want the gains, exercise is the key that creates the demand for new structure. Protein does nothing to stimulate growth. It simply provides the building materials.

Mo' Protein, Mo' Protein

I have watched big lads scarf down 24 egg whites at a sitting. Others tell me they have eaten protein to the point of vomiting, under the illusion that it will turn into muscle. Plain dumb! If you eat enough excess of protein to grow a hippopotamus, then that's what you'll become, a roly-poly lump with a burgeoning rump.

So, even if you train your brains out, don't fall for the muscle mania myth that you need to stuff protein *ad nauseum*. Despite magazine ads claiming "25 lbs of solid muscle in 12 weeks," most athletes furiously pumping the iron, and on the best nutrition, gain less than 10 lbs a year. The best we have measured in drug-free athletes at the Colgan Institute is 181/4 lbs.

Remember the principle of **physiological dynamics** from Chapter 1. You have to wait on Nature to grow muscle. Muscle proteins are replaced about every six months. The limiting rate of turnover of muscle cells indicates that it is impossible, even in the biggest men, to grow more than about *one ounce* of new muscle per day. That's 23 lbs a year. Oh, you can use all sorts of tricks to make muscles hold more water and *look* bigger, but growth of new muscle **tissue** is absolutely controlled by physiology.

Let's be generous and set the *maximum* one-year gain at 25 lbs of new muscle. That's less than half-a-pound a week, about an ounce a day. Human muscle is only 22% protein, so the maximum amount of new muscle most folk can grow in a day, requires less than a quarter-of-an-ounce additional protein to grow it - about a tablespoon. Athletes do need quite a bit of extra protein, but most of it is used to combat protein losses caused by training and protein used for energy. For the protein required for new muscle *structure,* you can grow Tarzan from a tablespoon a day.

Your Personal Protein Program

Space in this book permits me to cover only a tiny fraction of the research. But the evidence I do cite is representative of nearly two decades of work with thousands of athletes, and analyses of all existing studies. From this database, the Colgan Institute has evolved a simple method of assessing individual protein needs. The criteria are type of sport, intensity or stage of training and bodyweight. They are pretty well in line with the research.

First, we classify sports by their need for strength, speed and endurance. Class 1 is sports that demand strength first, then speed, then endurance. It includes weightlifting, shot-put, javelin, discus, and men's gymnastics. Class 2 is sports demanding speed first, then strength, then endurance. Sprints of all kinds, jumping, boxing, wrestling, karate, judo, sprint swimming, women's gymnastics, and ball games fall in this class. Class 3 is sports where endurance dominates. These include middle and long distance running, triathlon, cross-country skiing, cycling, and tennis.

The protein needs for each class are shown in Table 15. They are based on protein levels of 2.0 g/kg/day for Class 1, 1.7 g/kg/day for Class 2, and 1.4 g/kg/day for Class 3. That is a range of nearly 2-3 times the RDA.

Your training program also influences protein needs.

Table 15. Daily protein requirements for athletes (grams).

| Bodyweight | | Sports/Training Category* | | |
kg	lbs	Class 1	Class 2	Class 3
40	88	80	68	56
50	110	100	85	70
60	132	120	102	84
70	154	140	119	98
80	176	160	136	112
90	198	180	153	126
100	220	200	170	140
110	242	220	187	154
120	264	240	204	168

*See text for explanation of classes.

Source: Colgan Institute, San Diego, CA.

Examples give the best explanation. The Colgan Institute did the nutrition program for boxer Bobby Czyz from the time he was a club boxer in New Jersey until he won the world championship. At one stage, he was moving up from 6 round fights to 10 rounders. He needed more endurance. For six months, we moved him from Class 2 to Class 3, reducing his protein so that we could fit more complex carbohydrates into his diet.

Another example is skier Dr Harry Buzbuzian. He started a weight program during the off season to bring up his strength. Strength increase was accelerated by eating protein at a Class 1 level. But it did not help endurance. As soon as snow training resumed, we shifted him back to Class 3, to permit him to have the carbs essential for long practice days on the slopes.

You should also allow for intensity of training. Our system is for competition athletes and is based on maximum training

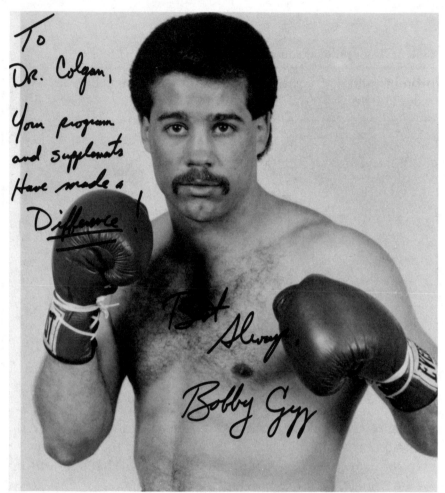

To
Dr. Colgan,
Your program
and supplements
have made a
Difference!

Best
Always
Bobby Gyy

Bobby Czyz used a nutrition program from the Colgan Institute from his club boxer days in New Jersey until he made world champion.

levels, 3 hours a day or more. If you put in only 1-2 hours you need less protein, so move one class to the right. If you are already in Class 3 move to the next *lower* bodyweight.

Testing Your Protein Intake

The table is pretty good, but because of biochemical individuality, it is not perfect. Dr Roger Williams at the University of Texas and other researchers have shown that individuals differ considerably in their needs for protein.[17] Champion bodybuilder Bill Pearl, for example, maintains his huge muscle bulk on a protein intake that would cause most big men to lose muscle fast.[18]

It's easy to know if you are getting too little protein. Your strength and muscle mass decline. But how do you know if you are getting too much? It is important to know because if you eat excess protein that is not used for structure, you put the body into a condition that hampers performance. When excess protein food breaks down during digestion, it fills your blood with more than the amino acids that make it up.

Excess amino acids are converted into non-toxic carbon dioxide and water plus highly toxic **ammonia**. Your body immediately protects itself by turning the ammonia into less toxic **urea**, which is then excreted by the kidneys. If you eat protein beyond their capacity to remove the toxic wastes, you overload the kidneys and poison your blood.

Chronic elevated urea is literally a pain in the butt. Inflamed kidneys generate a lot of low back pain, and general feelings of malaise. And unless your levels are really high, you will come out clean on all the expensive tests your physician decrees.

One biomarker that we use to identify this problem is the blood test for urea, called **BUN (blood urea nitrogen)**. The so-called "normal" range for BUN in the blood is 10-25 mg/dl. But back in the early '70s, Dr Richard Passwater was one of the first to suggest that a low BUN of 10-14 mg/dl is one measure of good health, and that a BUN level over 21 mg/dl indicates poor health.[19] Many sports medicine folk, including me, now agree with Passwater.

High BUN is also caused by dehydration. But if you are feeling off and your fluid intake is O.K., and you run a BUN over 21 mg/dl, then reduce your protein. Trust me, you will not lose muscle: you are only getting rid of the excess. BUN should drop within a month, and performance should perk up nicely.

Protein Sources

Your body can make most of protein's 21 amino acids from carbohydrate. It cannot make much of the nine *essential* amino acids, **isoleucine, leucine, lysine, methionine, phenylalanine, threonine, tryptophan, valine,** and in some people, **histidine.** A tenth amino acid, **arginine,** is essential for children, and probably for growth in a good many adults. All must be provided by your diet.[1,17]

The degree to which food provides the essential amino acids used to be measured by the Net Protein Utilization Index (NPU) or the Protein Equivalency Ratio (PER). Top of those measures are whey protein concentrate (lactalbumin) and egg white protein (egg albumin). Under ideal conditions they provide almost 100% of the amino acid mix needed by the body. Fish and meats are not as good, with scores around 80%, followed by casein and soy at about 75%. Many plant foods have scores below 50%.

But, with the new measure of protein described in Chapter 4, the Protein Digestibility Corrected Amino Acid Score (PDCAAS), the FDA has decreed that some vegetable proteins, especially soy protein, will show a score on food labels as high as whey or egg protein. Don't be fooled.

The usual food sources of proteins for athletes are muscles, that is, the steaks and chops and loins of sundry unfortunate beasts. The big problem with these sources is they come wrapped in fat - lots of fat. A lean beef steak, for example, has about 28 grams (1 ounce) of protein per 100 grams (31/2 ounces). But it has 31 grams of fat. A lean loin of pork has about 23 grams of protein per 100 grams. But it also has 29 grams of fat. Three slices of lean bacon contain only 12 grams of protein, but a whopping 70 grams of fat! And link pork sausages, beloved of the junk food breakfast, have only 9 grams of protein to 52 grams of fat. Might as well eat lard.

Apart from skinless chicken and turkey, especially the new

low-fat processed poultry described in Chapter 4, the only unprocessed animal foods that provide ample amounts of protein
without the fats are fish, shellfish, and egg whites. Table 16 gives
you the protein content of some low-fat animal foods that are
easily available. Some high-fat items you should avoid are
included for comparison. Some books show different figures
because they have not calculated the water content correctly. The
figures given here, compiled from our own food analyses at the
Colgan Institute, and from the world authority on food
composition, McCance and Widdowson, are the most accurate
you will find.[20]

Vegetable Protein

If you can't stomach fish every day, and you have run out
of creative ways to disguise egg whites, then vegetables and grains
are reasonable sources. Except for soybeans, however, proteins
in these foods are generally in the wrong ratios for human
nutrition. Rice, for example, although it feeds more than half the
world, will not maintain lean tissue, one reason that the rice eaters
are almost all small, small muscled people.

A common myth that needs deep burial is that plant
proteins are incomplete. McCance and Widdowson confirms our
own tests at the Colgan Institute that *all* common grains, nuts,
seeds, and legumes contain *all* the essential amino acids.[20] Grains
tend to be low in tryptophan and lysine while legumes are high.
But if you combine plant foods in the diet, your body gets
sufficient of each amino acid to maintain health.

Some grains are poor sources by themselves. Though it has
excellent carbohydrate qualities, brown rice is very low in the
essential amino acids, worse than white flour. Coconut, a "health
food" staple, is also a poor source, in fact a poor food all around
because of its high fat content. Don't eat it or any other nuts; they
are all high fat. All refined grains have lost a lot of their amino
acids. Don't eat them either. Leave refined foods for the supermarket rodents. If you are a vegetarian athlete, or tend that way,

Table 16. Protein, water, and fat content of common animal foods per 100 grams (3 1/2 oz.) serving.

Food (100 grams)	Protein (grams)	Fat (grams)	Water (grams)
Egg whites (scrambled)	9	0	89
Flounder (grilled, dry)	21	1	77
Orange Roughy (grilled, dry)	20	1	76
Shrimp (steamed)	17	1	81
Albacore Tuna (water packed)	24	1	74
Clams (steamed)	12	1	84
Mussels (steamed)	17	2	79
Turkey breast (skinless, roast)	23	2	74
Lobster (steamed)	22	4	73
Trout (grilled, dry)	24	4	71
Chicken breast (skinless, grilled)	26	4	69
Duck (skinless, roast)	19	5	75
Crab (steamed)	20	5	73
Venison (roast)	35	6	57
Rabbit (roast)	27	8	64
Salmon (poached)	20	13	66
High-fat Foods for Comparison (Don't Eat These!)			
Beefsteak (lean, grilled)	25	15	57
Pork Loin (roast)	23	29	46
Fatback bacon	12	70	17
Butter	0.5	82	16

Sources: McCance and Widdowson, Reference 20, and the Colgan Institute.

the best plant sources of protein are given in Chapter 4.

Another myth needing burial is that you have to combine plant proteins at the same meal. Nature made the human body a lot cleverer than that. Your amino acid pool is designed to accept needed additions any time they arrive. Numerous studies show that vegetable proteins taken even 24 hours apart combine in the body to provide all the protein amino acids.[21,22] It can take a gram of lysine from a midday mug of lentil soup and wait for its methionine (low in lentils) until whole grain rolls at dinner.

Calculate your protein needs from Table 14, then use the widest variety of low-fat protein food you can to try to fill them. It's a difficult job, impossible if you are on the road a lot, like many sports teams. We have reluctantly concluded that athletes cannot get optimum protein intake without a protein supplement. The best ones to use and some special amino acids you will need to fill in the gaps are detailed in the next chapter.

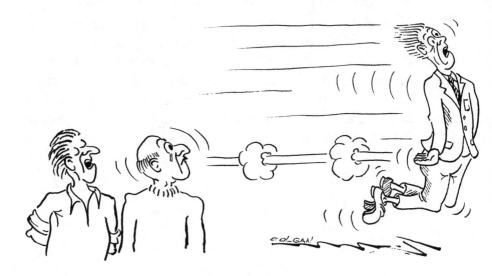

"He's been to that new tofu restaurant."

Chapter 13

Protein Supplements

Protein supplements come in three basic forms. First, there are **intact proteins**, such as casein, the main protein in milk. Intact proteins are all **polypeptides** (many amino acids joined together). Second, there are **hydrolysates**, made by putting intact proteins through an enzyme digester bath to break them down into single amino acids, **dipeptides** (two amino acids joined together) and **tripeptides** (three amino acids joined together). Third, there are **free-form amino acids** made by fermentation of a food base in the guts of specialized bacteria.

There is a continual war going on between supplement manufacturers about which form is the best. Intact proteins are the same as protein foods. Most of the powders and meal replacement drinks use casein, whey protein, egg protein, or soy protein in various combinations. Your digestion has to break these down into single amino acids, dipeptides and tripeptides for absorption.

The best argument for intact proteins is that the human gut evolved over millions of years to digest protein in that form. Consequently, the gut initiates all sorts of essential physiological activities in the body in response to intact proteins. The best argument for hydrolysates is that they are already pre-digested and can be absorbed more easily. Proponents claim that hydrolysates are the same as intact proteins after digestion, simply more easily bioavailable.

The amino acid ratios in intact protein powders and hydrolysates are fixed by the amino content of the protein used. So the best argument for free-form amino acid mixes is that the ratios of amino acids are not fixed: you can mix them in any ratios you like. If there is an ideal mix for different kinds of athletes, you can make it exactly.

These arguments are all valid, but the real question is, which form of protein supplement works best? Since 1974, the Colgan Institute has tracked all the studies comparing the three forms. The edge for absorption lies with hydrolysates. They are absorbed faster than intact proteins.[1,2] They are also absorbed better than free-form amino acids because the human gut has a special transport system for dipeptides and tripeptides that single amino acids cannot use.[3]

Hydrolysates are also better retained. I used to favor the free-form amino acids, but numerous recent studies of burn and surgery patients have shown that nitrogen retention and recovery from injury is faster with hydrolysates than with intact proteins[4] or equivalent free-form amino acid mixtures.[5,6]

Hydrolysates work best in healthy guts too, at least in animals. Dr Gary Zaloga and colleagues at Bowman Grey School of Medicine in North Carolina, compared a hydrolysate formula with intact proteins and with an equivalent free-form amino acid formula. The hydrolysate subjects grew 50% faster than the free-form amino subjects and 30% faster than the intact protein subjects.[3]

Dr Marie Poullain and colleagues at the prestigious INSERM Research Unit at Le Vesinet in France did a similar study. Nitrogen retention, a measure of increase in lean tissue, was highest with a whey hydrolysate. Animals grew 7.5% compared with 3% on intact protein, and 1% on free-form amino acids. The hydrolysate was more than twice as effective as the next best form of protein supplement and *seven times* as effective as free-form aminos.[7]

Until very recently, scientists couldn't understand why a

free-form mixture that has exactly the same ratios and amounts of amino acids as a hydrolysate, just doesn't work as well. As my friend, leadership guru Stephen Covey says, "You were looking in the wrong jungle." We were examining every triviality about amino acid structure, when the answer lay not in the amino themselves but in Nature. During evolution humans developed the separate gut system to absorb dipeptides and tripeptides for very special reasons. When two or more aminos are joined together they carry information. That information causes physiological responses that do not occur to single (information-less) aminos. New studies show that dipeptides and tripeptides signal the liver to produce somatomedin C, the anabolic growth factor that stimulates muscle growth.[3,8]

The carrying of information to the body by dipeptides raises another problem for makers of commercial amino acid supplements. Many of them trumpet the RDA, saying that their formulas contain all nine essential amino acids. They neglect the eleven non-essential amino acids that the body can make. Anticipating the research, Dr Roger Williams, nutrition genius at the University of Texas, first explained to me in 1975 why protein formulas should also contain all the non-essential aminos. Sounds like a contradiction but it works this way. Information from the essential and non-essential amino acids linked together as dipeptides signals the body to accept the protein into its store. If you leave out the non-essential amino acids from a protein formula, studies show that the human body can't hold onto it.[5]

So when you buy protein supplements, go first for hydrolysates (predigested proteins) rich in dipetides and tripeptides. That way you get an anabolic response along with your protein, and you also get maximum nitrogen retention. Intact proteins and protein concentrates are second choice. They do provide the dipeptide information, but the studies show they are only about half as good as hydrolysates for retention.

For protein sources, egg white (egg albumin), and whey protein (lactalbumin) are the sources used successfully in most studies. As we will see in Chapter 22, there is evidence that lactalbumin also boosts immunity, whereas casein (milk protein) and soy protein have little effect.[9] Excellent commercial mixes of lactalbumin and egg albumin are the Mass Fuel supplements by Lee Haney and Gainers Fuel by TwinLab.

Sad to say, free-form aminos are out. I used to be a fan, but have to bow to science as the only yardstick. The new studies we examined above show that free-form aminos don't measure up. The only exception is three special amino acids, the essential branched chains.

Branched Chain Amino Acids

Brilliant studies of protein use, especially those by Dr Peter Lemon at Kent State University, Ohio, show that exercise gobbles some amino acids much faster than others. It took 20 years of scientific detective work to ferret out the truth, but it is important for all athletes who want to optimize their protein nutrition. So it bears telling.

It took from 1970 to 1990 to establish that exercise causes muscles to release large quantities of the non-essential amino acids, **alanine** and **glutamine**, in much larger quantities than any other amino acid.[10,11] These amino acids are then mostly excreted from the body and lost. There is insufficient alanine and glutamine in muscle to provide the quantities lost during exercise. So much of what is released must be made in the muscles from other amino acids *during* the exercise.

The three **branched chain amino acids (BCAA), leucine, isoleucine, and valine** make up one-third of muscle protein. So they were likely candidates to supply the material to make alanine. But leucine is the only one that is relatively easy to measure. By the early '80s, studies showed conclusively that exercise uses up more leucine than any other amino acid.[13] This rapid loss of leucine occurs during both endurance exercise [14] and anaerobic exercise.[15]

World authority on protein, Professor Vernon Young at

MIT and colleagues, examined just how much leucine can be lost. They measured leucine oxidation in subjects made to ride for two hours on an ergometer bicycle at an easy 55% of VO_2max. They found that leucine oxidation increased by 240%, even during such a moderate level of exercise.[16] The leucine oxidation during this exercise period was almost 90% of the total daily requirement for leucine given in the RDA handbook.[17] Athletes need a lot more than that.

It is likely that there are similar losses of isoleucine and valine, but they are much harder to measure. Nevertheless, recent studies show that exercise directly increases the activity of an enzyme called **branched-chain keto-acid dehydrogenase**, the controlling enzyme in the degradation of all three BCAA.[18]

The possible sources of the BCAA loss during exercise are three:
1. Increased uptake of free BCAA from the blood
2. Reduced use of BCAA in muscle protein synthesis
3. Breakdown of muscle protein

All athletes want to avoid the reduced muscle size and strength consequent on reduced protein synthesis and muscle breakdown. The smart strategy, therefore, is to ensure an adequate supply of free BCAA in the blood. Studies suggest that eating BCAA easily increases blood levels.[10,19] So BCAA supplementation seems a sensible "insurance" to save your muscle.

How Much BCAA

There are no direct studies with athletes to determine BCAA requirements. But excellent recent studies in Dr Vernon Young's laboratory at MIT have shown that even *sedentary* men require much more leucine than the RDA handbook recommends.

Even at leucine intakes of 20 mg/kg/day, 40% greater than the RDA figure, the men were found to be in negative leucine balance. In this state optimum muscle maintenance is not possible, and because of the principle of synergy, the status of all other amino acids is comprised. The MIT researchers conclude:

> Current values for leucine requirements may under-
> estimate significantly intake levels actually needed to
> maintain protein nutritional status.[20]

Their data indicate that leucine requirements for healthy young, sedentary men are in the range 20-40 mg/kg/day. For athletes exercising 3 hours per day or more, we estimate requirement to be at least 60 mg/kg/day. For an 80 kg (176 lb) athlete, that is 4.8 grams of leucine a day.

The MIT team also examined the kinetics of valine requirements. They concluded that valine intake could be inadequate at below 40 mg/kg/day.[21] This figure is four times the RDA recommendation. We estimate that athletes in intense training require at least 50 mg/kg/day. For a 80 kg (176 lb) athlete, that is 4.0 grams of valine a day.

Similar studies have not yet been done for isoleucine. It seems likely, however, that athletes in intense training could require 20 mg/kg/day, twice the current RDA recommendation.[17] For an 80 kg (176 lb) athlete, that is 1.6 grams of isoleucine per day.

From current science we can't get any closer than that. For athletes of different weights the daily amounts are given in Table 17. Remember you get a lot of these in your protein food. Straight BCAA supplements are just an experimental top-up.

If you use BCAA, make sure to buy only those that specify singular, free-form L-amino acids on the label. Amino acids come in L for levo and D for dextro, denoting the direction of rotation of the chemical spiral. The body can use only L-amino acids to make proteins. D-amino acids are useless, and DL forms only inhibit the use of the L form. Buy only capsules in dark glass bottles with expiry dates and lot numbers. Light exposed BCAA, or old, oxidized BCAA, are hell on your gut and have no nutritional value at all.

Amino acids, like all proteins, should be eaten in small

Table 17: Estimated daily requirement of branched-chain amino acids (BCAA) for athletes in intense training.

Bodyweight kg lbs	Leucine (grams)	Valine (grams)	Isoleucine (grams)
40 88	2.4	2.0	0.8
50 110	3.0	2.5	1.0
60 132	3.6	3.0	1.2
70 154	4.2	3.5	1.4
80 176	4.8	4.0	1.6
90 198	5.4	4.5	1.8
100 220	6.0	5.0	2.0
110 242	6.6	5.5	2.2
120 264	7.2	6.0	2.4

Source: The Colgan Institute, San Diego, CA.

meals throughout the day. Most athletes can't digest more than about 30 grams of protein at a sitting. That's six large egg whites, or a chicken breast, or a can of albacore, or more conveniently a protein shake. Take your additional BCAA at the same time for maximum absorption and retention.

One last wrinkle. There is some new evidence that BCAA taken 1-2 hours before intense training spare muscle BCAA and spare testosterone during training, and increase testosterone levels after training.[22] The amounts of BCAA found effective are about the 80 kg line in Table 17. This evidence is discussed in more detail in Chapter 32. BCAA supplementation taken at the right time may have a real anabolic effect.[23,24]

Chapter 14

Vitamins Are Nuts And Bolts

Yesterday, the top tennis coach in California asked me, "What combinations of vitamins should I give the guys before a match?" His conception of the function of nutrients as one-hit performance boosters is all too common. And the myth is continually fueled by supplement ads that promise to turn you into Arnold Schwarzenegger overnight.

Let's get it straight: **The business of nutrition is to build a better body.** Any one-hit, slam-bam, immediate ergogenic boost is a drug effect. You can use mega-doses of some vitamins to produce a drug effect. But they are very inefficient as hot-shot ergogenics, because the body recognizes them as building and maintenance department and treats them accordingly.

That's the way you should treat them too. Vitamins are essential components of structures and functions in the body that take years to develop to their full capacity. You feed them in *every day* in the right amounts, train *regularly* and *consistently,* week in-week out, and gradually your body will change to match your dreams. I've done it with young lads and lasses a thousand times: watched them grow from fumbling, stumbling, no particular talent, until their muscles, their bones, and their brain, became one unified, focussed structure of grace and power that seized Olympic Gold.

You can do it too. The human body is so malleable that, with the right nutrition and training, even meager talent can be fashioned into a champion. So forget the quick-fix. Ben Johnson couldn't hold onto his drug-boosted body. Without the drugs it declined into an also ran at the Barcelona Olympics. You want a body that continues to improve. Vitamins are some of the building materials that make it happen. We will look at each one in terms of nine criteria:

1. What does the vitamin do?
2. What are the best food sources?
3. Is it deficient in foods?
4. Do athletes need more than foods provide?
5. Are athletes deficient?
6. How do you measure your vitamin status?
7. How much do you use as a supplement?
8. Is it toxic?
9. Does it have any ergogenic effects.

Vitamin A (Retinol)

Like all the vitamins, retinol has multiple functions. It is essential for vision, skin and mucous membranes, cell growth, reproduction, and normal immunity.[1] Retinol (named after the retina of the eye), is fat-soluble, meaning that it works in lipid (fat) complexes in the body. It makes the visual purple of your eyes that is essential for night vision.

Best food sources of vitamin A are liver and fish liver oils. Best sources of beta-carotene, the precursor of vitamin A, are carrots and dark green leafy vegetables. It's a common myth that all yellow and orange vegetables are rich in beta-carotene. Most of them contain other carotenoids (there are over 500 types) that are not used at all by the human body.[2] In contrast, one large carrot can contain 18,000 IU of active beta-carotene. That's 3,000 mcg RE, three times the RDA. No worries, you can't O.D. on carrots. After a few too many, your gut becomes persuasively explosive.

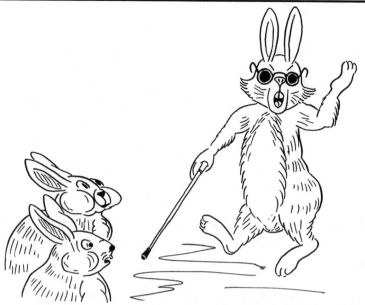

"Bugsy gave up carrots when he heard vitamin A could be toxic."

As we saw in Chapter 11, studies have found numerous athletes deficient in vitamin A.[3] And nationwide surveys have found widespread vitamin A deficiency in the general population.[4]

Vitamin A in its various forms, including it precursor beta-carotene, used to be measured in International Units (IU), an obsolete, inaccurate measure that still appears on labels and product literature. The correct measure now used in nutrition science for more than a decade, is **micrograms of retinol equivalents (mcg RE)**. To help you translate, 1 mcg RE equals 3.3 IU retinol.[2] The current RDA for vitamin A is 1,000 mcg RE, which equals 3,333 IU.

Beta-carotene is one of the few carotenoids that is converted to vitamin A by the body. But it is a poor source. It takes 6 mcg of beta-carotene to yield 1 mcg RE of vitamin A. Beta-carotene, however, has antioxidant functions independent of its vitamin A functions, and should be considered a separate nutrient. Apart from turning your skin yellow, it is not toxic in any reasonable amount.

You can get a reasonable estimate of your vitamin A status from a **plasma retinol** test. An acceptable level for athletes is above 20 mcg/dl.[6] You can also measure beta-carotene with a **plasma carotene** test. An acceptable level for athletes is above 40 mcg/dl.[6]

At the Colgan Institute we use vitamin A supplements of 1,000-5,000 mcg RE with athletes in heavy training. Vitamin A can build up in the body, and in rare individuals can cause obvious symptoms of toxicity with supplements of 8,000 mcg RE (25,000 IU) per day.[5] So watch your retinol intake. There is no evidence that mega-doses of vitamin A or beta-carotene have any ergogenic effects.

Vitamin B₁ (Thiamin)

Thiamin (not thiamine) is a water-soluble vitamin that enters and leaves the body daily, so you have to eat it daily for optimal health. Vitamin B₁ helps to maintain normal energy metabolism. If you want to impress someone, thiamin is required for the **oxidative decarboxylation of alpha-keto acids** and for **transketolase activity in the pentose phosphate pathway.** That's biochemical gobbledegook for, thiamin works to burn carbs.

The best food sources of thiamin are whole grains. To evaluate the thiamin content of American grains, the United States Department of Agriculture measures the content in fresh, raw, unprocessed samples. But the food we eat is rarely like that. We have found that the thiamin content of grains varies up to 6-fold depending on age, quality, storage, and processing.[7] And losses of thiamin from grains and flour during commercial baking can be 100%.[8] So the thiamin in your food may be only a fraction of its original content.

Even at conservative RDA levels, USDA surveys of 38,000 people have found deficient thiamin intake in 45 out of every 100.[9] With their much higher turnover of energy, athletes require more thiamin than the general population, so are even more likely to be deficient.

You can get a reasonable estimate of your thiamin status from the old reliable **erythrocyte transketolase thiamin pyrophosphate stimulation** assay. An acceptable level for athletes is below 10% TLPP stimulation.[6]

The RDA for thiamin is only 1.5 mg/day. You can safely use a lot more than that. Zero toxicity is reported at intakes of 500 mg per day.[2] At the Colgan Institute, we use 50-200 mg to maintain thiamin status in athletes.

More than that does you no good or harm, but is simply excreted from the body. Professor Melvin Williams of Old Dominion University, Norfolk, Virginia, has reviewed all studies in existence on possible ergogenic effect of thiamin. His conclusion and mine is, you can eat excess vitamin B₁, till it comes out your ears, but you won't boost performance a whisker.[7]

Vitamin B₂ (Riboflavin)

Another of the in-and-out of the body water-solubles, riboflavin functions especially to help the mitochondria (furnaces) of your muscle cells produce energy. Meats, poultry, fish, and dairy products are all good food sources. But we have found that content varies 3-fold in different samples of the same fresh, raw food.[7] Food-processing can also destroy up to 80% of riboflavin.[8]

With their greater energy turnover, athletes require additional riboflavin. Dr Daphne Roe and her group at Cornell University, have shown that even moderate exercise increases riboflavin requirements in healthy women.[10] So, it is not surprising that apparently well-fed athletes are sometimes found to be deficient.[11]

You can measure your riboflavin status reliably by use of the **erythrocyte glutathione reductase activity coefficient (EGRAC)** assay. An EGRAC of more than 1.25 signals deficiency.

The RDA for riboflavin is 1.7 mg/day. The Colgan Institute uses 25-200 mg per day with athletes. No case of riboflavin toxicity has ever been reported.[12] Ergogenic effect of mega-doses -- nil.

Vitamin B₃ (Niacin, Niacinamide)

Niacin is another water-soluble vitamin partly supplied by the tryptophan in your diet which the body converts to niacin. It functions as part of two enzymes, **nicotinamide adenine dinucleotide (NAD),** and with an additional phosphate, **(NADP).** They work in the glycogen energy cycle, the oxidation of fatty acids for energy, and in the tissue respiration.[2] Best food sources of both niacin and tryptophan are meats and fish. Niacin is highly resistant to food processing, so most of the original content remains intact in processed and cooked foods.

Because of their high use of niacin-linked processes in energy production, athletes require more niacin than sedentary people. But at the level of the RDA, they are rarely deficient. The old reliable test for evaluating niacin status is **urinary excretion of N-methylnicotinamide,** expressed as **mg/gram creatinine.** An acceptable level for athletes is 3.0 or greater.

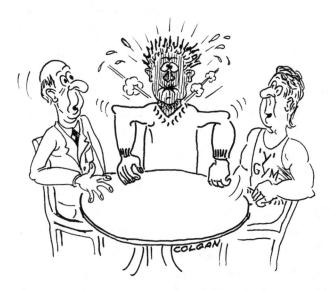

"Fred believes mega-doses of niacin really help his training."

The RDA for niacin is 19 mg. The Colgan Institute uses 30-100 mg mostly as nicotinamide. In the niacin form, above 30 mg causes vascular dilation with flushing, burning, and itching, the "niacin flush. " Apart from that discomfort, toxicity is low up to 1,000 mg per day.[5]

Because niacin increases the use of glycogen, studies have tried large amounts as ergogenic aids. Results show that megadoses (3-10 grams) of niacin do cause glycogen to be used more quickly. But they also block the use of fatty acids for fuel.[13] So glycogen depletion occurs very fast. Definitely an *anti-ergogenic* effect. Despite the evidence, we still get some very red-faced gentlemen who swear that niacin improves their performance. Pity they can never demonstrate it.

Vitamin B$_6$ (Pyridoxine)

Pyridoxine coenzymes function at all levels of protein and amino acid metabolism, and in making of hemoglobin and all new proteins.[2] It is also essential for the enzyme **glycogen phosphorylase** that breaks down muscle glycogen for fuel. So the right amount of vitamin B$_6$ is very important to athletes.

Best food sources are wheat germ, chicken, fish, and eggs. You would think that these common foods would make pyridoxine deficiency rare. Not so. The Nationwide Food Consumption Survey found that pyridoxine intake is deficient in 33% of households.[14] In a recent study we did at the Colgan Institute, 58% and 73% of two groups of runners were pyridoxine deficient.[15]

You can measure your pyridoxine status using **erythrocyte glutamic oxaloacetic transaminase (EGOT) activity in the presence and absence of pyridoxal-5-phosphate.**[16] It's a mouthful to say, but pretty simple for blood labs to do. An activity coefficient less than 1.25 is an acceptable level for athletes.

Requirements for pyridoxine increase as protein requirements increase, and as energy expenditure increases. So an athlete who is eating to put on muscle, and who is also training

3 hours or more daily, has a much higher need for pyridoxine than a couch potato. The RDA is 2.0 mg. Some studies have estimated requirements of athletes at double that figure. The Colgan Institute uses 10-50 mg per day with athletes. Acute toxicity is low up to 2,000 mg,[5] but intakes over 100 mg for months or years can cause nerve damage. This damage heals itself within 6 months following cessation of supplements.[17]

Because of its involvement in glycogen use, excess pyridoxine is likely to be *anti-ergogenic*. One careful study concluded that, like niacin, mega-doses of pyridoxine cause the body to deplete glycogen stores more quickly.[18] If you are in for the long haul, ditch pyridoxine loading.

Pantothenic Acid (Vitamin B₅)

Also called pantothenate, pantothenic acid belongs to the B-complex of water-soluble vitamins that has multiple roles in energy metabolism. It forms part of the important **coenzyme A,** and part of one of the carrier proteins for the enzyme **fatty acid synthetase.** Essentially, that means it is necessary for making of glucose and fatty acids, the main fuels of the body. It is also essential for making steroid hormones and brain neurotransmitters.[2] Pantothenic acid deficiency puts you in real bad shape.

Fortunately, it occurs widely in foods with an average intake in America of 6 mg a day.[19] No surprise that 6 mg is exactly the amount deemed a safe and adequate daily intake by the RDA Committee.[2] Without pussyfooting around, that amount will not work for athletes. Many athletes in intense training use four times the daily energy of couch potatoes. Their need for pantothenate increases accordingly. Consequently, the average diet is highly deficient for athletes.

Some athletes make up the pantothenate deficit by eating royal jelly, the diet of queen bees, and the richest natural source of pantothenate. Big waste of money. Pantothenate in pills costs pennies: in royal jelly it costs a dollar a dose.

There are no controlled studies on pantothenate deficiency in athletes. I have found some individual cases. Most of these were accompanied by disturbed sleep and the "burning feet" syndrome. If you see athletes with circles under the eyes who kick off their shoes during rests in training, and complain of "hot spots," then pantothenate deficiency is worth investigating.

You can measure your pantothenate status easily and fairly reliably by **24-hour urinary excretion**. Standards have not been widely established, but based on a number of sample studies [5] we have developed a standard of **greater than 9 mg/day excretion** as acceptable for athletes. To achieve and maintain this standard, in some cases requires a pantothenate intake of 100 mg/day. We use 20-200 mg pantothenate daily with athletes. Pantothenate is very low in toxicity. Ten grams/day of calcium pantothenate given to young, healthy men for six weeks produced no adverse symptoms.[20]

The best evidence that athletes often get insufficient pantothenate comes from positive studies of the vitamin as an ergogenic aid. An experiment by Dr D. Litoff and colleagues is representative of a number of studies showing positive effects on performance. They gave elite distance runners 2.0 grams of pantothenic acid or a placebo for 2 weeks. Subjects were tested on the ergometer bicycle at 75% VO2max.

Supplementation reduced lactate build-up by 17% and reduced oxygen consumption by 8%.[21] Two grams is far above anyone's pantothenate requirements. From our own case studies of what seems to be pantothenate deficient in athletes, we suspect that part of the dose in mega-dose studies is simply used by the athletes' bodies to bring their pantothenate status up to par. Performance benefits accordingly.

Folate (Folic Acid, Folacin)

Folate, a B-complex vitamin, forms part of vital transport coenzymes that control amino acid metabolism. Insufficiency of folate inhibits growth of new cells, especially the rapidly changing muscle cells and blood cells of athletes.

Although folate is widely available in fresh, dark-green, leafy vegetables, legumes, and egg yolk, it is one of the most commonly deficient vitamins. Folate is fragile. Food storage and processing destroys up to half of this vitamin in our food.[2] We have measured a 5-fold range of folate in different samples of stone-ground whole-wheat flour, from a low of 33 mcg/100 grams to a high of 149 mcg/100 grams. So even with minimally processed food, you cannot trust its folate content.[22]

Comprehensive government surveys show widespread folate deficiency in America.[22] Over the last 30 years, folate intake has dropped badly, as our food has become more processed. In keeping with the hidden food industry lobby agenda to set vitamin requirements to match the vitamin content of American food, in 1989 the RDA was down-graded from 400 mcg, which it had been for 20 years, to a mere 200 mcg/day. The latest RDA handbook does admit, "RDAs are neither minimal requirements nor necessarily optimal levels of intake."(p.8)[2] 'Nuff said!

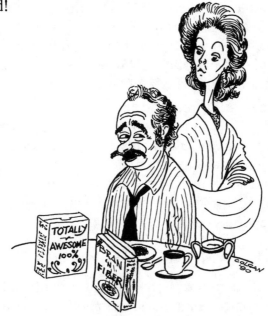

"OK. I've eaten 100% of the RDA's. Now can I have some real food!"

The RDA of 200 mcg is woefully insufficient for athletes, especially for those intent on growing new muscle and increasing their red blood oxygen-carrying capacity. Even in sedentary people, long-term studies show that 211 mcg of folate per day put them in serious deficit.[23] There are no studies of folate deficiency in athletes. At the Colgan Institute, however, we have found that folate supplementation increases body folate stores in multi-supplement studies that have improved performance.[15]

You can measure your folate status reliably using a microbiological assay, **red-cell folate/***Lactobacillus casei.*[24] To derive a norm for athletes, the Colgan Institute has used the work of Dr A.V. Hoffbrand and colleagues as a base,[25] plus the folate levels we have found in athletes in top condition. An acceptable level for athletes is above 220 ng/dl.

Folate supplements are restricted to 400 mcg/day by the FDA, because greater intakes tend to mask tests for the serious disease of pernicious anemia. In athletes who test negative for pernicious anemia, we have tracked the use of 800-4,800 mcg of folate daily for periods of 2-4 years. We observed no side-effects.

Toxicity is certainly low. Dr Charles Butterworth found no adverse effects in women given 10,000 mcg of folate daily for 4 months.[26] That level of folate will not boost performance, however. Evidence for ergogenic effects of folate is a fat zero.

Vitamin B$_{12}$ (Cyanocobalamin)

Cobalamin forms part of coenzymes essential for all cells, particularly rapid-turnover cells, including red blood cells, the lining of the gastrointestinal tract, and bone marrow cells. Deficiency of vitamin B$_{12}$ causes pernicious anemia, which wipes out your nerves and sends you raving mad before killing you.[2] So it's fortunate that severe deficiency is uncommon.

This B-complex vitamin is available only in animal foods. Vegetarians are the most commonly deficient. Average intakes in America are about 8 mcg/day in men and 5 mcg/day in women.[2] About 3 mcg/day is sufficient to offset a vitamin B$_{12}$ deficiency, but there is little evidence on how much is optimal. Athletes with their higher turnover of blood cells may require more than sedentary folk. But very few athletes we have measured show any sign of deficiency.

You can measure your cobalamin status reliably using the microbiological assay, **serum cobalamin/***Lactobacillus leichmani.*[28] An acceptable level for athletes is above 250 pg/ml.

A persistent myth surrounds vitamin B12 in sports. Numerous champions, such as New Zealand Olympic gold medalist John Walker, who had one of the longest running careers at the elite level, receive regular, massive B12 shots before races. Even 10,000 times the RDA appears to be non-toxic. A lot of athletes have copied the practice. Yet the studies on such supplementation are uniformly negative.[28] The only effect we have found in athletes given B12 shots is a reported euphoria and belief they can do better. That belief is shattered every time you test their performance. Yet the little buzz they get from the shot, like most stimulant pseudo-ergogenics, keeps bringing them back for more.

Biotin

Biotin is the last of the B-complex vitamins. By forming part of two enzymes, **pyruvate carboxylase** and **acetyl-coenzyme A carboxylase,** biotin is essential for **gluconeogenesis** (formation of new glucose) and fatty acid synthesis, two major fuels for human energy. Another biotin dependent enzyme, **3-methylcrotonyl coenzyme A carboxylase** is essential for catabolism of branched-chain amino acids. In plan language, this means that without adequate biotin you can't use fat or glucose for fuel properly, and you can't break down and subsequently build up new proteins. That leaves you with very little. Your hair and skin fall off, your muscles disappear, and you are too weak and confused to move. Biotin deficiency reduces you to a bald, skinny vegetable.[29]

Best food sources are liver, sardines, egg yolk, and soy

flour.[2] Bodybuilders who use raw egg whites in protein shakes are often marginal for biotin because raw egg white contains a substance called **avidin** that binds biotin and prevents the body using it.[30] Successful treatment requires 200-300 mcg of biotin a day.

Biotin in the US diet ranges 28-42 mcg/day.[31] Biotin is also synthesized in the human gut. Amounts are uncertain, but unlikely to be more than 20-40 mcg. Members of the RDA Committee have fought like Tweedledum and Tweedledee over biotin requirements. The 1980 Committee recommended a daily intake of 100-300 mcg. But when they found out in 1985 that the usual diet contained only 35 mcg, the new Committee quietly revised the requirement in 1989 down to 30-100 mcg/day.

Such shenanigans don't help when trying to determine an athlete's needs. We know that increased biotin levels promote protein synthesis.[29] We also know that athletes have increased needs because of their higher turnover of glucose, fatty acids, and branched-chain amino acids. Some researchers report low biotin levels in athletes,[32] but it's a real problem to determine what level is low.

You can measure your biotin level reliably using the microbiological assay, **serum biotin/***Ochromonas danica*. After reviewing all the available studies, the Colgan Institute has developed a tentative norm for athletes. An acceptable level is above 1,000 pg/ml. Coaches may be surprised at the number of athletes who fall below this level.

Biotin deficit is easy to fix. Oral supplements raise blood levels promptly. The Colgan Institute uses 300-5,000 mcg daily with athletes. Expensive stuff. Intakes of 10,000 mcg daily don't cause any toxic side-effects.[2] But they don't cause any ergogenic effects either.

Vitamin C (Ascorbate)

Like the B-complex, vitamin C is water soluble (except for the ascorbyl palmitate form), and quickly in and out of the body.

The function of this vitamin stressed in college textbooks is its essential use in **hydroxylation of the amino acids proline and lysine** in forming **collagen**, the protein of the white fibers of your skin, bones, and connective tissues. With inadequate ascorbate, your skin quickly disintegrates, which happens as a first sign of scurvy. But these functions of vitamin C are not as important for athletes as its antioxidant functions. It takes only 30 mg of vitamin C a day to prevent scurvy,[2] but as we see in Chapter 20, it can take grams a day to combat oxidation.

Chapter 20 on antioxidants also covers the amounts in the human diet and athlete's needs. Your serum vitamin C status can be measured easily by the **2,6-dichlorophenol-indophenol** assay.[33] An acceptable level for athletes is above 0.50 mg/dl. If you want to get fancy and expensive, you can measure **leucocyte** ascorbate levels using **high performance liquid chromatography (HPLC)**. Tests for most vitamins can be done more accurately on HPLC. But, the technology is ve-r-r-r-r-ry pricy.

Throughout this book, I have tried to give you methods that are accurate enough, while keeping costs to a minimum. Most scientists and coaches are like me, continually reduced to penury by the cost of research. And most athletes have barely enough to live on. So many of my recommendations aim to get the information in the cheapest way possible. But if you go the HPLC route, then leucocyte ascorbate is a much better measure of the body pool of ascorbate than the old serum method.[34] An acceptable level of HPLC leucocyte ascorbate of athletes is 4.0 mg/gram, wet tissue.

Because of the antioxidant effects of vitamin C, the Colgan Institute uses 2-12 grams of vitamin C with athletes. The rationale is explained in detail in Chapter 21 along with methods to estimate your personal intake. Toxicity is very low.

Double Nobel Prize winner, Dr Linus Pauling, got dumped by most of the scientific community as a has-been, when he recommended multi-gram doses of vitamin C in the early '70s. All his major critics are now dead, while he goes on into his '90s lecturing vigorously. In my last discussion with him, he was still sharper than a tack. We will see in Chapter 18 that many of the syndromes that attack athletes are very similar to the syndromes of aging. Mega-doses of vitamin C have no direct ergogenic effect,[35] but in combating illness and injury the effect is profound. Pauling is one little bit of living proof.

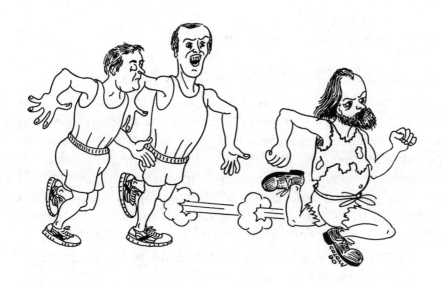

"So what if he's faster. At least we're properly dressed."

Vitamin D (Cholecalciferol)

One of the fat-soluble group, vitamin D is essential for bone growth and mineral balance in the body. Sunlight enables you to synthesize vitamin D on your skin. In healthy athletes, 30 minutes per day of summer sun produces a lot more vitamin D than the RDA of 10.0 mcg. The old IU units still appear in labels and product literature as a measure for vitamin D. To help you translate, using the new measure, 1.0 mcg equals 40 IU.

Vitamin D used to be deficient in food until milk and dairy

products were fortified. Now almost everyone on a reasonable diet gets plenty. There is no evidence that athletes need supplementary amounts. Nevertheless, because we cannot rely on food content or sunlight induction of vitamin D, the Colgan Institute uses 10 mcg/day with athletes. We have not measured vitamin D status, a task that presents many problems.[6] Vitamin D can be toxic if taken in amounts only five times the RDA.[2] Studies using 37.5 mcg for two months showed no ergogenic effects on the physical performance of children aged 10-11. Nor did a massive single dose of 10,000 mcg.[36]

Vitamin E (D-alpha-tocopherol)

The main function of vitamin E is as an antioxidant. We cover food sources and requirements in detail in Chapters 20 and 21. The RDA is 10 mg-alpha TE. This measure has been used in science for decades, but the obsolete IU measure is still prominent in popular literature. To help you translate, vitamin E is correctly given as **milligrams of alpha-tocopherol equivalents (alpha TE).** Each 1 mg-alpha TE equals 1 IU of alpha-tocopheryl acetate. Different forms of tocopherol have different values.

A lot of the vitamin E in foods is destroyed by processing.[2] The amount in American diets approximately equals the 10-mg alpha TE of the RDA.[2] No surprise there. Athletes require a lot more than that, as we see in Chapter 21.

Many sports medicine facilities (and hospitals) still try to determine vitamin E status from blood or serum levels. These measures are next to useless because they depend on the level of circulating blood lipids.[37] A much better measure is the **stability of erythrocytes in hydrogen peroxide** popularized by Dr Philip Farrell from the Department of Paediatrics of the University of Wisconsin.[38]

Vitamin E is of very low toxicity. Even 3,000 mg-alpha TE daily, that is 300 times the RDA, produces no side-effects in most subjects.[39] The Colgan Institute uses 400 to 2,000 mg-alpha TE daily with athletes. As with vitamin C, there is little evidence of a direct ergogenic effect of mega-doses of tocopherol, although numerous studies have tried to find one.[28] But the indirect effects are another story. As I have stressed before, the business of nutrition is to build a better body. Vitamin E is one of the basic components.

Vitamin K (Phylloquinone)

The last of the fat-soluble vitamins, **phylloquinone**, is essential for formation of **prothrombin** one of the compounds that enables your blood to clot. When vitamin K is low, you bleed like a stuck pig. So it is an important vitamin for athletes because of their continual hemolysis caused by exercise.

Fresh, green leafy vegetables are the best food source, providing 50-800 mcg of vitamin K per 100 grams of food.[2] An average American diet contains 300-500 mcg of vitamin K.[41] The flora in the human gut also produce some vitamin K. Your gut contains 2-3 lbs of flora and fauna, a wide variety of bacteria, yeasts, molds, etc. (about the same weights as your brain), all working busily 24 hours a day. Without them, you couldn't survive.

Physical trauma, such as the intense muscle contractions and effort of training, increase the need for vitamin K.[40] But there are no studies that have measured this need in athletes.

You can get a reasonable estimate of your vitamin K status from the **Quick plasma prothrombin time** assay.[42] An acceptable level for athletes is less than 15 seconds. Longer than that is a sign you bleed too easily. The RDA for vitamin K is 80 mcg. That should be provided easily by your diet. At the Colgan Institute, we use 80-100 mcg of vitamin K with some athletes. Even mega-amounts of phylloquimone have no reported toxicity,[2] but no ergogenic effects either. Do not take vitamin K in the **menadione** form. That is toxic, and in large doses can cause a host of problems.[43]

Choline

Choline is not a vitamin because the body can make it. But most of your choline still comes from the diet. It forms part of phosphatidyl choline (lecithin) which is an essential component of all cell membranes for every one of the thirty trillion cells in your body. It is also what is called a **methyl donor** in energy metabolism. In the brain, choline forms part of the neurotransmitter **acetylcholine**, intimately involved in your anabolic drive (see Chapter 32) and in memory. Mega-doses of phosphatidyl choline are used with moderate success to improve memory in elderly folk.[44]

Choline is widely available in foods from eggs and soybeans to numerous vegetables.[45] Estimates of the amount required by humans are confined to infants and related to the amount of choline in human breast milk (about 7 mg per 100 calories).[46] Some researchers rationalize that athletes need the same amounts as infants because of their similar rapid tissue turnover. That idea puts daily choline requirements at about 200 mg for a 3,000 calorie diet. The average daily dietary intake in America is 400-900 mg. So athletes are unlikely to be deficient.[2] Nevertheless, plasma choline levels are sometimes depleted in marathon runners after races,[47] which might impair performance. The Colgan Institute uses 50-500 mg/day with some athletes.

Choline in its various forms is not toxic. But mega-doses (15-25 grams) used with athletes in vain attempts to find ergogenic effects do produce much gas and diarrhea. And the recurrent myth that supplementary choline is lipotropic (a "fat-burner") is just promotional codswallop. There is no evidence at all that choline improves performance or reduces bodyfat. But it does tend to make you smell like a week-old fish. So the stink might help you disturb your competiton.

Inositol

Dubbed a co-factor in the health food marketplace,

inositol (more correctly **myo-inositol**, the form used by the body) forms part of the lipids in your cell membranes. Myo-inositol used to be damned by mainstream nutrition scientists as a pseudo-nutrient. But recent discoveries show it is essential for normal calcium metabolism and insulin metabolism.[48,49]

Inositols are provided by food and also made in the body. No one knows how much is in the diet or how much humans need. Animals put on a zero myo-inositol diet develop abnormal fatty acid metabolism and other problems.[50] The Colgan Institute uses

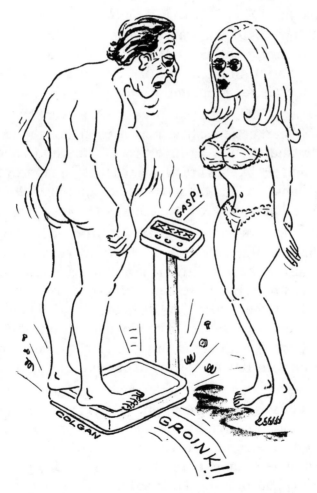

"I told you those lipotropics wouldn't work darling."

50-500 mg of myo-inositol with some athletes.

Doses in the gram range do not appear to be toxic,[2] but no one has done any studies with athletes to see whether inositol acts as an ergogenic. I doubt it, seeing that some nutritionists use inositol as a sedative.[51] Snake oil merchants also sell inositol as a fat-burner. I think they're the same folk that sell pixie dust to attract the Tooth Fairy.

Coenzyme Q10 (Ubiquinone)

Coenzyme Q10 (CoQ10) is essential for virtually all energy production. It works to help transfer electrons in the energy cycle in the **mitochondria** (furnaces of the cell). It is also intimately involved in maintaining immunity,[52] and in normal heart function.[53] It is also a potent antioxidant.[54]

In Japan, CoQ10 is used successfully to treat hundreds of thousands of heart patients. In America, even though there are a host of new studies showing its efficacy,[53] the Food and Drug Administration (FDA) has branded CoQ10 an "unapproved food additive." Thanks to Senator Orrin Hatch and his **1992 Health Freedom Act,** that nonsense may soon disappear.

CoQ occurs very widely in food, especially in polyunsaturated vegetable oils.[55] The body converts CoQ to CoQ10 and also makes some from the amino acid methionine. So deficiency is unlikely for sedentary people. No one knows whether athletes need more CoQ10, but it is a good bet because of their high energy turnover. The Colgan Institute uses 10-60 mg/day of CoQ10 with some athletes. No toxicity has been reported even with 100 mg of CoQ10 per day for 4 years.[56]

The best evidence that athletes need extra CoQ10 comes from studies of this coenzyme as an ergogenic. The first studies reported increased exercise tolerance in heart patients.[54] Then the reports on athletes began to roll in. In one of the latest studies, well-trained male runners at the University of Bologna in Italy were run to exhaustion on the treadmill. Then for the next 7 weeks, they were given 100 mg CoQ10 per day or a placebo. Then they were run on the treadmill again. Subjects receiving CoQ10 ran 12% further and 8% longer than the placebo group.[57] CoQ10 is an essential nutrient worth investigating if your goal is optimal performance.

Other Co-factors

Bioflavonoids are a big family of chemicals including rutin and **hesperidin** that have numerous, but still undefined functions, in the human body. They help maintain the strength of capillaries and they are linked to vitamin C functions.[59] There is some evidence that bioflavonoids can inhibit bruising.[60] They are widely used for this purpose by clinical nutritionists. The Colgan Institute uses 100-500 mg of bioflavonoids daily with some athletes.

Pyrolloquinolone quinone (PQQ) is a recently discovered nutrient required for the enzyme **lysyl oxidase**, essential for normal collagen metabolism. Animals fed a zero PQQ diet grow poorly and develop disorders of collagen metabolism affecting skin, connective tissues, and bone.[61] These studies indicate that PQQ may be an essential nutrient. That is, we have to get it from our diet. No one knows how much we may need, but there is a flurry of new research on PQQ as an anti-aging compound. Until some of those studies are complete, the best food sources are unprocessed citrus fruits.

Para-amino-benzoic acid (PABA) is best known for its ability to prevent sunburn and skin damage by ultra-violet B. But it offers little protection against ultra-violet A. To protect you against UVA, you need a benzone compound such as oxybenzone or benzophenone. Check that your sunscreen contains protection against UVA and UVB. With our reduced ozone layer and increased risk of skin cancer,[58] I hope you use a sunscreen. Sunburn does more than cook your skin, it whacks the hell out of your immune system.

There are hundreds of other substances touted as vitamins and co-factors. We get asked to examine so many that our laboratory hello is "What's today's wonder drug." Most of them turn out to be duds. The vitamins and co-factors reviewed in this chapter are the whole bag that have any reasonable evidence to back them up. So if you hear someone say that we missed colostrum, or lipoic acid or succinic acid, or biopterin -- we didn't. Either they were dumped down the plug for wasting our time, or they are exposed as snake oil in Chapter 31.

Chapter 15

Minerals Are The Framework

The five macroelements, **oxygen, hydrogen, nitrogen, carbon,** and **sulfur,** make up 96% of the total weight of your body. Fortunately, we don't have to consider how to get them. They are well supplied in breathing and in the other nutrients. Water (H_2O), for example, supplies large amounts of hydrogen, and sulfer forms part of the amino acids methionine and cystine, and the vitamins thiamin and biotin. Nitrogen is provided by all proteins, and carbon is part of all foods. The carb bit of carbohydrate stands for carbon. The hydrate bit stands for hydrogen and oxygen which are usually present in the proportions to form water. Nutrition science is pretty logical.

When we look at the next level, the macrominerals **calcium, magnesium, phosphorus, potassium,** and **chloride,** dietary supply becomes crucial, because they are not so universally distributed. It gets even worse when we look at the trace elements. Dietary supply is just as crucial, but there are 16 of them, some very scarce in food.

Because we need only a few thousandths of a gram of some trace elements, and a few millionths of a gram of others such as **iodine** or **selenium**, some folk think they are less important than say calcium, which we need in gram amounts. Big mistake! Remember the principle of **synergy**. Recent science shows conclusively that if even one of the essential minerals is inadequately supplied, then the others cannot do their proper work.

I emphasized this principle in my first book for the public in 1982, **Your Personal Vitamin Profile,** and got a lot of arrows in the back from sports medicine folk who thought that total synergy was still unproven. Now, hundreds of studies later, they are coming round. Cheers to running guru, physician Dr George Sheehan, for example, who emphasized in 1991 that he takes a mineral supplement to ensure adequate supplies of trace elements.[2] His huge following of athletes will be the better for it.

Like we did for vitamins, this chapter considers each mineral in terms of nine criteria.

1. What does the mineral do?

2. What are the best food sources?

3. Is it deficient in foods?

4. Do athletes need more than foods provide?

5. Are athletes deficient?

6. How do you measure your mineral status?

7. How much do you use as a supplement?

8. Is it toxic?

9. Does it have any ergogenic effects.

Calcium

The body of a 70 kg (154 lb) athlete contains about 1.3 kg (2.85) lbs of calcium. About 99% of that is in his bones. The remaining 1% moves about controlling conduction of impulses along nerves, contraction of muscles, and a myriad of other functions. The big problem is that, in order for life to continue, the level of calcium outside your bones has to be maintained within very narrow limits. If your calcium intake is inadequate for even a day, then your body cannibalizes its own skeleton to make up the deficit.[3]

Optimal bone strength is essential for all athletes. Look what happened to decathlete Dave Johnson at the Barcelona

Olympics. He got a stress fracture in his foot, and years of training and hopes for gold went out the window. Stress fractures from weak bones are almost epidemic in American athletes. The first step to combat them is to get your calcium nutrition right.

Best food sources of calcium are dairy products and leafy green vegetables. Don't use bone meal supplements. Livestock bones in America today are heavily contaminated with lead.[1] Some other foods to avoid when you take your calcium are breads and cereals because the **phytates** in grains bind with calcium and inhibit absorption.[3] So do the **oxalates** in spinach, rhubarb, cocoa, chocolate, and coffee.[3] Drinking chocolate milk to get your calcium, is just plain dumb.

Take your main calcium supply at night, because calcium flux in the body is greatest during sleep. A large glass (14 oz.) of milk (low-fat), taken by itself, provides 500 mg of elemental calcium. Of that, about 150 mg is absorbed.[4] Like Mom says, milk before bed does build strong bones.

Bone is fascinating stuff. Unless you continually stress it, the structure disintegrates. And if you stress it in only a particular direction, all the new molecules grow and align themselves only in that direction to resist the stress. The heavier you stress bone in all directions without breaking, the stronger it gets.[5] But only if you have *all* the necessary elements available in the blood to build it.

Just to remind you, calcium by itself won't build a molecule of bone. That's why all the hundreds of calcium supplements have not made a dent in the burgeoning epidemic of osteoporosis, which now affects 6.3 millon Americans.[6] To use the calcium, your body has to have adequate supplies of at least, **magnesium,**[7] **silicon,**[8] **fluoride,**[9] **zinc,**[10] **copper,**[11] **boron,**[12] **manganese,**[13] **phosphorus,**[3] and **vitamin D.**[14] This mass of supporting evidence is from mainstream nutrition science, yet the idea that multi-nutrient synergy is essential for bone growth, is still virtually unknown to the public. You should learn it good, because optimal bone growth is crucial for athletes.

The average intake of calcium in America is 743 mg/day.[3] That is way below the RDA of 1,200 mg. Calcium intake in America is deficient in all groups. Maximum bone mass and bone strength is achieved between ages 18 and 35. Two women in every three between those ages get less than the RDA for calcium.[6]

Over a span of 20 years, numerous studies have found that athletes in a wide variety of sports, including such diverse disciplines as basketball, hockey, skating, swimming, and gymnastics, have deficient intakes of calcium.[15,16,17] It is getting better, hopefully because of books like this, but we have a long way to go.

Athletes may be doubly calcium deficient because bone mineralization increases tremendously in response to the stress of exercise.[18] This increased density of bone requires greater calcium intake in order to make it. Female athletes are especially vulnerable because their bone metabolism is always on the edge of disaster. **Amenorrhea** (loss of periods) caused by the detrimental affects of intense exercise on hormone balance, occurs in up to 40% of elite female athletes. Unless mineral intake is absolutely optimal this hormonal imbalance causes significant excretion of body calcium cannibalized from their bones.[19] The high protein intakes of many athletes also cause increased excretion of calcium, often resulting in a negative calcium balance.[20]

Measurement of calcium status is difficult. The usual measure on a blood screen, **serum calcium**, is useless for athletes. The body can continue to live only if calcium in the blood is kept within narrow limits. So it has many control mechanisms to adjust blood calcium levels. Because survival is more important than strong bones, in otherwise healthy athletes, the body will pull calcium from bone into blood to maintain blood calcium levels until the skeleton collapses. So your serum calcium can remain within normal limits (8.7-10.7 mg/dl) even with minuscule calcium intake.

Following our own findings of low calcium intake in many

athletes, the Colgan Institute uses supplements of 400-1,600 mg to correct deficits. There is no reported toxicity for calcium intakes up to 2,500 mg/day. Higher intakes than that stress the kidneys and may result in kidney stones.[3] Mega-calcium intakes also inhibit the absorption of iron and zinc, and disrupt the synergy of mineral use by the body.[21]

There is some recent evidence that calcium supplements can be ergogenic for both anaerobic and endurance performance. Dr T. Nishiyama reported increases in maximum power.[22] And Dr J.H. Richardson and colleagues found, in animals, that calcium supplements prolonged time to exhaustion.[23] Given the high incidence of calcium deficient in diets, and the high calcium demands of exercise, it is likely that such ergogenic effects simply reflect correction of an imbalanced mineral status in the body. Don't pop calcium pills, go for the whole enchilada.

Magnesium

Your body contains 20-30 grams of magnesium, 60% in the skeleton and 40% in soft tissue.[24] Magnesium forms part of over 300 enzymes in the body. It is essential for burning of glucose for fuel, transmission of the genetic code, muscle contraction, and a zillion other functions you can't exist without.[3] Best food sources are legumes and whole grains. But over 80% of the magnesium in food is lost by removal of the germ and outer layers of cereal grains in making white and so-called "enriched" flours.[25]

Every time you eat white or "enriched" bread and baked goods, you retard your athletic development. Biochemists established more than 30 years ago that magnesium is one of the eight nutrients required for proper metabolism of carbohydrate.[26] If most of the magnesium is missing (it is *not* added back in "enriched" flours), then your body has to rob other tissues of magnesium in order to deal with the junk carbs.

With the degradation of our food supply, average intakes of magnesium in America have declined proportionately. Americans today get only 329 mg/day for males, and 207 mg/day for females. That's only 80% of what we got early in this century,[3] and well below the RDA of 350 mg for males, and 280 mg for females.[3]

Because of the use of magnesium in energy metabolism, and in muscle contraction, athletes probably need more than sedentary folk. They also lose a lot of magnesium in sweat.[27] Studies show deficient magnesium intakes are common in many sports including wrestling, triathlon, endurance running, and dancing.[28-30]

Magnesium status is difficult to measure in athletes in training. Red blood cells contain three times the magnesium of blood serum, and hemolysis (destruction of red cells) in athletes caused by exercise, falsely elevates serum magnesium levels. In athletes not training, a **serum magnesium** level below 1.9 mg/dl may signal a deficit. Other clues to magnesium deficit are cramps, muscle tics and tremors, and muscle weakness.

The Colgan Institute uses magnesium supplements of 400-1,200 mg/day with athletes. If your kidneys are sound, there is no evidence of toxicity of magnesium up to 6,000 mg/day.[31] There is no evidence that mega-doses of magnesium have any ergogenic effects, beyond correction of a deficiency.

Phosphorus

You have about 800 grams of phosphorus in your body, 700 grams of which is in your bones.[3] The rest is essential for so many other processes, from the making of **adenosine triphosphate (ATP), creatine phosphate,** and many other steps of the energy cycle, to the metabolism of red blood cells, that just to list them would take pages. We deal more with the importance of phosphate in Chapters 23 and 25.

Phosphorus is everywhere in foods, and a lot more is added during processing in America. Average intake is about 1,500 mg for males and 1,000 mg for females. Best sources are meats, milk, fish, and whole grains. The only sedentary people likely to suffer phosphorus deficiency are those who regularly use antacids containing **aluminum hydroxide**. This chemical inhibits phosphorus absorption.[32]

As we see in Chapter 25, athletes may need more phosphate than the general population. Status is hard to measure in athletes in training, because hemolysis caused by exercise releases phosphorous from red blood cells, and falsely elevates serum levels. In athletes who are not training, **serum phosphorus** provides a reasonable measure. An acceptable range is 3.0-5.0 mg/dl.

Apart from phosphate loading for an ergogenic effect, the Colgan Institute rarely supplements athletes with phosphorus. Phosphorus is not toxic in any reasonable amount, but megadoses cause the body to lose calcium, because of its interaction with calcium metabolism. It has pronounced ergogenic effects which deserve full explanation and are covered in Chapter 25.

Sodium

Sodium, potassium, and chloride are the three main electrolytes in the human body. They perform myriad essential functions without which the whole electrochemical machine of man would stop working in a second. Sodium is the main **cation** (positively changed electrolyte) outside the cells. It is everywhere in food, and so much is added to foods during processing that the average American gets up to 5 grams daily, 10 times the minimum amount recommended in the RDA handbook.[3]

From all the ads for electrolyte replacement drinks for use during and after exercise, you would think that athletes need more sodium. Except for some ultra-distance athletes (Ironman length triathlons, 100-mile running races) that's just promotional flapdoodle. *The human body conserves its electrolytes.*

Sweat may taste salty, but it is a lot less salty than you are. At the end of a marathon race or a 3-hour marathon training session, you have lost much more water than electrolytes.[33] You are in **electrolyte overload.** You need water first, then carbs, never sodium. Giving athletes salt tablets on a hot day is a great way to make them *lose.*

Because sodium levels are to tightly controlled in the body, **serum sodium** levels are pretty stable. An acceptable range for athletes is 135-145 mcg/l. The Colgan Institute does not supplement athletes with sodium. Just the opposite. We recommend all athletes to toss the salt cellar entirely. Supplements are definitely anti-ergogenic. Salt pills make you retain water, and swell up like the Michelin Man. Take them a few hours before performance, and your salt-edema feet may not even let you get your shoes on.

Potassium

Potassium is the main **cation** (positively charged electrolyte) inside your cells. It interacts with sodium and chloride in conduction of nerve impulses and a host of other essential functions. The ratio of potassium to sodium in the body reflects our evolution. Mankind evolved on a high potassium/low sodium diet. Most fresh food is built that way. Seafood, even though it grown in a medium where the ratio of potassium to sodium is 1:24, is still a high potassium/low sodium food.

Fresh salmon, for example, is 100 parts potassium to 17 parts sodium. Fresh tuna is 100 parts potassium to 20 parts sodium. Stone-ground whole wheat flour is 120 parts potassium to 1 part sodium. And fresh milk is 100 parts potassium to 36 parts sodium.

Processing reverses these ratios in the most unhealthy way. Lox is 100 parts potassium to 200 parts sodium. Canned tuna is 100 parts potassium to 330 parts sodium. Commercial whole wheat bread is 100 parts potassium to 570 parts sodium. And butter is 100 parts potassium to 3,600 parts sodium.[35]

Overall, the average ratio of potassium to sodium in fresh foods is about 1:7.[35] In the American diet, that ratio is reversed to about 2:1.[3] If you want optimal performance, stick to fresh foods with enough potassium to suit your body structure, and deep-six the salt.

If you have to have that salty taste, there are plenty of substitutes, such as Morton's Light Salt, that use a potassium salt instead of most of the sodium. Average potassium intake in America is about 2,500 mg/day.[36] The recommend intake in the RDA handbook is 3,500 mg/day.[3] So even couch potatoes are considerably short.

Because of hemolysis and consequent losses of blood cell potassium, plus potassium losses in sweat, athletes may be shorter than most. Potassium deficit has devastated performance for some marathon runners.[37] A comprehensive study of 554 athletes for 4 years indicates that it is a common dietary fault. The study covered wrestlers, bodybuilders, rowers, footballers, gymnasts, track and field athletes, swimmers, and dancers. One of the most frequent problems was low potassium intake.[38]

Potassium deficit in the body is hard to measure in athletes in training, because potassium levels in blood are kept within narrow limits by multiple mechanisms, and hemolysis, caused by exercise, releases red cell potassium which falsely evaluates serum potassium levels. In athletes not in training, **serum potassium** is a reasonable measure. An acceptable level is 4.5-5.5 mcg/l.

The Colgan Institute uses potassium supplements of 100-500 mg/day with some athletes. Potassium is not toxic up to 5 grams per day, but do not take it on an empty stomach unless you like vomiting. Ergogenic effect of mega-doses -- nil.

Chloride

Chloride is the main **anion** (negatively charged electrolyte) outside your cells. It works with the two main cations, sodium and potassium, to control fluid and electrolyte balance. It is the chloride bit of sodium chloride (table salt).

Because we get too much salt, we also get too much chloride, about 6 grams daily.[3] Minimum requirements are only 750 mg/day. If you eat low on sodium (as you should), you will also keep down your chloride. Overload, not deficiency, is the problem.

Chloride overload or deficit in the body is hard to measure. Tightly controlled **serum chloride** levels range from 99-110 mcg/l.[39] The Colgan Institute does not use chloride supplements. Chloride has all the toxicity problems of sodium, and definitely no ergogenic effects.

Iron

The main job of iron is to form part of **hemoglobin,** the red pigment that carries oxygen in the bloodstream from lungs to muscles and brain. Iron also forms part of numerous essential enzymes.[3] About a third of your iron is in storage form as **ferritin** and **hemosiderin,** stored mainly in the bone marrow and liver. It is the loss of this store that plagues many athletes. We cover this problem in detail in Chapter 21.

Iron is widely available in whole grains, vegetables, meats, and eggs, and is added to many processed foods. **Heme iron,** mainly from meats, is the most bioavailable. With all this iron about, you would think that everyone gets ample. Not so. Iron deficiency is common throughout America,[39] and especially common in athletes (see Chapter 21).

One reason for the high incidence if iron deficiency is the problem of absorbing it from food. The best heme iron from meats is only 10% bioavailable. Non-heme iron from vegetables may be only 1% bioavailable. Calcium, fiber, and antacids all inhibit absorption further, whereas vitamin C helps you to absorb iron.[40]

More women than men are iron deficient. In the 1980s, surveys established the mean iron intake of young women as 10.7 mg/day.[41] Until that time, the RDA for women was 18 mg of iron/day.[42] A standard of 70% of the RDA is widely accepted as a cutoff point for serious deficiency. After it was established that the young female population was receiving only 60%, which made the US food supply look bad, the RDA for women was quietly reduced to 15 mg/day, so that they were above the 70% cutoff again. Politics!

Measurement of iron status is covered in Chapter 21. The Colgan Institute uses iron supplements of 10-25 mg daily with athletes, depending on their status. Iron intakes above 100 mg per day increase your risk of infections, and have multiple toxic side-effects (see Chapter 21). Don't take excess iron. Mega-doses of iron are definitely anti-ergogenic.

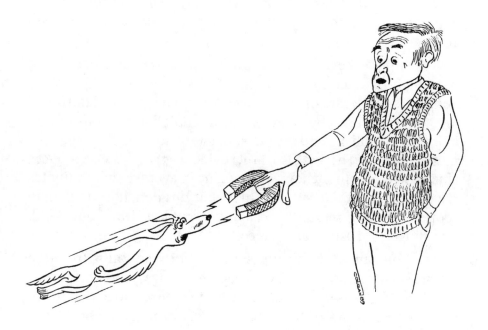

"Martha! I've found your iron pills."

Zinc

Zinc forms part of numerous essential enzymes for a thousand different functions in your body, from cell growth to testosterone production. The body pool is small and has to be constantly replaced from the diet. Inadequate zinc, even for one week, retards muscle growth and weakens immunity.[43]

Best sources of zinc are meats, eggs, and seafood. The

average zinc level of a 2,850 calorie American diet is 13.2 mg, 88% of the male RDA of 15 mg.[3] But studies of actual zinc intake in adults reveal a daily level of only 8.6 mg.[44] Zinc deficiency is probably widespread.

Because adequate zinc is essential for normal testosterone levels and sperm counts, some researchers suggest that the high incidence of impotence in American men is partially caused by chronic zinc deficiency.[45] Perhaps that's why oysters are so popular as an aphrodisiac: they are loaded with easily absorbed zinc.

Athletes certainly need more zinc than couch potatoes, for their high production of red blood cells to replace cells lost by hemolysis, for losses of zinc in sweat, for the increased fatty acid metabolism caused by exercise, for multiple interactions of zinc in iron metabolism, and for the added testosterone they need for muscle growth. There is also direct evidence that exercise reduces zinc status.[45] With the low level of zinc in average diets, athletes are doubly at risk. No surprise then that zinc deficit is rampant in sports including marathon running, triathlon, track and field, wrestling, gymnastics, and dance.[16,28-30,46-48]

You can get a fair measure of your zinc status from the simple **serum zinc** assay.[49] An acceptable range of serum zinc for athletes is 80-140 mcg/dl. Better measures are the more complicated assays of the zinc transport proteins **albumin** and **alpha-2-macroglobulin**.

The Colgan Institute uses supplements of 15-50 mg of zinc daily with athletes. Toxicity of zinc is low up to 500 mg/day.[31] But large doses of zinc interfere badly with copper metabolism.[50] They have no ergogenic effects. Remember synergy and avoid excess zinc.

Copper

You need copper for many enzymes, including those that produce nor-adrenalin,[51] one of your get-up-and-go hormones. Best food sources are organ meats and seafoods. Average

American diets provide a daily copper intake of 1.2 mg for males and 0.9 mg for females.[52] Copper requirements for humans are still unknown. The RDA handbook recommends a safe and adequate intake of 1.5-3.0 mg/day. The average intake is only two-thirds of the lower end of this scale.

Because of their greater use of copper to form nor-adrenalin, athletes may need more than the general population, certainly more than the amount in the average diet. There is no clear evidence, however, of copper deficiency in athletes.

Evidence is hard to gather because simple assays of copper in blood do not reflect tissue status. Some researchers have used the level of the copper-containing enzyme **ceruloplasmin** as a measure, and have found significant reductions caused by long, intense training.[53] But ceruloplasmin is altered radically by hormonal changes that also occur during exercise, so it is a poor measure.[54] The most accurate measure, which has not yet been used on athletes in controlled studies, is the **erythrocyte superoxide dismutase** assay.[55]

The Colgan Institute uses copper supplements of 0.5 mg to 3.0 mg with athletes mainly to bring copper intakes up to the recommended level. Daily intakes up to 10 mg, and occasional intakes up to 100 mg have not shown toxicity.[31] Large doses of copper have no ergogenic effects.

Manganese

You need manganese for proper formation of bone and cartilage, for normal glucose metabolism, and as part of the endogenous antioxidant **superoxide dismutase.**[13] Whole grains and black tea are the best food sources. Average intake in America is 2.7 mg/day for men and 2.2 mg/day for women.[51] The amount needed by humans is uncertain. The RDA handbook recommends a provisional daily intake of 2.0-5.0 mg.[3]

Because of their greater bone and soft tissue turnover and their higher metabolism of glucose, athletes may need more manganese than sedentary folk, but there are no controlled studies of effects of exercise on manganese levels.

As there are no norms for humans, you can't measure your manganese status. The Colgan Institute supplements athletes with 2.0-5.0 mg/day of manganese. Ergogenic potential is untested, but highly unlikely. Manganese is considered one of the least toxic of the trace elements if taken by mouth. But don't breathe manganese dust. Steel and chemical industry workers exposed to manganese dust, develop **locura manganica**, permanent insanity.[13]

Chromium

Many nutrition discoveries crucial to athletes are very recent. Until recently, chromium was considered more appropriate for car fenders than human nutrition. In the 1968 edition of the RDA handbook, it merited only the comment that studies on chromium, "are suggestive of a possible role in human nutrition."[56] By the 1989 edition, chiefly through the efforts of Dr Walter Mertz of the USDA, chromium was shown to be essential for normal glucose metabolism, insulin metabolism, fatty acid metabolism, and muscle growth, and merited three pages.

Chromium and its elusive **glucose tolerance factor (GTF),** which still has not been isolated, is widely dispersed in foods. Whole grain and shellfish are good sources. But it is easily destroyed by food processing.[57] From sugar cane to white sugar, for example, over 90% of the chromium disappears. The human body evolved with sugar cane including its chromium. It cannot handle sugar without it. Consequently, a high-sugar diet depletes body tissues of chromium in order to deal with the sugar.[57]

Because of degradation of our food, mainly by long storage and processing, the average daily intake of chromium in America is only 25 mcg in a 1,600 calorie diet, and 33 mcg in a 2,300 calorie diet.[57] The recommended safe and adequate daily allowance in the RDA handbook is 50-200 mcg. Consequently, chromium is one of the most deficient minerals in the American food supply. Because chromium is rapidly depleted by exercise and is so important to optimal performance, needs of athletes are discussed in more detail in Chapter 29.

Chromium status is difficult to measure. No human norms have been established, and no controlled studies have yet been done on normal levels in athletes. As explained in Chapter 29, the Colgan Institute uses 200-800 mcg/day of chromium picolinate with athletes.

Trivalent chromium, the kind that occurs in foods, is not toxic even in amounts 1,000 times the recommended intake.[57] **Hexavalent chromium** or **chromate** is highly toxic and a known carcinogen.[3] Mega-doses of chromium are not ergogenic, but Chapter 29 shows that correct daily intakes may indeed be anabolic.

Selenium

After 40 years of trying, selenium finally made the RDA table of essential minerals in 1989. Among other functions, it works as an antioxidant in conjunction with vitamin E. It forms part of an enzyme called **glutathione peroxidase** that destroys damaging free radicals called **hydroperoxides.**[58] Many diseases including heart disease result from selenium (and vitamin E) deficiency.

Selenium is widespread in foods. Seafood and meats are the best sources. Grains, produce, and food animals grown on selenium-poor soil are poor sources. In 1981, I did an analysis showing that selenium deficiency in soils occurs in 10 states in America plus the District of Columbia.[59] Average daily intake in America is about 108 mcg.[3] The RDA is 70 mcg for males and 55 mcg for females. As we will see in Chapter 20, on antioxidants, athletes have special needs for selenium beyond those of the sedentary population.

Selenium deficiency is often assessed in medicine by the level of **glutathione peroxidase activity.** But that assay is useless in athletes because it is sensitive only to severe deficiencies.[60] In

18 years, I have never found an athlete with severe selenium deficiency. The Colgan Institute uses selenium supplements of 200-400 mcg/day of L-selenomethionine with athletes. This form is not toxic up to 1,000 mcg per day.

Selenium can be very toxic, especially in high amounts. And thereby hangs a tale. One famous macho movie star turned up in my office wanting a nutrition program to save his hair. After voluminous testing we found he was suffering from selenium poisoning, one effect of which is to make you hair fall out in bunches. He had been reading a well-known book on life extension that advocates selenium. He was taking 5-6 times the big dose recommended, because Hollywood knows so well that bigger must be better. It took me hours to persuade him that his "anti-aging" nutrition supplement was the cause of his hair loss. Mega-doses of selenium are definitely anti-ergogenic.

Iodine

You need dietary iodine to make your thyroid hormones. Because they control all energy in the body, you better get it right. Inadequate iodine causes the thyroid in the neck to grow massive, trying to provide more cells that produce thyroid hormone, so as to make up the deficiency. In areas where iodine is deficient in the soil, and therefore in the produce and food animals grown on the soil, the disfigurement of a huge goiter (enlarged thyroid), hanging from the neck used to be commonplace. So did the mental retardation of cretinism, also caused by iodine deficiency. Iodized salt turned that problem around, though goiter and cretinism still occur in remote areas of Kentucky, Louisiana, Texas, and South Carolina.[61]

Seafood of any kind is the best food source. Even breathing sea air every day will give you sufficient iodine to prevent goiter. Iodine intakes in the general population, however, have been declining steadily since 1980, presumably because people are cutting down on salt. The average intake in America is about 250 mcg/day for males, and 170 mcg/day for females.[52] That is well above the RDA of 150 mcg.

Athletes may need more iodine than the general population because you lose a lot in sweat. One study showed a loss of 146 mcg per day from very moderate activity in a hot environment.[62] There are no simple tests for iodine status. A thyroid panel is sometimes an indication, but low thyroid levels in otherwise healthy athletes are seldom caused by iodine deficit. The Colgan Institute uses supplements of 50-200 mcg/day with some athletes. Iodine is not toxic up to 2,000 mcg daily,[3] but may exacerbate acne. Ergogenic potential -- nil.

Boron

Before 1981, the mineral boron was considered unimportant for human nutrition. Then Drs Curtiss Hunt and Forrest Nielsen at the USDA Human Nutrition Research Center in Grand Forks, ND, showed that boron is essential for normal growth in chicks.[63] By 1990, together with other scientists, they showed that it is probably an essential nutrient for humans too. Boron seems to provide biochemicals called **hydroxyl groups**, essential for manufacture of the active forms of some steroid hormones; especially hormones involved in calcium, phosphorus, and magnesium metabolism in bone, and in muscle growth.[64] Hence the popular interest in boron as a possible anabolic supplement for athletes.

There are no studies yet with athletes, but clinical research suggests that adequate boron status is necessary for normal testosterone production. Post-menopausal women supplemented with 3 mg per day of sodium borate showed increased blood levels of testosterone and 17-beta-estradiol, the most active form of estrogen.[61] In some of the women, the increase in estrogen levels was as large as is achieved with estrogen replacement therapy. But remember, in these women past menopause, hormone production was below par to begin with.

The hormonal demands on the bodies of both male and female athletes, indicate that their nutrition should be optimal in every nutrient that is involved in hormone production. The real question is, does the average athlete's diet contains sufficient boron to meet those demands. The answer is, probably not.

In 1987 the Colgan Institute did an analysis of the boron content of the American diet, based on extensive chemical analysis of over 200 foods by other researchers. We reported that the average boron intake of a good mixed diet in America is only 1.9 mg per day.[66] This figure agrees with the 1.7 mg per day found in a recent analysis of the average diet in Finland.[67]

Individual diets can be much lower, however, because high boron foods, soybeans, almonds, peanuts, prunes, raisins, dates, and unprocessed honey, may be seldom eaten. A recent precise analysis of the self-selected diets of adults showed boron intakes of only 0.42 mg and 0.35 mg per day.[68]

No one knows exactly how much boron you need. The women in the above study who showed a big response to boron supplementation, were fed a diet containing 0.25 mg boron per day for 17 weeks before the study began. So that is not enough even for sedentary folk. Dr Forrest Nielsen, the leading expert on boron, suggests from his animal studies that 2.0 mg may be sufficient for the average person. When you add the hormonal demands of exercise, an athlete's requirement for boron may be higher.

The Colgan Institute supplements athletes with 3.0-6.0 mg/day of boron citrate and aspartate. The only brand we trust is TwinLab. Toxicity of boron is low, but intakes above 50 mg/day may interfere with phosphorus and riboflavin metaboslim.[69] So don't take large doses.

Boron supplements of up to 10 mg per pill, are currently being sold to athletes as anabolics, with wild claims that they increase testosterone levels. Give me a break! Boron may be an essential part of the process, but it doesn't cause the body to produce testosterone. As explained in Chapter 32, testosterone levels are tightly controlled by multiple mechanisms. If you are getting sufficient boron, then adding a mega-dose more does nothing but interfere with your metabolism of other nutrients.

Molybdenum

You need dietary molybdenum as part of three essential enzymes, **xanthine oxidase, aldehyde oxidase,** and **sulfite oxidase.**[70] Molybdenum content of food varies widely even in different samples of the same food.[70] Whole grains and legumes are the best sources. Average dietary intake in America is about 109 mcg/day for males and 76 mcg/day for females.[3]

No one knows how much molybdenium you need, nor how to measure molybdenum status. The provisional RDA recommendation is 50-250 mcg/day. The Colgan Institute uses 40-150 mcg/day of molybdenum with athletes as part of complete multi-nutrient supplements. Toxicity starts at a huge 10 mg daily, causing gout-like disease.[71] Molybdenum has no ergogenic potential.

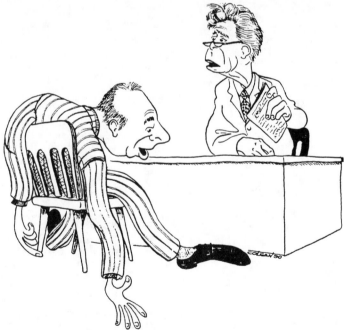

"Its either a severe calcium deficiency or you mislaid your skeleton somewhere."

Other Trace Elements

There is evidence for the essentiality of silicon for normal bone growth.[8] Cobalt forms an essential part of vitamin B_{12}.[3] Fluoride is essential for both teeth and bones.[9] Nickel is essential for normal growth.[64] Beyond that, science knows little about them.

In addition, arsenic (believe it or not) is essential for normal animal growth.[64] And the evidence is mounting that tin, germanium, and vanadium are essential for animals also.[64] But, apart from health marketplace hype, there is no evidence to recommend their use with athletes. As Chapter 31 shows, supplements of germanium and vanadium now being touted to athletes, are simply modern versions of carpetbaggers' snake oil.

Chapter 16

The Right Supplements

How do you know the supplements you are buying are the right stuff? How do you know which ones among the myriad of bottles lining the shelves of health food stores and pharmacies are genuine, potent, true-to-label, and made of the best forms of vitamins, minerals, and other nutrients? You don't. This chapter gives you the clues to separate the good from the bad from the ugly. And there are plenty of ugly.

A few months ago, for example, the Colgan Institute was asked whether a new 500 mg L-carnitine pill was any good. The athletes who asked were surprised when our lab technician pronounced it a dud without even bothering to open the bottle. He knew immediately it was not up to specs, because you can't fit 500 mg of L-carnitine into one pill and still keep it small enough to swallow.

L-carnitine is very hygroscopic (attracts water), and has to be mixed with two or three times its weight of a dry, neutral excipient, such as tricalcium phosphate, in order to prevent it turning into a pool of water. It also has to be made into pills in a special low humidity environment. The pill in question weighed 1008 mg, yet claimed to contain 500 mg of L-carnitine, plus 350 mg of other vitamins and amino acids. Not possible to make.

With the recent acceptance of vitamins into mainstream medicine, and the hundreds of new studies showing their efficacy in the treatment of disease, there has been huge growth of public use of supplements. This burgeoning $4 billion a year market, has encouraged a lot of companies to switch their operations into the supplement area, and a lot of new companies to enter the field. The Colgan Institute has recently investigated 21 different vitamin companies. All of them have lots of shiny equipment with all the bells and whistles. But only two have the essential qualified people and expertise to do a quality job.

How To Choose Vitamins

Multi-vitamins are some of the worst offenders. In a recent study, Linda Shaffer and Michelle Fairchild of Yale New Haven Hospital, evaluated 257 brands of vitamins bought off the shelf at pharmacies, grocery stores, and health food stores. Many were incomplete or had too little or too much of one or other nutrient. Only 49 were considered adequate.[1]

The Colgan Institute has done a continuing similar analysis of nutrient supplements for the past 12 years. We have a hotline used by thousands of athletes on which we give advice about brands and products we have tested and found adequate. This service is free as part of our nutrition education function. We buy the samples like you do, off the store shelf. No manufacturer pays us a dime to test their products, or to approve them. And we receive no federal or other grants for this work. Our recommendations are not for sale. The hotline number is (619) 632-7722.

There are other laboratories that test supplements, but the manufacturer pays big bucks for the testing program. It costs between $50 and $100 to test each single ingredient of a vitamin pill. That's just time and materials, no profit. For one 40-ingredient multi-vitamin/mineral, a decent test at a decent lab, plus the lab's profit, runs about $6,000. A company might have 20 such pills. You be the judge of the lab results you might expect, when they are being paid $120,000 or more, and the pills are being supplied by the supplement manufacturer.

Wrong Ingredient

Pills being potent and true to label is only the first problem. By law, the pill only has to be true to label *chemically*. That is, when you analyze it by **high performance liquid chromatography (HPLC)** or other chemistry procedure, it only has to show the required spikes on the chart for the ingredients claimed. But many legal forms of nutrients are hardly bioavailable at all.

Magnesium oxide, for example, a common source of magnesium in multi-vitamin/mineral pills, is only one-tenth as bioavailable as magnesium aspartate. But the aspartate form takes up far more room in a pill than the oxide form. You can't use nearly as much and still keep the pill to a size that can be swallowed. So on the label, the amount of magnesium you can put in a pill in the aspartate form is much less than you can put in the oxide form. Consequently, pill makers continue to use the oxide so that their label potency can be as high as possible. They know that consumers go for the biggest numbers, and have no understanding that 100 mg of magnesium aspartate is far better than 400 mg of cheap magnesium oxide.

It goes the other way too. **Pyridoxal-5-phosphate (P-5-P)**, for example, is an expensive form of pyridoxine (vitamin B_6). Some supplement makers tout it as the form used by the human body, and therefore superior and meriting a higher price. They neglect to tell you that every molecule of P-5-P is broken down in digestion to plain old pyridoxine, and transported that way through the intestinal wall. The body then turns all the pyridoxine into pyridoxal-5-phosphate again. So inexpensive **pyridoxine hydrochloride** is every bit as good as P-5-P in a vitamin pill.

The same goes for the prohibitively expensive **dibencoside** form of vitamin B_{12}, being falsely touted as an anabolic. This coenzyme **(5,6-dimethylbenzimidazolyl cobamide)** is the form in which the human body uses vitamin B_{12}. But your body converts vitamin B_{12} to the dibencoside form very efficiently. There is no reason to pay 100 times the price for it when your body does the job for free.

Some distinctions between forms of vitamin are more subtle. Many supplements use the synthetic **dl-alpha-tocopherol** as their vitamin E. Yet clinical studies show unequivocally, that the natural source form of vitamin E, **d-alpha-tocopherol**, raises serum vitamin E levels 40% higher and red blood cell levels 300% higher than the synthetic form.[2,3] The public does not know these things, but you should know them good if your goal is optimal performance.

Some forms of carotene used in vitamins, and claimed to be beta-carotene, have zero biological activity. The **menadione** form of vitamin K can be toxic, whereas the **phylloquinone** form is non-toxic in any reasonable amount.[4] With a tip of my hat to Dr Luke Bucci for pointing me in the right direction, fat-soluble forms of thiamin, called **allithiamins**, are superior to water-soluble thiamin.[5] Calcium or magnesium ascorbate are better forms of vitamin C than regular ascorbic acid. The list is endless.

The same goes for every one of the minerals. Iron as iron sulphate or oxide is useless compared with iron as **ferrous fumarate** or **iron picolinate**. Selenium as **L-selenomethionine** is better absorbed than sodium selenite. Silicon from the **horsetail herb** (*Equisetum arvense*) is superior to silicon dioxide. **Chromium picolinate** is far superior to chromium chloride or chromium nicotinate. **Zinc picolinate** is far and away better than zinc sulphate. Unless you know what forms of the minerals actually work in the human body, you may be religiously taking mineral supplements every day that have virtually no affect.

Hundreds of other compounds, including vitamin B15, pangamic acid, *Ammi magjus*, lipoic acid, polylactates, glycosaminoglycans, royal jelly, bee pollen, wheat grass, spirulena, Mexican wild yam, *Yucca schidigera*, have no evidence whatsoever to support their inclusion in supplements. Many of these are exposed in Chapter 31. But new compounds, some good, some bad, come down the pike every month. I hope what we cover here whets your appetite for more of the truth, because you need to know it to build that optimum body.

You can keep up to date by reading the Colgan Institute magazine, **NUTRITION & fitness,** or you can call our hotline, (619) 632-7722. I promise you will always get the straight facts uncontaminated by federal grants, food industry lobbies, university policies, or other commercial or political biases.

There Are No Natural Vitamins

One of the most frequent questions asked on our nutrition hotline concerns natural versus synthetic vitamins. Because the word "natural" sells, many supplement makers use it in their advertising and product labels. But the pill ingredients themselves are about as natural as a polyester suit.

All vitamins today are predominantly synthetic. That is, they are pure chemicals created out of a food base. Most vitamin C, for example, is made from corn. First, the corn is chemically converted to sugar (d-glucose) and crystallized. Then it is chemically converted to pure, synthetic L-ascorbic acid. There is not a molecule of the natural corn left in it.

How about vitamin A? Many folk think that has to be natural because it is extracted from cod liver oil. Unfortunately, the stubborn cod will not cooperate by standardizing their livers, so that 5,000 IU of the vitamin A therein will fit neatly into a No 2 gelatin capsule. Vitamin makers have to dice and slice every batch with synthetic vitamin A or vegetable oil to adjust the potency. To these some companies add butylated hydroxytoluene (BHT), sodium benzoate, methylparaben, propylparaben, sorbic acid, and a host of other chemicals.[6] Is that synthetic enough for you?!

What about so-called "natural" rose hip or acerola vitamin C? Look carefully at the label. If it is honest it will state, "*with* rose hips" or "*with* acerola vitamin C." The best rose hip powder contains only a few milligrams of vitamin C per ounce. A 1,000 mg rose hip vitamin C tablet has to be 99% synthetic ascorbic acid, because a 1,000 mg pill made of pure rose hip vitamin C would be the size of a baseball.

Acerola powder from the acerola cherry is the most potent and expensive commercial source of natural vitamin C. It contains about 200 mg of vitamin C per gram of powder. So a 1,000 mg tablet of vitamin C would weigh 5 grams of powder plus 1 gram of excipients, 6 grams in all. Far too big to swallow. The biggest pill that most people can deal with is 1.5-2.0 grams. Consequently, an acceptable acerola vitamin C pill would be of very low potency. Even then, few people would buy it because acerola is 12-20 times the cost of plain ascorbic acid.

One more example. Some months ago, we received a "natural B-complex" supplement stating on the label that it was made from organically grown yeast. Each pill claimed to contain 100 mg of niacin, plus other B-vitamins. We tested them: there was 100 mg of niacin per pill. But it could not be natural. The best yeast contains less than 40 mg of niacin per 100 grams.[7] The biggest yeast tablet that anyone could swallow would contain less than 1 mg of natural niacin. The pills we received were almost totally synthetic.

Such mixing of synthetic vitamins with a sprinkling of natural vitamins, then calling them "all natural," is a mild deception of the marketplace. Let's move on to some of the more serious problems.

False Claims

There are hundreds of shiny supplements on the market that make completely false claims. Many of them are exposed in Chapter 31. It's no wonder Dr David Kessler, new head of the FDA, is cracking down so hard. Unfortunately, he does not have sufficient qualified staff in nutrition, so they often crack in the wrong direction. Until they get better aim and focus, you have to protect yourself.

Vitamin C is a big seller so it gets a lot of attention from fast buck operators. Take the sago palm vitamin C fiasco.

Everyone wants their vitamins to be non-allergenic, so if you have an anti-allergy story as a selling hook, you will get more customers. Some companies put it about that sensitive people react to vitamin C from corn because they are allergic to corn. (Chemists laugh right here but let's go on.) The Japanese company Takeda began producing vitamin C from Indonesian sago palm. Few people are allergic to sago, so "sago palm vitamin C" began sweeping the market. But, as I explained previously, when vitamin C is made, the food base used goes through so many chemical transformations and purifications, that not a molecule of it remains in the final ascorbic acid.

That's fortunate because sago palm is gathered by unwashed natives in steaming jungles, where they squat on the sago trunks, sweating freely into their work, scraping sago starch into balls, complete with tree maggots, flies, fungi, viruses, yeasts, and molds. By the time this mess is chemically converted to pure crystalline ascorbic acid, not a molecule of the organic ordure remains. All the high-priced sago palm vitamin C products are simply plain old synthetic ascorbic acid.

The sago palm scam has no scientific backing, and is easily exposed because it contradicts principles of chemistry. But there are many claims apparently backed by scientific studies that are much harder to refute. The expensive Ester-C form of vitamin C is a good example.

In 1987, Drs Marilyn Bush and Anthony Verlangiari at the University of Mississippi, reported that, in rats, Ester-C was about twice as well absorbed and twice as well retained as ascorbic acid.[8] In 1991, they published a second study reporting that Ester-C was about four times as potent as ascorbic acid at preventing scurvy in rats.[9] These studies led to market claims that Ester-C is four times as effective as ascorbic acid. Like many scientists, I was almost convinced.

Then Ester-C was analyzed independently by Dr Assad Kazeminy of the Irvine Analytical Laboratory, Irvine, California. It was composed of ascorbic acid, dehydroascorbic acid, and calcium.[10] That is, it is mainly regular calcium ascorbate, which is well known to be more effective than ascorbic acid. Ester-C contains no exotic compounds that might make it superior.

In September 1991, the Food and Drug Administration sent a distributor of Ester-C a regulatory letter telling them to cease and desist their claims as "false and misleading." The FDA's own analyses found that one dose of Ester-C provided 1,096 mg of vitamin C, about the same as a 1.0 gram tablet of ascorbic acid.[11] World expert on vitamin C, Dr Linus Pauling agrees. When asked about Ester-C he replied, "it isn't an ester...it's mainly calcium ascorbate."[12] Shows you that in the vitamin market, you often pay more for the sizzle than the sausage.

Then there are the dreaded dilutions. You can buy many "complexes" of nutrients on the wholesale vitamin market. A retail label may read "Each pill contains 500 IU of mixed tocopherol complex." The complex can be anything from 50% tocopherols, plus 50% vegetable oil filler, to 95% tocopherols and 5% filler, depending on how much you are prepared to pay. But the consumer can't tell the difference, so you know which grade he gets from unscrupulous pill makers.

The Colgan Institute receives hundreds of unsolicited samples of new products, each one claiming to be the best. Among last week's crop was a bottle of vitamin E oil. It contained 4 oz. of oil. The label proclaimed in big print, "Vitamin E Oil. 20,000 IU of vitamin E." Sounds like a lot unless you know that 1 IU = 1 mg of commercial vitamin E.[4] That's 28,400 IU per ounce. If the bottle was really vitamin E oil, it should read 113,600 IU of vitamin E. On the back in tiny print it read, "in a base of wheat germ oil," as if it was an unimportant constituent. The true analysis of this mix is 83% wheat germ oil and 17% vitamin E.

As the consumer becomes more educated, some companies are starting to cite their suppliers' **Certificates of Analysis** in retail product literature to convince you about product composition. Buyer beware. Recently, we bought some linoleic acid in oil-filled capsules from a big supplier. My lab tech noticed that the Certificate of Analysis was dated three years ago. On ringing the company, we were nonchalantly told that not every batch is analyzed, but the extraction method is standard, and the material is fresh, so it will be near enough the same potency as on the certificate. That's like saying that the flowers from a particular florist will be as good as you got three years ago, even though it has changed hands twice and is now a dry cleaners.

I have laid out these examples, to show you that we do our homework. The most blatant scams are dealt with in detail in Chapter 31. There are many others I have no room to include. Before you waste $50 on some new wonder supplement, call our hotline for the straight answers.

"Elementary My Dear Watson"

You need the sleuthing power of Sherlock Holmes to find out the levels of minerals in many supplements. I am holding a bottle that says on the label:

Two pills contain: calcium gluconate.......1,000mg

To many folk that looks like a good dose of calcium, 83% of the RDA of 1,200 mg. Not so. RDAs, and all discussion of minerals in this book, and in any scientific book on nutrition, refer to *elemental* quantities, the actual amount of the mineral element itself. Calcium gluconate is only 9% elemental calcium.[13] So the two-pill dose contains only 90 mg of calcium, an insignificant amount. You would have to take 26 of these pills to get the RDA.

Become an avid label reader. If the amount given on the bottle refers to the source material of any mineral, then the elemental mineral content is meager. The most potent source of calcium, and one of the best absorbed, is calcium carbonate, which is 40% elemental calcium.[13] So if the above pills had used the calcium carbonate source, they would contain 400 mg of calcium, requiring only 6 pills to get the RDA.

Other common sources are calcium acetate (23% calcium), calcium citrate (21% calcium), and calcium lactate (14% calcium). For comparison, milk is less than 1% calcium.[13]

Those sources put those percentages of calcium in the pill, but that's not the amount that gets into your body. Some manufacturers claim a 60% absorption rate. But controlled studies yield, carbonate (39% absorbed), acetate (32% absorbed), citrate (30% absorbed), and milk (27% absorbed).[13] More calcium is excreted than ever gets into your tissues.

Let's do the numbers to see what you get from a good calcium supplement, a pill containing 1,000 mg of calcium carbonate. Amount of elemental calcium is 400 mg. Amount absorbed is 39%, that is only 156 mg. Most supplements are a lot worse than that. Now you know why so many American women are chronically short of calcium.[4]

The same scenario goes for all the minerals. To calculate how much is getting into your body, you have to know the source material, its elemental content of the mineral, and the absorption rate of that source. With more than 500 sources of minerals used in the supplement market, I can't cover them here. The calcium example alerts you to the problem. You can get the answers for other minerals by calling our hotline.

The Right Stuff

Decent supplement manufacturers use the best forms of vitamins and minerals, bought from the top chemical manufacturers. **Hoffman LaRoche**, Nutley, NJ makes the best bulk vitamin C, and the best of most of the b-vitamins. **Henkel**, La Grange, IL, makes far and away the best vitamin E in the world. **Nutrition 21**, San Diego, CA makes the best minerals in picolinate form. If you know the material sources used in a supplement, you have a pretty good idea of its quality.

Decent pill makers always state the elemental quantities of minerals. They always put in real amounts rather than token amounts of expensive compounds. They give full disclosure of all ingredients including excipients, and they test true to label. They also have proper batch numbers and expiry dates, and have their full address on the bottle.

Real supplement companies do not have post-office box addresses or worse, show no address at all. Real companies do not claim secret ingredients, which incidentally, is against the labelling laws. Nor do they add glitzy ingredients that are current market buzzwords, such as yohimbe bark, orchic glandulars, or colostrum.

In Chapters 14 and 15, I have given you the ranges of amounts, and the best chemical form for each nutrient. One excellent source of most of them is the **TwinLab** brand. We have tested their vitamins, minerals, and amino acids extensively over the last decade, and have yet to find them wanting.

Nutrition Nirvana

With the exploding use of supplements in medicine, there are tremendous new developments that will really enhance athletic performance. In the past, the best science has done is to test supplements on animals and men, usually by challenging them with a disease or trauma, or by producing a severe nutrient deficiency, then treating it. That was the era of minimal nutrition to cure deficiency disease: the minimal intake of vitamin C to stop scurvy, the minimal intake of protein to maintain nitrogen balance in a couch potato , or the minimum amount of niacin to prevent pellagra.

Now we are entering the era of optimal nutrition. A new scientific journal, **The Journal of Optimal Nutrition**, published its first issue in July, 1992.[14] A few years ago responsible scientists scoffed at the idea of nutritional optima. The general view was that we were still 50 years away from that level of research. Now scientists are clamoring to write about it.

On the research front, the latest development will yield nutrient supplements superior to anything that has been made before. Respected microbiologist Dr Myron Wentz of Gull Laboratories, Salt Lake City, Utah, is starting to test for nutritional optima by growing human cells *in vitro* (in the test tube). By feeding the cells different nutrient combinations, he aims to determine which combinations produce the best growth, the best resistance to disease, and the longest life. It is an advance in nutrition science that coincides well with the dawn of the third millennium.

Chapter 17

What Nutrient Toxicity?

Since 1974, the Colgan Institute has used vitamin and mineral supplements with more than 31,000 people. Some of these have been taking the supplements regularly for the last 18 years. During that whole period, we have had reports of 229 cases of possible toxicity.

Analysis of each of these cases has shown that most reported symptoms resulted from coincidental infections, injuries, foods eaten, emotional stress, and other events. These events were mistakenly attributed to the supplements by users. In 161 cases, symptoms disappeared over time, despite continued use of supplements. In 38 cases, symptoms disappeared promptly on cessation or reduction of supplements. Twenty-eight of the remaining 30 cases were real and continuing reactions to nutrients. They involved gastrointestinal upsets, skin rashes, headaches, nausea, and fatigue. None was serious. In all 28 cases, symptoms cleared up over time after cessation of supplement use, or after adjustment of the supplement mix. The two last cases remain a mystery

Two out of 31,000 seems a pretty good safety record for nutrients. If you assess your **biochemical individuality** and your **lifestyle dynamics** and pay attention to **complete nutrition** and to **synergy of nutrients**, then use of reasonable amounts of nutrient supplements must be one of the safest ways on Earth to improve your body.

But the media love to engage in vitamin bashing and gleefully pounce on any reported case of nutrient toxicity. At various times, vitamin A poisoning has been highlighted, as if eating a carrot puts you at terrible risk. Vitamin C has been accused of causing rebound scurvy when you stop using it, and of destroying vitamin B_{12} in the human system. Vitamin B_6 has been solemnly indicted by humorless churls in academic offices as a cause of nerve damage. And mega-doses of any nutrient have been denounced as poisoning in tones reminiscent of the Salem witchcraft trials. Let's see if these charges are true or false.

Vitamin A

Any substance can be toxic, even water if you take enough of it. Eskimos don't eat polar bear liver. Even their sled dogs avoid it.[1] The dogs know it makes them sick. One pound of polar bear liver can contain 2,000,000 mcg RE (6,600,000 IU) of vitamin A. That is enough to poison anyone.

The medical literature contains about 600 cases of vitamin A poisoning.[2,3] A lot of these cases have been with women given daily *prescribed* mega-doses of over 330,000 mcg RE (1,000,000 IU) of cis-retinoic acid for skin complaints. Such mega-doses of vitamin A are especially dangerous because they build up in your bodyfat.

World expert on the toxicity of nutrients, Dr John Hathcock of Iowa State University and the Food and Drug Administration, concludes that toxicity of vitamin A does not occur for most people in normal health until they take a dose above 1,000 mcg RE per kilogram bodyweight.[1] That's 70,000 mcg RE (230,000 IU) for a 70 kg (154 lb) athlete. He does cite some reports of headache, intracranial hypertension, and skin lesions in children and sick individuals at intakes of only 10,000-15,000 mcg RE, but none with normal adults.[15] In any case, sensible supplementation does not even approach such figures. We have never found an athlete that needed more than 5,000 mcg RE (16,500 IU) per day.

Vitamin C

Every so often the media resurrect the old bogey that vitamin C destroys vitamin B_{12}, and can make you anemic. This notion arose from a flimsy report by Dr Victor Herbert in 1974 of low serum vitamin B_{12}, in 4 out of 18 spinal cord injury patients prescribed high doses of ascorbate as a urine acidifier.[4] The media story was then bolstered by an even flimsier report of Dr J.D. Hines in 1975, that 3 out of 90 elderly people taking high doses of vitamin C had low vitamin B_{12}.[5] Herbert measured B_{12} in food, in the presence of high levels of ascorbate, and concluded it was bound by the ascorbate and no longer bioavailable.

The problem is he used the assay of Lau, a procedure appropriate only for measuring vitamin B_{12} in blood serum. This assay is far too weak to pull B_{12} out of food. This error has since been roundly criticized by a number of independent laboratories,[6,7] including mine,[8] but there is no news value in shamefaced retractions, so the media maintain the myth. The evidence shows clearly that vitamin C does not interfere with vitamin B_{12} metabolism.

A second claim for ascorbate toxicity is that excess vitamin C causes formation of kidney stones, because it degrades to **oxalate**, which is the base material of many stones. A third claim is gout because vitamin C metabolites might raise uric acid levels in the body.

Your body is much smarter than that. Even with multi-gram doses of vitamin C, control mechanisms keep oxalate levels and urate levels from rising too high.[9] Vitamin C has been used in medicine in multi-gram amounts daily, for decades, to acidify urine in various diseases. An international symposium of experts on the subject, concluded there was no evidence of stone formation nor gout with multi-gram supplements of vitamin C.[10]

The final purported problem with vitamin C is that it causes rebound scurvy when you stop taking it. This media splash was based on an anecdotal report of apparent vitamin C dependency in two new-born babies, born to mothers who were taking high levels of ascorbate.[1] No confirmed case of rebound scurvy has ever been reported.[1,11] Serum levels of vitamin C do drop markedly on cessation of supplements, but then return to within the normal range within 21 days on an average American diet.[12]

Vitamin B₆

The third nutrient to receive a media thrashing for purported toxicity is vitamin B₆. Taken in large amounts (500 mg to 5 grams) for months or years, vitamin B₆ does cause severe nerve damage.[12,13] These huge overdoses are usually self-administered by women who have read popular articles on the use of vitamin B₆ to treat premenstrual syndrome. They are also sometimes *prescribed* for mental patients.[13,14] Some cases of nerve damage have been reported at an intake of only 117 mg/day. Fortunately, most of these cases clear up spontaneously within 6 months of stopping supplementation.[15]

Vitamins And Minerals Are Safe

One good way to assess the safety of vitamin and mineral supplements is to compare them with medicines. It's pretty simple to get at the truth. Just read the annual reports of the Poison Control Centers.[17] For the period 1985-1990, 2,251 people died from use of prescription drugs, including 640 from simple analgesics, such as aspirin. Nasty stuff!

In the same period the total deaths from use of vitamins - *one* - from overdose of niacin. Vitamin A is often cited in the press as potentially toxic. Total deaths in 1985-1990 - zero. Vitamin B₆ is often cited in the press as a neurotoxin. Total deaths 1985-1990 - zero. Vitamin C is used in mega-doses by millions of Americans every day. Total deaths 1985-1990 - zero. And so on down the list. Used in any sensible amounts, vitamins and minerals are about as toxic as lemonade.

Part IV

Performance

Those who have no time for nutrition and exercise had better reserve a lot of time for disease.

Michael Colgan, Continuing Medical Education Lectures, 1988

Chapter 18

Vitamins And Performance

With much scientific ado about nothing, hundreds of silly single-nutrient studies have been done and continue to be done on athletes, trying to show that this or that vitamin does or doesn't improve performance. And gaggles of silly professors review these studies, the pro-vitamin camp shouting 'tis, and the anti-vitamin camp shouting 'tisn't, without ever relating the results to basic principles of nutrition. With a hang of the head I have to admit I've sometimes been guilty myself. So you don't make the same mistake, here's the bottom line.

The typical study of vitamins in sport gives a self-selected group of undergraduates (participating for college credits), an arbitrary amount of a single vitamin or mineral for a few days, or at best, a few weeks. These studies (usually done with your tax money), break the rules of nutrition science so badly, they amount to scientific treason. The perpetrators should be taken out and shot.

All the random assignment, double-blind, repeated cross-over, super-controls, and fancy statistics cannot save them. First, they take no account of **biochemical individuality**. Different athletes have radically different nutrient needs. Champion cyclist Howard Dorfling, for example, soaks up B-complex vitamins like a sponge. But to feed the same doses to his teammates would put every one of them into overload. Megadosing athletes who already have adequate amounts of a nutrient, cannot do anything good. Unless you assess the nutrient status of athletes before you start supplementing (and here I don't mean those wishy-washy dietary analyses that pass for assessment in many journals), you might as well feed them bull pucky.

Second, we have seen throughout this book that nutrients work only in **synergy** with each other. Arbitrarily increasing one nutrient without increasing at least its principle synergists is useless. I show in Chapter 21, for example, that, even in iron deficient athletes, iron supplementation by itself hardly works at all. To get reasonable results you have to supplement with its principle synergists, folic acid, pyridoxine, ascorbate, tocopherol, cobalamin, and zinc.[1]

Third, the business of nutrition is to build a better body. That has to wait on the **physiological dynamics** of Nature. Unless there is a turnover of blood cells and muscle cells, so that superior cells can grow in the improved nutrient environment provided by the supplementation, you cannot expect improved performance. Blood cells take three months to turn over, and muscle cells six months.[2] The *minimum* study of vitamins should be at least six months long. Until recently, before this principle was understood, the average length of studies on vitamins in sport was about three weeks. That's like measuring the rainfall in Arizona for three weeks, and wrongly concluding that it doesn't rain there at all.

Of course you might luck out on a tropical storm and wrongly conclude that Arizona is wetter than Oregon. That sometimes happens with vitamins. In a 10-subject trial, one or two subjects might be really deficient in the nutrient under study. In a month their performance booms, dragging the statistics of everyone else into the highly significant zone. All the pro-vitamin buffs immediately shout "told you so," and vitamin X becomes the latest ergogenic fad. Hogwash and flapdoodle!

You have to get down to the nitty-gritty. What really counts is the individual athlete and his individual performance. If two out of ten athletes get a great result and eight do not, you have shown nothing by averaging the performance of the whole group.

The only way to know what's going on is to analyze hundreds of studies minutely, toss out the bad, keep the good, and look for trends in the evidence. That's what we've been doing at the Colgan Institute for the last 18 years.

In this book, I can review only a handful of the studies. What I offer you is representative of the trends of evidence. All that evidence points to one conclusion: vitamins and co-factors are building materials, precise nuts and bolts that fit exactly into pre-drilled holes. The number and size of the holes that you have are as individual as your fingerprints. If any one of the holes is left unfilled, or if there are excess nuts and bolts floating about, then growth, development, and function of your body is impaired, and performance cannot be optimal.

I have shown you that the Recommended Dietary Allowances of vitamins make no allowances for the nutrient demands imposed by exercise. I have shown you that athletes and the general population are deficient in many nutrients, even at the antediluvian levels of the RDAs. And I have shown you that athletes are often severely deficient in relation to the nutrient demands of their training.

Yet ignorance continues to abound. On one hand, conservative physicians and dieticians (often with hidden commercial agendas), continue to push the myth of the good mixed diet as optimal for everyone.[3] This delusion, as yet an unpunished form of malpractice in American medicine, does not occur in animal breeding, because sickness directly affects the bottom line. Breeders know that food is deficient. Supplementation is standard practice.

Dr Burton Kallman, chief scientist of the National Nutritional Foods Association, has calculated that the standard monkey diet in zoos is supplemented with 23 times the RDAs for vitamins and minerals.[4] That's what it takes to yield optimum growth and resistance to disease in animals that are our closest relatives. Yet some ignorant sods continue to bleat that humans don't need any of it.

We get plenty of the "good mixed diet" types coming to the Colgan Institute for help. They are the most deficient and the most unsuccessful of athletes. It sickens me to see a lad or lass with great athletic potential, who has wasted years under the influence of some ignorant nutritionist or dietician, who has restricted their development to the mediocre level permitted by our nutrient-poor American food.[5]

On the other hand, there are the vitamin freaks (again, often with hidden commercial agendas), who tout endless variations and combinations of vitamins as ergogenic rocket fuel.[6] It sickens me equally to see athletes popping handfuls of useless pills and powders in the days before competition. Usually they or their coaches have fallen for ads of muscular giants, proclaiming they were 95 lb weaklings and similar ballyhoo, until they took Brand X. All hype and dreams. To indicate how bad the marketplace can be, on 6 May 1992, the New York Department of Consumer Affairs charged six sports supplement companies with deceptive advertising.

Get both idiotic notions out of your mind. Food cannot provide sufficient vitamins to meet the demands of intense exercise. And taking vitamins beyond levels that are sufficient to balance their use during exercise, and tissue growth and maintenance, boosts only the cash flow of the supplement makers.

If you are serious about optimum performance, your job is to use this book to analyze your individual nutrient needs, and then precisely fulfill them. If the task gets too complex, call our hotline (619) 632-7722 for help.

Put nothing in your mouth unless it fits your individual plan. There are no overnight miracle foods and no overnight miracle vitamins. The miracle comes from matching your nutrient needs to your biochemistry and your training, then subjecting the mix to a daily dose of good, hard sweat.

Chapter 19

Minerals and Performance

We have seen in Chapter 15 that athletes can be seriously deficient in the essential minerals, calcium,[1-3] magnesium,[4-6] potassium,[7] iron,[8] zinc,[5,9,10] chromium,[11] and possibly boron.[12] For some other essential minerals, there are no human norms, and no good way to measure the status of the body. Nevertheless, working with the tools we've got can make a big difference to your performance.

As with vitamins, the first step is always to assess your mineral status, *before* you put any supplement in your mouth. As Chapter 1 shows, mineral overload is almost as detrimental to performance as mineral deficit.

Popping calcium pills, as I have seen some lasses do, because their training has made them amenorrheic, and they are scared of weakening their bones, is just plain dumb. But taking 500 mg of calcium daily, because your diet measures out at only 800 mg, is a smart move. That is, if you also check and correct your status on synergists of calcium for bone growth that may also be deficient: magnesium, zinc, manganese, copper, and boron (see Chapter 15). Unless you tackle supplementation with at least this amount of precision, you are wasting your time.

Some minerals, such as phosphorus, have pronounced ergogenic effects that are covered in Chapters 23-25. But, make no mistake, these are drug effects and should be reserved for an edge in competition. Keep always in focus that the business of nutrition is to grow a better body.

Other minerals have also been reported as ergogenic, including calcium[13] and magnesium.[14] In these cases, however, it is likely the minerals are correcting a deficit, not acting like a drug. With magnesium, for example, you only have to make the intake a tiny bit low to whack performance severely. A recent animal study made rats only marginally deficient in magnesium, but it reduced their endurance performance by a huge 33%.[15]

But don't believe for a moment that magnesium supplements will necessarily benefit your endurance. First check your intake and status as detailed in Chapter 15. If you check out O.K., more magnesium will not help you. And, remember, there are wide individual differences. Coming up to the '88 Olympics, swimmer Matt Biondi showed persistent low magnesium. But to feed the whole US Swim Team Matt's magnesium supplement, would have put them into detrimental overload.

Minerals may also have apparent anabolic effects. As detailed in Chapter 29, chromium in the form of chromium picolinate increases muscle growth and reduces bodyfat. But, chromium is one of the most deficient minerals in the American diet.[11] And athletes need a lot more chromium than couch potatoes, because it is used rapidly during exercise.[16] So the chromium picolinate effect is probably not a drug effect, but simply correction of a latent chromium deficiency endemic in athletes.

And that should be your focus. Ignore the ludicrous claims now pounding the marketplace, such as vanadium boosts performance, boron boosts testosterone levels, and germanium boosts everything. When you look at the science of it, they are all codswallop and mendacity. Listen to the marketplace and you will go nowhere.

Instead, let science be your guide. Use this book to patiently document your individual nutrient needs and deficits, and then fill them one by one. If you have problems or questions, ring our hotline (619) 632-7722. Do it right and train right and I guarantee you a high performance body.

Chapter 20

Antioxidants Combat Injury

The mail spat fire and brimstone after a recent article of mine was quoted in various sports magazines, advocating high supplements of antioxidants for athletes, to combat the inevitable health *damage* caused by exercise. Yes, *damage*! Readers just did not want to know that exercising without nutritional protection is downright unhealthy.

Some letters claimed I was knocking athletic training and destroying motivation to exercise. Others claimed I didn't really prove the case that exercise damages the body, or that antioxidants prevent injury. The best letters suggested that what I was saying would help performance and deserved elaboration.

So, I've been waiting to get this book out, in order to explain what happens in more detail. Here I will take you on a no-holds-barred tour of your muscles and show:

1. how exercise generates free radicals and causes muscle damage.
2. how antioxidants prevent damage and shorten recovery time.
3. how to design your own personal antioxidant program.

If you are not convinced by the end of this chapter that you need such a program, write to me and I'll eat my sweatshirt.

How Exercise Injures Muscle

Muscle power is generated by conversion of the chemical energy of a compound in your muscle cells called **adenosine triphosphate (ATP)**, to the mechanical force of muscle contraction. But your store of ATP is very limited. During exercise it must be regenerated continuously. The principle way your body does this, is by conversion of muscle stores of fat and sugar (glycogen).

We need to dip into a bit of biochemistry to understand how this happens, but stick with me. Once you get a handle on it you will know why some nutrient supplements work, and why a lot of others are just hype and dreams.

The conversions of fat and sugar to energy occur by oxidation. Pairs of hydrogen atoms (H_2) fire off from the fat and sugar like guided missiles, and hit the oxygen from your blood (O) to form water (H_2O). For 95% of your oxygen consumption, the conversion is pretty clean, and does not produce many free radicals.[1]

The scientific gobbledegook for this process is **the tetravalent reduction of oxygen with cytochrome C oxidase**. That is *the* energy production process explained in all college biochemistry texts. But many of the texts leave out the second chemical pathway by which muscles use oxygen, which explains why a lot of sports physicians and nutritionists know nothing about it.

Though it involves only 5% of your oxygen use, this recently discovered **univalent reduction pathway** is very dirty. That is, every time you exercise, it produces millions of **superoxide free radicals, hydroperoxides** and **hydroxyl free radicals**. These act like shrapnal, damaging every muscle cell they contact. The damage they cause is a major source of the continued muscle soreness and weakness you feel for days after heavy exercise.

There are now more than 100 studies supporting this discovery. I can review only a fraction of them here. If you need a complete A to Z of the research to convince you that exercise damages and ages the body in this way, then read, **Oxy-radicals**

in Molecular Biology and Pathology.[2] That text will oscillate the most skeptical sphincter.

Whenever you push your training, the scenario gets worse. Athletes in top gear use 12 to 20 times the oxygen of sedentary folk.[3] That's a ton of free radical potential.

We don't know yet how much their extra use of oxygen increases free radicals in athletes, but new work on animals gives us a pretty good idea. In 1989, in some of the first direct measurements, Dr Alexandre Quintanilha and colleagues ran rats on a treadmill for progressively longer periods. In a few weeks the rats could run for two hours nonstop every day. They were run at only 0.9 miles per hour, which is a jog for a rat. Once trained they did not appear too distressed by the exercise. But measurements showed a *three-fold* increase in muscle free radicals during exercise. And autopsies showed extensive muscle damage.[4]

The sheer volume of oxygen you use is not the only reason that exercise overwhelms your muscles with free radicals. The vital chemical **cytochrome C** also gets used up. Cytochrome C oxidase is the last catalyst in the chain that regenerates ATP, so your muscles can continue working. With any intensity of exercise beyond wimp level, cytochrome C activity can drop by 50% or more.[5]

This well established reaction is why some manufacturers put cytochrome C in sports supplements. But the notion that giving this chemical by mouth can increase cytochrome C oxidase activity in muscles, is pure hokum. Not a shred of scientific evidence. When I asked one manufacturer why he was doing it, he replied, "You have to keep an open mind." True, but not so open that your brains fall out.

When cytochrome C activity falls, another nutrient you've heard about, coenzyme Q (CoQ), comes to the rescue. But in completing the regeneration of ATP, CoQ itself may produce some superoxide radicals.[6] As we see throughout this book, whenever you push performance, the human body always seems to be shooting itself in the foot.

Despite the oxidation of CoQ itself, you need high muscle levels if you want to excel. Elite athletes show much higher levels than sedentary folk.[7] And long, intense training programs raise muscle CoQ.[8]

But you don't have to slog it out for years to get there. There is a simple nutritional shortcut. Dr Karl Folkers and colleagues at the University of Texas have shown that oral supplements of CoQ can easily increase muscle levels.[9]

More important, CoQ supplements also improve performance. In collaborative studies with Dr Folkers at the Free University of Brussels, Dr J. Van Fraechem gave a group of healthy, young men 60 mg of CoQ per day for 8 weeks. They did not change their usual level of daily exercise which was fairly minimal. Without any change in exercise, their maximum exercise capacity increased a whopping 28%.[9]

Sure, they were sedentary types with lots of room for improvement. I'm not suggesting athletes could gain 28%. But if you are out there busting a gut, it makes sense to supplement with coenzyme Q. The form to use in supplements is coenzyme Q10 which is the chemical transformation used by human bodies.

You even get a bonus because CoQ10 is also a powerful antioxidant, and neutralizes some free radicals as well as increasing the efficiency of the energy cycle. Researchers have found that the overall effect of elevated CoQ in muscle is a net *reduction* in free radicals.[9] I tend to favor this view but cannot support it in athletes yet, because the only reasonable study to date has been with rats.[10]

Nevertheless, CoQ levels decline rapidly with age after 25.[9] So for its multiple essential functions in athletic performance, the Colgan Institute uses daily supplements of 30-60 mg CoQ10 in all sports formulas. One good commercial brand that shows the same chemical profile as the research grade we use at the Colgan Institute, is made by TwinLab.

Free Radical Damage Persists

The free radical attack caused by exercise doesn't stop when you stop. The hydroxy radicals especially (made from busting up your body water), continue to injure you long afterwards. It works mainly like this. Hydroxy radicals react with fats inside your muscle cell membranes to make them go rancid, a process called **lipid peroxidation.**[11] This creates havoc for cell processes, leading to much pain and inflammation, and wailing and gnashing of teeth.

The rancid fats themselves then become free radicals called **peroxylradicals**, which in turn do more damage and spawn further radicals. With every bout of intense exercise, you literally get an inflammatory chain reaction that lasts up to 20 hours.

The combined muscle damage caused by the free radicals produced during exercise, plus the hydroxy radical chain reaction after exercise, is not the end of the story. The damage itself initiates another free radical sequence that goes on for days.

It happens this way. As with any bodily injury, as soon as free radical damage occurs, your immune system becomes active to combat it. The ground troops of the immune system, called **neutrophils**, move in to mop up the dead and dying muscle cells. But in doing so, they release masses of free radicals themselves, which cause further damage.[12] No one has yet explained why the body attacks itself in this way. Some researchers put it down to an evolutionary weakness in the human system.

The net result of this free radical circus, is that any bout of intense exercise, leaves you stiff and sore and unable to exercise properly for up to five days.[13] If you do force yourself, and continue to push it, then your risk of more serious injury goes through the roof.[14]

Most experienced exercisers have learned this sad fact many times over. Consequently, they are always working out below their potential, so as not to get too sore. If you work out below potential - you guessed it - the end result is way below potential.

After the first few years of training to get the kinks out, many athletes then spend years negotiating their way around free radical damage. If they work too hard, then training is set back by repeated injury. And the cells they kill cause losses of muscle and strength. But if they don't work hard enough, the muscles are not sufficiently stimulated, and they make no gains, or even lose because of atrophy. Catch 22! Antioxidants may just be able to help you do something about it.

Antioxidants Save Your Muscle

Free radicals are a sort of Saddam Hussein army, indiscriminately killing cells, poisoning enzymes, manufacturing toxic chemicals, destroying cellular membranes with lipid peroxidation, and even causing the body to shoot itself in the foot.[15] So they need a variety of defense mechanisms to outwit them.

The body fights back against oxidation with three main endogenous antioxidants, **catalase** which neutralizes hydrogen peroxides, **superoxide dismutase (SOD)** which destroys superoxide radicals, and **glutathione peroxidase** which detoxifies peroxides.

But trying to boost your muscle supplies of these beneficial chemicals is tricky business. You can't increase the first two with oral supplements, because they are slaughtered by your digestive system. Not a molecule survives. Studies show that oral SOD supplements do not raise blood or tissue levels.[16]

So don't waste your money on SOD supplements. Even if they could survive digestion, the molecule is too big to fit through cell membranes. So supplementary SOD could work only outside the cells. Not an effective position.

The weak effect of extracellular SOD is clearly shown by the experimental use of injectable SOD (a prescription drug called **orgotein**) to treat arthritis. Results are disappointing. If it doesn't work when you put it straight into the bloodstream, it's a betting certainty that SOD in pill form is just another profitable flapdoodle.

Boost Your Glutathione

One major endogenous antioxidant you can manipulate nutritionally is glutathione. Animal studies show that even one bout of intense exercise to exhaustion can reduce muscle glutathione by 40%, and liver glutathione (from which muscles increase their supply) by 80%.[17] After exercise, muscle and liver glutathione continues to decline, indicating continued use of this antioxidant to combat free radical attack. Autopsies on the animals show that their glutathione stores are eventually over-whelmed by free radicals, which then cause extensive muscle damage.

We don't usually work out *that* hard, but it gives you the general idea. Glutathione is a great defender of muscle. You cannot prevent muscle damage and maintain training intensity without an adequate store.

Glutathione is produced in the body from cysteine and other amino acids. And there is reasonable evidence that increased intake of cysteine can increase body glutathione production.[18] In addition, you can take preformed glutathione. Some of it gets through digestion intact. And recent animal studies show that preformed glutathione, delivered to the site of free radical attack, protects cells from injury.[19]

Taking supplemental n-acetyl cysteine (the preferred form) for the body to make more glutathione, and taking supplemental glutathione itself, are highly experimental strategies. No one knows the amounts required to protect human muscle. Clearly it depends on the individual's biochemical individuality, size, age, the type, intensity, and frequency of exercise, and the levels of other antioxidants in the body.

At the Colgan Institute, we have analyzed all the research to date to come up with this daily glutathione cocktail for a 175 lb young adult aged 20-30 years:

350 mg n-acetyl cysteine

200 mg L-glutathione

But, I stress, it is experimental. All we know so far is that our cocktail does boost bodily glutathione. Before trying any such strategy you should read the scientific references given and make your own decision.

One other point. Body glutathione declines rapidly with age.[20] In fact the decline in glutathione levels is so reliable, it is used as an index of human aging.[21] So, if you want a long athletic career, better eat your Wheaties (well sprinkled with glutathione).

Boost Nutrient Antioxidants

In addition to glutathione, you can increase your body's protective store with the nutrient antioxidants, vitamin C, vitamin E, selenium and coenzyme Q10. I have already noted CoQ10 above, so will focus here on the other three. Vitamin E is especially important.

The main areas of muscle cells protected from free radicals by glutathione are the surfaces of the cell membranes. But inside the fatty membranes, where the lipid peroxidation chain reaction occurs, fat soluble vitamin E is champ. Vitamin E breaks the chain reaction, by absorbing the free radicals to form what are called **tocopherol radicals** and **tocopheroxyl radicals.**

Breaking the chain reaction quickly uses up your store of vitamin E, leaving it as so much clinker clogging the membranes. Vitamin C then enters the picture. Dr Al Tappel, at the University of California, Davis, showed over 20 years ago that vitamin C neutralizes the tocopheroxyl radicals and regenerates the vitamin

E again, allowing it to return to the fight.[22] This cycle uses up vitamin C rapidly so you better have an ample supply, if you are getting into any serious exercise.

The mineral selenium also assists. In fact, selenium helps both glutathione and vitamin E. It forms what is called the **active site** where glutathione destroys lipid peroxide radicals. It also acts synergistically with vitamin E to improve its free radical killing efficiency.[23] To do an effective antioxidant job you need adequate supplies of all these nutrients, glutathione, vitamin E, vitamin C, and selenium.

Food Doesn't Cut It

The big problem is that American food does not provide enough of any of them. At first blush the food looks O.K. Five studies cited in the latest RDA handbook, show that the average male intake of vitamin E is 9 mg per day.[24] That seems as near as you need to the RDA level of 10 mg per day. Not so, for two reasons. First, the 9 mg is an average which means that half the population gets less then 9 mg. Second, and more important, recent research shows that *five times* the RDA of vitamin E may be required to prevent free radical damage.[25]

And that is in sedentary folk. From the studies above, athletes in intense exercise should expect to generate at least three times the sedentary levels of free radicals.[17] So their vitamin E requirement could run *10 to 15 times* the RDA.

Seems a lot, until you realize that the RDA is based on an obsolete assessment of vitamin E as a functional component of certain physiological reactions. In such assessments, excess intakes cannot confer any benefits. That's why the RDAs have stayed where they are in the face of massive evidence against them.

From all I have written above, it should be clear the major requirement for vitamin E is for its antioxidant action. The requirement for vitamin E antioxidant action for any individual, depends on the levels of fatty acids in his tissue that can suffer oxidation, and the levels of free radicals that he generates. If you carry a bit of lard, and work out like a madman, you better eat plenty of vitamin E.

No one knows how much is right. But at the Colgan Institute, we have used 1,200- 2,000 IU daily as d-alpha tocopheryl succinate, with athletes for the last 16 years. Before you jump on that figure, remember it is still an experimental strategy. So read the scientific references given and make your own decision.

What about toxicity? In my whole career in sports nutrition, covering supplementation of thousands of athletes, I have never seen vitamin E cause any side-effect. One weightlifter took 20,000 IU per day in mistake for 2,000 IU. We didn't discover it for months, until he complained how much his vitamin E was costing. But we couldn't find any sign of toxicity.

A recent review in the prestigious **American Journal of Clinical Nutrition** expresses it more scientifically. Vitamin E experts, Drs Lawrence Machlin and Adrienne Bendich, examined 49 separate studies on vitamin E, and concluded that, "oral vitamin E supplementation resulted in few side effects even at doses as high as 3,200 IU per day".[26]

Selenium, Vitamin C, Deficient

American food also lacks sufficient selenium and vitamin C. In the journal **Science** in 1981, I published a short report showing that selenium is deficient in the soils of ten states plus the District of Columbia.[27] Produce and livestock cannot manufacture selenium. If this mineral is not in the soil, it is not in your food and not in your body.

How could such a deficiency be allowed to happen, with all these nutrition professionals pontificating about how good the American diet is? Easy! As the RDA handbook admits, selenium was not considered essential in human nutrition until 1979.[24] It didn't make the RDA list until 1989. Health authorities didn't know it was deficient in the food supply, because they didn't even know you needed it.

At the Colgan Institute, we have been using selenium supplements with athletes since 1974. No one knows how much is right. Our best assessment is 200-400 mcg per day, which is twice the recommended amount, and four times the current RDA.[24] Don't use more than that. Beyond 800 mcg/day, selenium can become very toxic.[28] We use the selenomethionine form. It is better absorbed than the more common sodium selenite.

Vitamin C is also deficient in the American diet, for its function as a dietary antioxidant. It is true that the average amount available per person in our food is 114 mg,[29] which is nearly twice the RDA.[24] But, the requirement for vitamin C is still assessed by an obsolete method that calculates the amount required for certain enzymatic actions. This has little to do with the amount of vitamin C required for its equally important antioxidant action, which, in any individual, is dependent on the level of free radicals he generates. Thankfully, the Food and Drug Administration has finally recognized that the RDAs have little value, and is ditching these figures from food labels and dietary descriptions.

How much vitamin C? For its multiple antioxidant functions, not just to combat exercise free radicals, the Colgan Institute uses between 2 and 12 grams daily with athletes. The amount varies widely with the athlete. Ways to estimate your need are given below.

We use a mixture of calcium ascorbate, magnesium ascorbate, and the fat soluble ascorbyl palmitate, as well as ascorbic acid. We pay special attention to limiting acidic reactions of ascorbic acid in sensitive individuals, and in endurance athletes. Overdosing on ascorbic acid will produce urgent diarrhea in anyone. So don't take 10 grams of ascorbic acid before a triathlon to combat free radicals. Like one good lad and true of my acquaintance, you will not even make it from the bathroom to the start line.

Your Personal Antioxidant Program

Nutrient requirements are highly individual. And the long-term safety of using high doses of antioxidants is not yet proven for humans. So, although we have used them safely and successfully with athletes for 18 years, you should read the scientific references given, before making any decision to adopt an antioxidant program.

If you do decide, some variables that can help you design a personal program are: duration of training, intensity of training, bodyfat, age, and size. The longer you train per session, the more antioxidants you need. The more intense the training, the more antioxidants you need. The higher your bodyfat, above 10% for males and 15% for females, the more you need. The older you are above 30, the more you need. And the bigger you are, the more you need.

These are the basic variables we use at the Colgan Institute. We score them on the table below. We score one point for each **Low** category, two points for each **Middle** category, and three points for each **High** category. We then apply the total score to the second table. A score of 5-8 gives antioxidant requirements at the low end of the ranges. A score of 9-12 gives requirements in the middle of the ranges. A score of 12-15 gives requirements nearer the top of the ranges.

We do use other variables to decide requirements for individual athletes, including blood tests, type and phase of training, medical history, and level of environmental pollution in the athlete's home area. But these require complex testing. The table given is simple to use and provides a good basic guide.

We start everyone at the low end. If an athlete has not used antioxidants before, or has stopped using them more than three months previously, then his system has to adjust numerous enzyme counts in order to deal with them. This adjustment takes around three months. Even after adjustment is complete, antioxidants should always be taken in divided doses, and always

Table 18. Basic variables used to estimate antioxidant needs of athletes and ranges of antioxidants used with athletes by the Colgan Institute.*

Estimating Antioxidant Need			
Variable	**Low**	**Medium**	**High**
Training per day	below 1 hour	1 to 2 hours	above 2 hours
Intensity of training	50% of max	70% of max	80%+ of max
Bodyfat			
Male	below 10%	10-15%	above 15%
Female	below 15%	15-20%	above 20%
Age	20-30	30-45	above 45
Size	80-150 lbs	150-200	above 200

Antioxidants Used in Studies With Athletes	
Antioxidant Nutrient	**Daily Amount**
n-acetyl cysteine**	50 - 350 mg
L-glutathione	100 - 200 mg
Vitamin E	1,200 - 2,000 IU
Coenzyme Q10	30 - 60 mg
Vitamin C	2.0 - 12.0 gms
Selenium†	200 - 400 mcg

** N-acetyl cysteine should be used only with at least three times its amount of Vitamin C, so as to avoid the possibility of it precipitating in the kidneys as cystine, and possibly causing kidney stones in sensitive individuals.

† Selenium can become very toxic above 800 mcg per day.

Consult text for preferred forms of the nutrients in this table.

*Source: Colgan Institute, San Diego, CA.

with food. To jump in with high levels of antioxidants from the first day, is a great way to an upset gut and expensive and uncomfortable urine.

In this chapter I reviewed a little of the evidence showing that supplementary antioxidants can protect muscle from free radical damage during exercise, and thereby reduce injury and shorten recovery time. Although the evidence is strong, most of the studies are very recent. So use of these antioxidants is still a highly experimental strategy. At the Colgan Institute we have been studying it for 18 years, and still have only a few of the answers. Nevertheless, our record of success with athletes suggests we may just be on the money.

Chapter 21

Good Red Blood

In 1984 I got a call from sports medicine folk at the University of Oregon. Alberto Salazar, then world marathon champion and one of the best marathon runners of all time, had serious iron deficiency. The problem had not shown up in any blood tests used by Salazar's medicos, because they were relying on the wrong tests - serum iron and hemoglobin.

These tests are still wrongly used today by thousands of physicians to diagnose iron deficiency. For Salazar both were within the normal range. His problem was actually spotted by the wife of Canadian sports physician Doug Clement while watching the athlete's lack-lustre performance on television. Clement, an expert in iron-deficiency, phoned Salazar's coach, the great Bill Dellinger, and suggested he test **serum ferritin**, an accurate measure of iron store. The test showed near zero iron.

They gave Salazar iron supplements and he improved sufficiently to make the Olympic team. But he was still not right, and the sports medicine folk at the University of Oregon called me for advice. I outlined a supplement program of hematopoietic (blood-forming) nutrients, and warned them that unless Salazar was put on them immediately, he would have a permanently reduced capacity to make red blood that would damn his performance forever. The conservative medics overruled my advice and, despite years of trying, Salazar has never come back. Sub-optimal nutrition cut short the run of the best American marathoner in history.

Some folk object to this "experiment of one" whenever I write about it. But this famous case only illustrates what I have seen many, many times ruin the careers of top athletes. Unless you take care of your red blood nutritional needs, detrimental changes occur, probably in the bone stem cells that grow into blood cells, and probably in muscle cells themselves, that *permanently reduce your performance.*

I have tracked over 100 cases of this syndrome since world cross-country champion Doris Brown Heritage broke her foot in the 1972 Olympics. After trying unsuccessfully for years to make a comeback on inadequate nutrition, she said,

> I don't know if it was because of age or what, but my iron levels never went up where they were, my endurance never came back, I never had the strength again.

Don't let it happen to you. If you want optimum performance, study this chapter well, read all the references, and close your ears to the obsolete and incorrect advice of anyone who ever tells you that you will pick up again on a hefty dose of iron.

Making Red Blood

The red cells that carry your oxygen, called **erythrocytes**, make up 35-50% of your blood. The rest is mostly plasma fluid with a sprinkling of the white cells of the immune system. The proportion of your blood made of red cells is measured by the **hematocrit**. A hematocrit of 50 provides 25% more red blood cells than a hematocrit of 40, with a similar increase in the maximal oxygen delivery to muscles. So athletes of every stripe are always trying to hike their hematocrit.

Each red cell is 25% - 35% **hemoglobin**, the red pigment made from iron and other nutrients, that carries almost 100% of your oxygen. The greater the amount of hemoglobin per cell, the greater the possible amount of oxygen delivered to muscles. So athletes are always trying to adjust their nutrition to hike their hemoglobin.

But many of them make a terrible job of it. Studies of male distance runners show they have hemoglobin levels below those of sedentary controls.[1,2] And the iron status of both male and female endurance athletes is below that of the general population.[3] I have reviewed more than 50 studies that show low iron stores, low hemoglobin, low hematocrit, and reduced performance in athletes from recreational to Olympic status.[4]

In this land of plenty, how can that happen? I have to put the answer hot and heavy. Many American athletes have poor hematological status, because the standard advice they receive on nutrition to support the red blood system is 50 years out of date, and actually *detrimental* to their bodies.

Studies attempting to raise deficient iron stores and low hemoglobin and hematocrit levels in athletes, typically use 200 mg or more of iron per day.[4-6] That level of iron overload does force hematology up a bit. But it's not the healthy way to do it. Side-effects of gastrointestinal pain, constipation, nausea, and heartburn reduce compliance to a minimum.[7] Most iron pills over 100 mg per day prescribed for athletes, are dumped quietly down the plug. It's fortunate that the side-effects of excess iron cause athletes to dump the pills, because they are a serious and continuing cause of infection.

Excess Iron Causes Infections

No animal organism can live without iron. The sole exception to this rule is lactic acid bacteria. This odd deviation of Nature has a well defined purpose. In discussing that purpose, we can lay to rest the idiotic medical practice in America of feeding large amounts of iron to athletes, pregnant women, and even babies.

Let's start with babies because they give you the right perspective about iron. When a human or animal baby is born, its gastrointestinal tract is sterile, that is, contains zero bacteria. It also contains zero iron. So, the only bacteria that can grow in it are lactic acid bacteria, and they start infiltrating the gut within minutes of birth. That's a nice trick of evolution, because lactic acid bacteria are essential to digest the mother's milk that is the first food of animals and almost all humans.

Nature allows only lactic acid bacteria to grow in the newborn gut in order to protect it from harmful bacteria that could otherwise multiply and kill the baby. *All other bacteria grow greedily in the presence of iron.*

But what happens when the mother feeds the baby from the breast. Doesn't that put iron into the gut. You might think so if you look at all the stupid iron-fortified baby formulas that are supposed to substitute for human breast milk. Let's get it straight. *Mother's milk, far and away the best food for babies, contains virtually no iron.*[8]

Most physicians still seem unaware that infants do not need iron. A human baby is born with a reserve supply of iron in its tissues of approximately 75 mg per kilogram bodyweight. That's about twice the iron level found in healthy athletes. An infant can grow healthy and normal for at least a year without requiring any external iron. Nature designed it that way to allow the immune system to develop before the onslaught of bacteria that occurs once the baby is weaned onto iron-containing solid foods.

Why then do physicians still recommend iron for infants? Plain pig ignorance! Why then do baby food manufacturers fortify baby formulas with iron? Plain market greed! Old medical texts, ignorant of the intricacies of nutrition, taught physicians only that iron is an important nutrient needed for making red blood cells and that pregnant women often become near anemic as blood is taken by the growing fetus. So they still feed pregnant women huge amounts of iron, 300 mg a day is commonplace, to try to boost their hemoglobin levels. Doesn't work, never has. And it doesn't put iron into the mother's milk either.

The illogical extension to this nonsense is then to feed the newborn with iron-supplemented formula, presumably to continue the iron the mother was getting. What it amounts to is that some academic physicians decided they were smarter than Nature and could design a better formula than mother's milk, putting in iron (and other nutrients) in amounts that devastate the infant's gut. Uninformed sports physicians then carry on the nonsense and advise excess iron for athletes to put them in the same predicament.

Professor Eugene Weinberg of the University of Indiana has warned repeatedly how iron fortification of food in America leads to increased disease.[9] And there is a whole new medical text, **Iron and Infection**, that cites hundreds of recent studies showing that excess iron in the body enables infections to flourish.[10] I have no space to cover them so I will give just one example from my home state of California. In 1979 there was an outbreak of cases of infant botulism. Researchers compared breast-fed babies (therefore receiving virtually no iron) with babies fed iron-supplemented infant formula. The breast-fed babies all had milder cases of the disease and *none* died. The formula-fed babies all had severe cases of the disease and *10 died.*[8]

What have babies to do with athletes? Athletes don't usually die of iron-promoted infections, nor even get really sick. So it is more difficult to point the finger at iron. Because they are more fragile, babies provide a good model of just how much damage iron can do.

Yet because of ignorance of the advances in nutrition science, iron is still the most widely prescribed nutrient supplement. There are enough iron pills on the shelves of bathroom cabinets across this country to rebuild the Titanic. A lot of disease in America can be attributed directly to the overuse of iron.

How Much Iron?

But you can't skip iron either. It's essential for making hemoglobin. A mere 10% drop in hemoglobin levels can decimate endurance performance by 20-25%.[11,12] A boost in normal hemoglobin levels by the practice of blood doping can increase performance by 20-25%.[12,13] So the right amount of iron is an essential component of every athlete's diet.

But how much is right? The RDAs provide no reliable guide. To be generous to the Committee that set the RDA for iron, they must have stopped following advances in science somewhere about 1950. They even have an RDA for infants from birth of 6 mg per day. No wonder that America is 16th in the world for infant mortality rate. Nor can you rely on the common practice of coaches and sports physicians, who often give athletes iron pills of 300 mg a day. Great way to recurrent infections and a griping gut.

The best way to get the iron requirement of an athlete is to assess how much he uses. For starters, *sedentary* males use about 1.0 mg of iron per day for a wide variety of bodily functions. Because of monthly menstruation losses, *sedentary* females use an average of 1.5 mg per day.[14] Athletes use those sedentary amounts too - plus a lot more. We sweat a bunch and iron pours out in sweat. We break down blood cells in every workout. And working out to the max we also frequently bleed into the gut.

If you heat subjects in a dry sauna to about the same temperature that an endurance athletes experiences in training on a medium sunny day, they sweat 1.3 liters per hour. In that sweat they also lose about 0.5 mg of iron per hour.[15] If you train real heavy 3 hours a day, iron loss can be 1.5 mg.

Then there is iron loss by **hemolysis** (destruction of red blood cells). Heavy exercise breaks blood cells, the blood leaks and is then excreted from the body. Many studies have found this blood loss in runners.[16,17,18] It was termed **footstrike hemolysis**, because they thought it occurred because of the foot impact on the ground breaking blood cells as they flowed through the underside of the foot.

At the 1984 Olympic Scientific Congress, however, I reviewed evidence that hemolysis occurs in cross-country skiing where there is little impact [19] and in bodybuilding. The Colgan Institute proposed the concept of **compression hemolysis,** that is, the crushing of blood cells by intense muscle contraction.[20] Since then, compression hemolysis has been confirmed in numerous sports where there is no impact, including swimming and rowing.[21,22] It is a potent source of iron loss in athletes.

Other sources of hemolysis and therefore iron loss in athletes in heavy training include, gastrointestinal bleeding,[23] acidosis,[24] and peroxidation of cell membranes by free radicals.[25] The total losses from these sources adds to compression hemolysis to make an iron loss of at least 1.0 mg per day.

If we add all the causes of iron loss for an athlete training heavy, 3 hours a day, we get

	Males	Females
Bodily functions	1.0 mg	1.5 mg
Sweat	1.5 mg	1.5 mg
Hemolysis and Bleeding	1.0 mg	1.0 mg
Totals	3.5 mg	4.1 mg

That doesn't sound like much until you understand that only 10% of the iron in a good diet is bioavailable.[14] So to get sufficient iron, a male athlete in heavy training needs to eat a minimum of 36 mg of iron, and a female athlete 41 mg - every day.

Average intakes of iron by athletes are much below these figures. Analysis of athletes' diets show that they contain about 6 mg of iron per 1,000 calories.[26,27] So, to make the cut for iron, males would have to eat 6,000 calories a day, and females almost 7,000 calories, way too much food for most of us.

The only good answer is supplementation. At 6 mg per 1,000 calories, a 3,000 calorie diet provides 18 mg of iron. So a 20-25 mg iron supplement each day will keep you in iron balance. Don't take a lot more than that or you increase your risk of infection. And excess iron is difficult for the body to excrete.

Other Hematopoietic Nutrients

There is only one problem. Iron by itself hardly works at all to raise your hemoglobin or hematocrit. As we saw in Chapter 1, it needs to link in **synergy** with a whole lot of other hematopoietic (blood-building) nutrients.[28]

As we will see, these nutrients - **folate, zinc, cobalamin, pyridoxine, ascorbate, and tocopherol** - are also likely to be poorly supplied by the athlete's diet. Yet, they are as important as iron stores in maintaining hematological status. We will take them one at a time.

Folate. There are no controlled studies of folate intakes of athletes, but in the general population they can be well below the RDA.[29] Inadequate dietary folate reduces erythrocyte (red blood cell) formation. Moreover, demand for folate increases in accord with the increased **erythropoiesis** (making of red blood cells) caused by the loss of blood cells through hemolysis and bleeding during exercise.[30]

Because the average intake of folate in sedentary people has now declined to about 200 mcg, in the latest handbook the RDA was revised downwards to 200 mcg, half the value used for 20 years previously.[14] This new RDA, which represents the amount of folate now provided by American food, is insufficient for athletes. Even in *sedentary* males, an intake of 211 mcg of folate per day for six months causes a big decline in folate status.[31]

Folate intake also affects performance for another reason. Folate status affects iron status and vice versa.[32] In the folate study above, for example, there was also a large decline in iron status, with subjects losing about half their iron stores over six months. This loss occurred despite a daily iron intake of 16.8 mg of iron, that is, 168% of the RDA for adult males.[31] So if you are supplementing with iron, you had better supplement with folate also.

Zinc. The average zinc *content* of a 2,850 calorie mixed American diet is 13.2 mg (88% of the RDA).[33] A more precise study of free-living adults shows that the actual zinc *intake* can be a lot lower than that. Subjects on "good mixed diets" were getting only 8.6 mg of zinc per day.[34] Such a level is inadequate for anyone. A long-term investigation of sedentary males and females on 10 mg of zinc daily in a mixed diet, showed them to be in negative zinc balance throughout the length of the study.[35]

These amounts of zinc are almost certainly insufficient for athletes. Additional zinc is required for increased production of erythrocytes, for increased free fatty acid metabolism during exercise, for replacement of dermal losses of zinc during sweating, and for the interactions of zinc in iron metabolism.[28,36]

But most athletes take vitamin/mineral supplements. They should get enough zinc - right? Wrong! A recent study of 71 competitive triathletes, for example, showed that 60% of them had zinc intakes below the RDA, despite their supplements.[37] And there is now considerable evidence, that athletes from runners to wrestlers, also have poor zinc status as a direct result of the increased demands for zinc imposed by intense training.[38] No use at all taking extra iron if you don't have enough zinc to make it work.

Cobalamin. Body stores of cobalamin (vitamin B_{12}) required for optimal health are uncertain, although intakes of 3 mcg/day will prevent vitamin B_{12} deficiency in most sedentary people.[14] There are no data on the cobalamin requirement of athletes, but it is likely to be higher because their increased demand for erythropoiesis requires vitamin B_{12} to make the blood cells. Also, adequate cobalamin is essential to normal folate metabolism.[39]

Pyridoxine. The US Nationwide Food Consumption Survey found that pyridoxine (vitamin B_6) intakes were deficient in the diets of one-third of households.[40] Pyridoxine deficiency is also common in normal, sedentary subjects serving as controls in nutrition research.[41,42] The average pyridoxine intake in the US is 1.87 mg/day for males, and 1.16 mg/day for females.[14] These levels are below the RDA of 2.0 mg/day for males and 1.6 mg/day for females.

Athletes are likely to be at greater risk of pyridoxine (vitamin B6) deficiency, for three reasons. First, pyridoxine plays a pivotal role in the formation of **heme**, one bit of the hemoglobin molecule.[43] Demand for heme is increased with increased erythropoiesis. Second, animal studies show that pyrodoxine deficiency impairs cobalamin absorption and reduces tissue levels of that nutrient.[40] Third, exercise increases the excretion of pyridoxine, an effect related to its function in making new glycogen.[43,44]

Ascorbate. Ascorbate (vitamin C) deficiency by itself produces anemia, no matter how much iron you have.[45,46] Ascorbate also functions to protect folate from oxidation by free radicals. So, insufficient ascorbate results in reduction of your folate store.[47]

Ascorbate needs of athletes are unknown, but are certainly higher than the RDA, because requirements rise sharply when the body is subjected to heat stress (such as the body temperature elevation caused by training).[48] Dr M. Visagie and colleagues found that mineworkers working in high temperatures required 200-250 mg/day of ascorbate to maintain serum vitamin C in the normal range.[49] Latest figures for the mean daily dietary ascorbate intake of adults in the US are: males - 109 mg, females - 77 mg.[14] These levels are insufficient to maintain the ascorbate status of athletes in heavy training. Consequently, red blood status of athletes on an average diet will be suboptimal.

Tocopherol. There is new evidence that athletes need more tocopherol (vitamin E) than sedentary folk, not only because of its antioxidant action to prevent oxidation, but also because a lot of vitamin E is used *during* exercise. In one recent study of athletes running on the treadmill at a very moderate pace, vitamin E in the quadriceps decreased by 30%.[50]

Tocopherol status of athletes is also especially important in combating hemolysis. Tocopherol deficiency increases hemolysis because it leaves erythrocytes more fragile and easily damaged.[51] Tocopherol deficiency can also result in anemia even if your iron supply is ample.[52] And adequate tocopherol is also essential for normal metabolism of vitamin B$_{12}$ and zinc.[53] Taken together, these effects of tocopherol indicate that any inadequacy will damage your red blood status.

The tocopherol intake of athletes is unknown, but it varies widely in foods, and the RDA handbook admits that large losses occur in food-processing. Because of these losses, the average daily intake in America is below the RDA for both males and females.[14]

Such intakes are highly inadequate for athletes, not only because of the increased demand for vitamin E to maintain red blood status, but also because of the increased demand to combat free radical damage to muscle during and after exercise.[54]

As you can see, the above studies present good evidence that if you supplement with iron, then, to promote synergy, you should also supplement with folate, zinc, cobalamin, pyridoxine, ascorbate, and tocopherol. But you don't just scarf down nutrients on the off-chance. Your biochemical individuality and your training and lifestyle dynamics dictate the levels of nutrients you need. Before you use any supplements, make every effort to measure your personal nutrient status. Whenever that seems like a drag, re-read Chapter 1, and the principle of **precision** and remember, God dwells in the details.

Measuring Hematological Status

The first problem you will have with measurement of iron status is uninformed sports medicine folk who think they can tell you from a standard SMAC 26 blood screen. They can't. Usually they rely on hemoglobin, and serum iron levels. A hemoglobin level less than 13 g/dl in males, and less than 12 g/dl in females is an identifying sign of iron-deficiency anemia. And so is a serum iron level below 40 mcg/dl. But neither test gives you much information about your iron status. And these tests were developed to measure disease in sedentary sick people. So you can't use them in the same way to measure nutrient needs in healthy athletes.

Iron stores can be virtually exhausted before hemoglobin or serum iron register any abnormal level.[55] Dr Doug Clement and his group in Canada found that 80% of a group of female athletes were iron deficient, but not one of them showed hemoglobin levels below 12 g/dl.[56] The hemoglobin test is useful to show how much of your iron is being converted into hemoglobin. In conjunction with hematocrit and erythrocyte count, it is also useful to show how much oxygen-carrying capacity you have. But it is useless for determining your iron store.

Because of these problems, in 1983 the Colgan Institute developed the model for iron status of athletes shown in Table 19. After four years of trials, I presented it at the World Athletics Cup Medical Congress in Canberra in 1987.[57] Since then it has become widely used.

Reliable measures for the other hematopoietic nutrients are given in Chapters 14 and 15 on the vitamins and minerals. Use these in conjunction with Table 19 to determine your individual needs. Some of the tests given are old reliables, listed because they are available in many blood labs. New tests are now available using the superior technology of **automated high-performance liquid chromatography**. But only large blood-testing organizations can afford the equipment to do them.

Whatever blood lab you use, choose it carefully and stick to it. Coaches and physicians turn up in my lab all the time waving blood tests from half a dozen different labs, unable to make sense of them. Different labs use different tests, different norms, different procedures, different reagents, different personnel. It would be a miracle if they got comparable results.

If you are going to do blood, do it right. The Colgan Institute advises all coaches and athletes to use a big automated blood lab, such as Metpath, with blood-draw facilities across the country. Only then can you compare this week's tests with those of six months ago to see how your nutrition program is improving your body.

Table 19. A model for iron status of athletes.*

Assay	Reference Range Males (M) Females (F)	Iron Depletion	Iron Deficient Erythropoiesis	Iron Deficiency Anemia
Serum ferritin (ng/dl)	M 30-160 F 25-100	< 30 ● < 25 ●	< 20 ● < 12 ●	< 20 < 12
Transferrin saturation (%)	30-45	< 30	< 16 ●	< 16
RBC proto-porphyrin (mcg/dl)	35-50	35-50	> 100 ●	> 200 ●
Serum Iron (mcg/dl)	M 60-200 F 60-200	60-200 60-200	< 60 ● < 60 ●	< 40 ● < 40 ●
TIBC (mcg/dl)	300-350	300-350	300-350	> 400 ●
Whole blood hemoglobin (g/dl)	M 13-18 F 12-16	> 13 > 12	> 13 > 12	< 13 ● < 12 ●
Erythrocytes		Normal	Normal	microcytic ● hypochromic ●
Hematocrit (%)	M 40-52 F 36-46	40-52 36-46	40-52 36-46	40-52 36-46
RBC (mil/mm^3)	M 3.9-6.8 F 3.6-5.8	3.9-6.8 3.6-5.8	3.9-6.8 3.6-5.8	3.9-6.8 3.6-5.8

● Identifying tests at each stage of depletion.

*Developed from models of Cook and Finch, and Colgan, et al. Reference 57.

Supplements Boost Red Blood

An increase in hemoglobin on a blood test is all fine and dandy, but the real question for athletes is - do hematopoietic nutrients make me go higher, faster, further? Some new evidence indicates that indeed they do.

The most recent study was done at the Colgan Institute in San Diego, California. Fifteen male and 12 female well-trained, endurance runners committed to an intense program of marathon training for 24 weeks. The study was done as a double-blind crossover. In this study design neither the researchers nor the subjects know who is getting the real nutrients and who is getting placebos, until after the study is over and the packet codes are broken. That's so no one can cheat. At 12 weeks, half-way through the study, the subjects were crossed-over, so that those getting packets of supplements stamped with one code are switched to packets stamped with the other code. That's so every subject got time on supplements and time on placebos. Then, if there was an initial difference between supplement and placebo groups, the crossover cancels it out.

The status of subjects on iron and other hematopoietic nutrients was measured by blood tests before the study, at 12 weeks, and immediately after the study. To ensure complete nutrition, both groups were given daily packets of supplements containing 100% of the RDA for all nutrients throughout the 24 weeks. In addition, the experimental group were given another daily packet containing 2.4 mg of folic acid, 100 mcg of cobalamin, 150 mg of pyridoxine, 500 mg of ascorbate, 48 mg of iron, and 60 mg of zinc. Tocopherol was not studied.

Results showed that blood levels of hematopoietic nutrients increased significantly throughout the high supplementation periods, and declined significantly throughout placebo periods, despite subjects receiving 100% of the RDA for all nutrients along with the placebo. More important, VO_2 max increased by 8-18% during high supplementation periods. And time to exhaustion on the ergometer bicycle increased by 7-19%.[4] That's a helluva an edge.

This study bears out our discussion that RDA levels of nutrients are insufficient to maintain red blood status. It also indicates that additional amounts of hematopoietic nutrients, even if they are not individually designed, and therefore not ideal, can improve hematological status, increase VO2max, and boost performance. If anyone tells you different, don't try to convince them by words, just show them how you can kick their butts.

Chapter 22

Strong Immunity

At least 52 elite American athletes missed selection for the Barcelona Olympics because of infections and illnesses. And during the Games, dozens more sick athletes performed poorly. Every one of those infections occurred because of weakened immunity.

At the Olympic Trials, Carl Lewis failed to win selection for the 100 meters because of an infection. Yet when we saw him at the Games winning the 4 x 100 relay, accelerating away from the best sprinters in the world with a smile on his face, we realized that a healthy Carl Lewis is still the fastest man in the world. I predict he will trounce the 100-meter gold medalist, British champion Linford Christie in the 1993 season.

Many more athletes at the Barcelona Games failed to medal because of injuries. "Part of the game," some coaches say. Not at all. Not part of any properly played game. As we will see, the seriousness of an injury, and the time it takes to heal are also intimately linked to immunity.

One of the first questions we ask athletes going on nutrition and training programs at the Colgan Institute is, "What are your training goals." The most frequent first answer is, "To stay healthy." They know that to improve your body to elite level, you have to have many months of consistent training, day in, day out, uninterrupted by illness or injury.

But often they do not appreciate how crucial a strong

immune system is for that continuing good health. And rarely do they have any idea that the latest discoveries in nutrition can be used to strengthen immunity.

That's surprising because the detrimental effects of intense exercise on immunity were first recognized at the St. Moritz Winter Olympics in 1928,[1] and have been studied intensively ever since. Sports medicine experts are coming to realize that athletic success requires more than optimal training and optimal nutrition. It also requires optimal immunity.[2] Science now offers many clues on how to achieve it.

The Immune System

To build a strong immune system, first you need a thumbnail sketch on how it works. That involves a little dip into biochemistry. Stay with me: it's worth its weight in gold.

The immune system is a body-wide network of specialized cells and processes. There are two divisions: **humoral immunity** and **cell-mediated immunity**. Humoral immunity produces **antibodies** in response to a vast array of invading viruses, bacteria, chemicals, and other substances foreign to your body.

All these invaders are called **antigens**. The humoral immune system makes a specific antibody for each antigen, capable of recognizing and attacking only that one. As you become exposed to more and more antigens, you build a huge library of thousands of different antibodies, a lifelong **immunologic memory** encoded in proteins. With proper maintenance, it will protect you very well.

Cell-mediated immunity is concerned with specialized cells. The most important are the **T-cell** and **B-cell lymphocytes** that differentiate into many different subsets with different reactions. We will cover only the few that you need to know in order to follow the research on sport and immunity.

Lymphocytes use the antibodies to enable them to recognize and attack invading antigens. When they do this, their numbers multiply rapidly. This is called the **lymphocyte proliferative response.** The stronger it is, the stronger your immunity.

Natural killer cells are large lymphocytes that do not need an antibody response in order to recognize many foreign cells. They can attack unknown invaders immediately without waiting up to 10 days for antibodies to form or be activated.[3] Natural killer cells are crucial to athletes, because they are the first line of defense that wards off a new virus or other invader, until the antigen-specific immune response can occur.[3]

The **phagocytes** are the cannibalistic foot soldiers of the immune system. Whenever the body is injured or invaded by foreign particles, an inflammatory response occurs that brings phagocytes scurrying to the site where they busily ingest dead and dying body cells. They also engulf and kill invading cells, especially if the invaders have already been tagged and neutralized by antibodies. The two main phagocytes are called **macrophages,** which are formed from **monocytes,** and **neutrophils.** They will ingest a wide range of particles from viruses and bacteria to poisons and even tiny plastic beads.[4]

In the battle with foreign invaders, macrophages and neutrophils use a lot of oxygen. The oxygen use produces a ton of free radicals, toxic oxygen by-products explained in Chapter 20. This reaction is called the **oxidative burst,** and is damaging to the body.[5] The smaller the oxidative burst, the better your immunity.

The **delayed hypersensitivity response** is also used to measure immunity. This is a cell-mediated response in which T-lymphocytes release growth factors for recruitment and activation of more macrophages. It takes one day to several weeks to occur, in contrast to other immediate immune responses. The better your delayed hypersensitivity response, the stronger your immunity.

You can get a fair measure of your own immune status from the **differential** part of a regular blood screen, the **SMAC 26 with CBC and Differential.** The total immune cells in your blood are only a sprinkle, but 50%-65% of them are the phagocytes called segmented neutrophils. Elevated "segs" usually means a bacterial infection, because as soon as an infection starts, your bone marrow releases neutrophils in massive numbers to combat it.

The second most common type of immune cells are the lymphocytes (25%-40% of the total white cell count). These are elaborated in the spleen and lymph nodes. They build immunity primarily against viruses, but also some bacteria and other foreign cells, by producing antibodies. Elevation of "lymphs" usually signals a viral infection.

Then come the monocytes (4%-10% of total white cell count). They are transformed into macrophages that engulf and digest foreign cells and the dead and dying body cells that are causing the inflammatory reactions. They also suck up stagnant fluids that collect at sites of inflammation, so are crucial to reduce swelling and inflammation in sports injuries.

Eosinophils comprise 1%-4% of the total white cell count. They are specialized to protect the lungs and gastrointestinal tract, so are vital to athletes. They also protect the skin and fight allergic reactions. Eosinophils are elevated in infections and illnesses of lungs and gut. Tip: cortisone shots knock them out, one reason to avoid cortisone.

You will see other immune cells, such as **basophils** and **bands**, on your blood test. They are rarely relevant in sports medicine. They are hardly ever used in research on athletes. The items we have covered are all you need to understand and use the research necessary to build a strong immune system.

One final point about bodily invasion, and this is relevant to nutrition also. Many athletes do not realize that the tube that extends from your mouth to your anus is not *inside* the body. To be inside, nutrients and invading microorganisms have to penetrate the gut walls. The hole that runs through you is just that, a complicated hole around which your body is formed.

Exercise Can Damage Immunity

Hundreds of studies attest to effects of exercise on immunity, but most of them are useless as a general guide because they failed to control for exercise intensity in relation to the fitness status of the individual athlete.

Studies that have measured immune responses to light or moderate exercise report only mild and temporary changes.[6] But studies on immunity after intense exercise show profound effects. Monocyte concentrations in blood are increased threefold, indicating a big immune challenge.[7] The lymphocyte proliferative response is suppressed suggesting that the immune system is being overwhelmed by the trauma of exercise.[7,8] And the activity of natural killer cells is suppressed for hours afterwards.[9,10] Because natural killer cells are your first line of defense, their suppression leaves you prey to opportunistic infections.

If the training is matched to the athlete, however, the immune system reacts to the trauma of exercise by growing stronger.[11] Trained athletes in good health have a higher number of natural killer cells, and a higher level of killer cell activity than sedentary folk.[12] They also have a higher base level of monocytes.[12] Both animal and human studies show that training programs, carefully designed to provide sufficient stress to challenge the immune system but not enough to overwhelm it, result in stronger immunity.[13]

But the average study simply recruits a bunch of subjects and arbitrarily decides exercise level and duration. If it is too light, nothing happens. If it is too heavy, immunity bombs. One recent study, for example, took young sedentary men from their habitual level of virtually zero exercise, to 40-50 minutes of aerobic exercise daily for five days a week. To you that might be a doddle, but to these guys it was boot camp. After 15 weeks, their natural killer cell activity was very depressed.[14] Fifteen weeks of what was intense effort for them, damaged their health defenses and left them prey to infection.

When we first reviewed the evidence on sport and immunity in 1984, the Colgan Institute decided to track American, British, and Soviet athletes looking for evidence of immune suppression. We found plenty! Athletes from all three countries are more susceptible to infections than the general population. And as their training or competition intensity increases, so does their rate of illness.

Other researchers agree. Dr G. Asgiersson found that athletes are more subject to bacterial infections.[15] Dr L. Fitzgerald of St. George's Hospital Medical School in London, reports that the immune systems of athletes at the top level of competition are often severely depressed, and they are especially subject to viral infections.[16] Dr L. Salo found that elite swimmers become more susceptible to illness as the swimming season progresses and exercise intensity increases.[17]

And there's the clue: exercise intensity. For example, marathon runners may be wonderfully healthy coming up to a marathon race. But after the intense effort of the race, many of them become ill in the following weeks. In one study, a third of all marathon finishers suffered an upper respiratory tract infection within two weeks after the race.[18] In another just published study, Dr Gregory Heath and colleagues at the Centers for Disease Control in Atlanta and the University of South Carolina, counted upper respiratory tract infections in 530 male and female runners over 12 months. Frequency of infections was directly related to weekly mileage. The higher the mileage the more infections suffered by the athlete.[19]

Soviet researchers report similar findings. After four months of intense competition, Soviet athletes (now Unified Team athletes), suffered a significant drop in the number and function of T-lymphocytes.[11] Dr I. Surkina gives the example of one athlete from the Soviet ski team who showed the most severe depression of T-cell proliferation. During the five subsequent months, he suffered six different recurring infections.[11] Think how that would devastate your training.

The next year the Soviets reduced the competitive season by decree. The athletes' immunity remained high and none became sick. But American and British athletes are not subject to government decrees. As emphasized by the rates of infection and injury before and during the Barcelona Games, far too many of us are chronically overtrained, and have chronically suppressed immunity.

Research studies agree. Elite American and British athletes have many more days off for illness than club level athletes.[20] In runners, infections can cause more days off training than injuries.[21] In American marathon runners, the most elite and hardest training have the lowest lymphocyte counts.[23] Both male and female members of the US cross-country ski team have poorer immunity than control subjects.[23] Dr Rod Fry of the University of Western Australia, has just published an excellent review showing that elite athletes are often overtrained, immune suppressed, and prone to infections.[24]

That seems to leave you caught between the proverbial rock and hard place. If you don't train intensely, you can't reach your potential. If you do train intensely, you devastate your immunity. No worries! Recent advances in nutrition can do wonders to help you.

Vitamin E Stimulates Immunity

Premature babies have low vitamin E status and very poor immune responses. Injections of vitamin E raise immune strength to that of normal babies.[25] Vitamin E is so effective that it has become a standard treatment for "premies."

Vitamin E content of lymphocytes and neutrophils is 10-20 times that of red blood cells, indicating the importance of this nutrient to their function. The main job of vitamin E is to prevent **lipid peroxidation** in cell membranes. That is, it prevents oxidation of fats by free radicals. It is the main nutrient antioxidant inside the skin of each one of your 30 trillion cells. If you make animals deficient in vitamin E, the membranes of their lymphocytes become damaged and immunity becomes severely depressed.[26] Addition of vitamin E to the nutrient mix quickly corrects this problem.[27,28] Even in healthy animals supplementary vitamin E enhances immunity.[29]

The pioneers in this work are Dr Robert Tengerdy and his group at Colorado State University. In a representative case of their many studies, healthy mice were given supplementary vitamin E and then deliberately infected with pneumonia. Over 60% of the mice resisted the challenge and did not develop the disease. A control group given the normal mouse diet *all* developed the pneumonia.[30]

The relevant point for athletes is that the control group diet contained adequate vitamin E according to laboratory animal standards. It took supplementation with additional vitamin E to boost the immune systems of normal healthy mice so that they could resist the infection.

One mechanism by which vitamin E operates is to reduce the damage caused by the immune system itself. As I explained earlier, when macrophages and neutrophils attack infections and injuries, they use a lot of oxygen. This produces an **oxidative burst** which releases many toxic free radicals which then damage your tissues. When rats are given supplementary vitamin E, the oxidative burst is much reduced.[5]

There are now over 100 studies since 1980 showing the immune enhancing effects of vitamin E. In one recent report, diabetics with the depressed immunity that is a plague of their disease, were given daily vitamin E supplements of 25 mg/kg bodyweight for two weeks. The average daily vitamin E intake was 1,500 mg per patient. Immunity, measured by the monocyte response, returned to the normal range.[31] It works on healthy people too. Dr M. Chavance, for example, tracked 100 normal human subjects for three years. Those with high vitamin E levels got many fewer infections.[32]

Vitamin E supplementation can even improve normal immunity in the absence of infection. In a double-blind controlled trial, Dr Simin Meydani and his group at Tufts University School of Medicine, measured the immunity of normal, healthy subjects, then gave them 800 mg per day of vitamin E or a placebo, for a month. Then he measured immunity again. Delayed hypersensitivity responses and lymphocyte proliferative responses were significantly enhanced.[33]

This research on the immune enhancing power of vitamin E parallels the research on its antioxidant action to prevent injuries in athletes discussed in Chapter 20. Although it is still cutting edge, and many studies remain to be done, the evidence is strong enough to suggest use of 800-1,600 mg of vitamin E (800-1,600 IU of d-alpha tocopherol) every day during periods of intense training.

Use the differential of the SMAC blood screen to gauge your biochemical individuality. Its not much, but it's the best we have yet that is easily available. The test should be done during a period of light training so as to show base levels. If any of yours are at the low end of the normal range or below it, it may indicate the need for the high end of vitamin E intake.

Our own case records indicate that some athletes of elite to Olympic status following this procedure, have gone three years without a single infection while taking these daily doses of vitamin E and other antioxidants. Their immune tests show very healthy levels. I know some conservative sports medicine folk who will mumble, "Premature," at this use of supplements. Don't believe them! Read the scientific references and decide for yourself. Vitamin E is non-toxic in the amounts suggested, [34] and could save your health and your training.

Vitamin C Enhances Immunity

The concentration of vitamin C in neutrophils and macrophages is about 150 times its concentration in your blood plasma.[35] During their oxidative burst while killing infection, the neutrophils suck up vitamin C like a sponge. They then use it to inhibit some of the oxidation. Not surprising that neutrophil responses are suppressed in vitamin C deficiency.[36]

Vitamin C supplementation also reduces the tissue damage from the neutrophil oxidative burst.[37] And vitamin C supplementation enhances the neutrophil response in healthy individuals.[38] In another study, vitamin C supplements of 1 gram per day enhanced both the lymphocyte proliferative response and antibody responses.[38] Bigger doses, 10 grams per day also enhanced the delayed hypersensitivity responses of healthy young adults.[39] There is no longer any doubt that daily doses of vitamin C in the gram range can enhance your immunity.

Selenium Can Boost Immunity

Selenium functions in synergy with vitamin E as an antioxidant. As we saw in Chapter 20, vitamin E protects fats against lipid peroxidation within your cell membranes, including the cell membranes of all immune cells. New research by Dr Fulvio Ursini and colleagues at the University of Padua, Italy, has discovered a selenium dependent enzyme, **phospholipid hydroperoxide glutathione peroxidase**, that shares the work. It detoxifies peroxidized fats within the membrane, and therefore spares vitamin E.[40]

It has been known for many years that selenium also works to activate the antioxidant enzyme **glutathione peroxidase** inside the cell itself. Glutathione peroxidase destroys toxic hydrogen peroxides and lipid peroxides.[41] Adequate supplies of selenium are therefore crucial to strong immunity. In one series of studies, animals supplemented with selenium alone, increased their immune strength by 400%.[42]

Animal studies show that if selenium is deficient in the diet, the beneficial effect of vitamin E effect on immunity is also reduced. The strongest immune responses are found in animals supplemented with both nutrients together.[43] In one recent study, animals made deficient in both vitamin E and selenium developed severely depressed immunity. Supplementation with the two nutrients restored T-lymphocyte responses to normal levels.[44]

There are no studies of the effects of selenium supplementation on the immunity of athletes. From the chemistry of selenium, however, and from its effects on animals, it seems a prudent strategy to use this nutrient in synergy with vitamin E. The amount you should use can be calculated from the table in Chapter 20.

Zinc Can Boost Immunity

One function of zinc is to act as a co-factor of nutrient antioxidants. Animal studies show that zinc deficiency causes a rapid decline of T-lymphocyte function.[45] Immunity is equally rapidly restored by zinc supplementation.[46] In animals with normal immunity, supplemental zinc improves the lymphocyte response.[47]

In a carefully controlled human study, Dr Jean Duchateau and colleagues at the Free University of Brussels in Belgium, gave groups of normal subjects with normal zinc status and normal immunity, 220 mg of zinc sulfate three times daily for a month. Compared with a control group and with their own immune strength before supplementation, lymphocyte responses were significantly enhanced.[48] That is far too much zinc (and the wrong form of zinc) for any purpose but an experiment, but it illustrates that zinc can enhance immunity above normal levels. For the right form of zinc and the right amounts for athletes, see Chapters 15 and 16.

Beta-carotene Boosts Immunity

With the National Cancer Institute running large trials that are tending to show beta-carotene prevents cancer,[49] this nutrient has become big news. It used to be thought that beta-carotene was simply converted to vitamin A in the body. But now we know it has independent functions in disease prevention.[50]

One way it works is by boosting immunity. Studies on

animals published in the **Journal of the National Cancer Institute** show that supplements of beta-carotene increase immune system action against some form of cancer.[51] The most important finding is that this nutrient can reverse malignant and advanced cases of certain cancers, and cure some animals, without any other treatment.

The main reason for this powerful action is that beta-carotene causes the macrophages of the immune system to release a specific chemical called **tumor necrosis factor**.[52,53] If beta-carotene can beat the lethal trauma of malignant cancer, it is likely to do wonders for the much smaller trauma of exercise.

Numerous recent animal studies and *in vitro* studies show that beta-carotene increases lymphocyte responses and natural killer cell responses to a variety of challenges.[54,55] But the crucial evidence for athletes comes from supplementation of normal, healthy human subjects. As yet, there are only two good studies, but they are dynamite. In the first, young, healthy men with normal immunity were supplemented with 180 mg/day of beta-carotene. Results showed a significant increase in the base level of T-lymphocytes.[56]

In the second study, different groups of healthy men and women with normal immunity were given a placebo or 15, 30, 45, or 60 mg of beta-carotene a day for three months. The placebo and the 15 mg dose had no effect. The 30, 45, and 60 mg doses all increased base levels of T-helper lymphocytes and natural killer cells. There was no increase in vitamin A levels in the body, indicating that it was the beta-carotene that was causing the immunostimulation.[57]

These results suggest there is a threshold dose below which beta-carotene does not work to boost immunity. The 30, 45, and 60 mg doses that were successful correspond roughly to 30,000, 45,000, and 60,000 of the old International Units (IU). From this work plus the evidence of its antioxidant properties reviewed in Chapter 20, the Colgan Institute uses 25-50 mg (25,000-50,000 IU) of beta-carotene daily with athletes.

Coenzyme Q10 Improves Immunity

CoQ10 is a controversial nutrient in America. Despite two decades of successful research,[58] and despite its widespread use in treatment of heart disease in Europe and Japan,[59] the US Food and Drug Administration continues to call CoQ10 "an unapproved food additive." To scientists, their position is incomprehensible, but in medical politics it makes eminent sense. Restriction of non-patentable, inexpensive nutrients, maintains the patent-dependent bottom lines of US pharmaceutical companies.

The problem is, these political shenanigans send confusing messages to sports medicine professionals and to athletes. Is CoQ10 legit or not? Six volumes of scientific research from over 100 laboratories, edited by world renowned expert Dr Karl Folkers of the University of Texas at Austin, say it is.[58] As I wrote at the start of this book, science is the only measure you can trust.

Twenty years ago at the New England Research Institute in Connecticut, physician Dr Emile Bliznakov and his group first reported a series of studies showing that CoQ supplements enhance macrophage activity in animals.[60] These findings were confirmed and extended by other laboratories. Animals fed CoQ have improved cell-mediated immunity and improved resistance to bacterial infection.[61]

Humoral immunity is also boosted by CoQ. Antibody production is increased, and a single injection of CoQ10 of 4 mg/kg bodyweight, has been shown to reverse the age-related decline in antibody responses in mice.[62]

It also works in human subjects. Studies report reversal of the age-related decline in humoral immunity using supplements of 60 mg/day of CoQ10.[62] With these effects on humoral immunity, you would expect improved resistance to viruses. And there is, and it's strong. CoQ10 shows anti-viral activity in animals against the potent Friend leukemia virus.[64] It also protects animals against otherwise lethal doses of encephalomyocarditis virus.[65]

These are only a few of the many hundreds of studies on CoQ10. They are representative of the research that shows it to be a valuable nutrient to help improve immunity in athletes. The Colgan Institute uses 30-60 mg per day with athletes, of the TwinLab brand of CoQ10, the only one we have tested and found trustworthy. Together with the potent antioxidant effects of CoQ10 covered in Chapter 20, the evidence of its immune boosting effects amply justifies such supplementation.

Arginine Improves Immunity

Arginine plays so many roles in sports nutrition that I hesitate to give it another place, lest this simple amino acid sounds too good to be true. But the evidence is so strong that arginine improves immunity that I have to include it in this chapter too.

Some researchers may object that it was established 50 years ago that arginine is not even an essential nutrient in adults.[66] True for couch potatoes, but not true for anyone whose body is under the sort of stress that threatens nitrogen balance or immunity.[67] In studies of stressed animals, with impaired immunity, arginine supplements improve the action of T-lymphocytes and the delayed hypersensitivity response.[68]

Arginine also works with postoperative patients and intensive care patients to improve immune responses.[69] And in healthy volunteers, recent studies show that 30 grams of arginine per day for 3 days improved immune responses to various deliberate challenges.[69] This unique action of arginine is not related to deficient levels of arginine in these subjects but to another mechanism entirely.

Although not yet proven by controlled studies, I'll lay my money that arginine stimulates immunity by the same mechanism that it stimulates muscle growth, that is, its action in releasing growth hormone from the anterior pituitary. In animal studies arginine fails to stimulate immunity if the anterior pituitary is blocked.[70] That is not the whole story, however, as new research also shows unique actions of arginine in various immune pathways.[71] These findings make arginine an important nutrient for optimum sports performance. As you use Chapter 30 to help you determine the amounts of arginine you need for your personal sports nutrition program remember you are also getting a bonus in improved immunity.

Glutamine is Vital to Immunity

A pile of new evidence shows that all cell replication in the immune system requires glutamine.[72] Unfortunately, this non-essential amino acid cannot be made by immune cells. It is made almost exclusively by muscle cells.[73] But the immune system uses a ton of it.[74] So your muscles have to supply large amounts of glutamine continuously to the immune system.[73]

Therein lies the problem. As we will see in Chapter 32, glutamine is also the main anti-catabolic agent in muscle, that is, the compound that helps preserve muscle during and after exercise.[75] The heavier your training, the heavier the stress on muscles, and the greater your muscle use of glutamine.[73,75] There is now considerable evidence that traumatic catabolic conditions, such as the effects of intense training, overwhelm the body's ability to produce glutamine. So both muscle cells and immune cells get inadequate supplies, with a consequent loss of muscle and strength and a decline in immunity.[73,76] This effect is so strong that some researchers now call glutamine a "conditionally essential amino acid",[77] and others suggest that skeletal muscles should be included as an essential part of the immune system.[73]

But don't start scarfing down glutamine to try and make up the deficit. Supplemental glutamine loads the body with toxic ammonia. Ammonia is a definite downer for performance, as explained in Chapter 23. The right stuff to use is **alpha-ketoglutarate**, the ammonia-free carbon skeleton of glutamine.[78] Branched-chain amino acids help too, because they work in the body to provide a substrate for glutamine.[79] All is revealed about amounts and methods of use of these amino acids in Chapter 32.

Boosting Immunity

Studies reviewed indicate that intense training suppresses immunity and that you can improve your immunity with specific nutrients, vitamin E, vitamin C, selenium, zinc, beta-carotene, coenzyme Q10, alpha-ketoglutarate and branched-chain amino acids. But don't forget synergy. Many other nutrients are involved in immunity including folic acid,[80] vitamins B1, B2, B3, B6, and pantothenic acid,[81] and chromium.[82] Dietary fat reduces immunity,[83] and dietary protein in the form of whey enhances immunity.[84] You can use Chapters 20 and 32 to assess your needs for the specific immune-boosting nutrients covered in this chapter, but your focus should always be on **complete nutrition.**

Part V

Ergogenics

Use makes the organ. The strength and endurance of body structures follow exactly the habitual demands for strength and endurance made upon them.

Michael Colgan, University of Oregon Lectures, 1984

Chapter 23

Beating The Burn

I am reading a typical ad in the top muscle magazine. It vows that if you follow their system and swallow their glop you will "increase your endurance 300% in just 90 days. Guaranteed." Hogwash and flapdoodle! Such ads cram the popular sports literature, claiming impossible ergogenic effects from mysterious mixtures of chemicals that are supposed to be "metabolic optimizers," or "vital links in the energy chain," or similar meaningless buzz-words born of marketplace babble. Resolve never to be suckered again by such tomfoolery. Let's take a closer look at how muscles fatigue so you can learn some real ways to beat the burn.

Muscles Go Acid

Your muscles work well only in a narrow range of almost zero acidity. Your arterial blood works best with no acid at all. The measure of acidity is the **concentration of hydrogen ions (pH)**. A pH of 7.0 is neutral, midway between very acid (pH of 1) and very alkaline (pH of 14).

The pH scale is logarithmic, like the scale for earthquakes. So small changes in the numbers mean large differences in acidity or alkalinity. A pH of 6 is 10 times more acid than a pH of 7. At rest, muscle pH is about 6.9, arterial blood is about 7.4.[1] As you begin to exercise, the increased use of muscle glycogen for energy produces **lactic acid and pyruvic acid**. These acids contain a lot of hydrogen ions (H +), which drive muscle and blood pH down into the acid zone.

The harder you exercise, the quicker you go acid. As muscle pH drops below 6.5, the acidity disrupts all sorts of links in the energy chain.[2] To take two examples, the enzyme **phosphofructokinase** is the rate-limiting step in muscle use of glycogen. Below pH 6.5, it stops working altogether.[3] Acidity also reduces muscle power directly by inhibiting the contractile action of muscle fibers.[4]

So the first thing that a successful ergogenic supplement has to do is reduce the accumulation of acidity in exercising muscle. You can put all sorts of other chemicals into the bloodstream, but unless you reduce acidity during exercise, your muscles will tie up.

Ammonia Build-Up

Acidity is not the whole problem. Patients with several rare diseases do not produce lactic acid during exercise, therefore, do not lower the pH of muscle and blood. Yet their muscles fatigue very quickly.[2] Some sports medicine folk refer to these patients to claim that lactic acid is not responsible for muscle fatigue at all. They fall into the trap of the all-or-none fallacy. Human biochemistry is so complex, and our ability to nut it out is so limited, that we strive to categorize effects into discrete little pigeonholes. If it is not x, it must be y. I hope by this far into the book, you are realizing that human bodies do not function by this *or* that discretely. They function by this *and* that *and* that *and* that, and a lot of other mechanisms we don't even know about.

A second inhibitor of exercise, happening simultaneously with the accumulation of acidity, is accumulation of **ammonia.** All anaerobic and endurance exercise produces oodles of the stuff.[5] Bad news! Ammonia is toxic to all cells, reduces the formation of glycogen, and inhibits the energy cycle. It has devastating effects on brain function.[6] We still don't know how much it contributes to fatigue, but we do know that the higher your blood ammonia, the poorer your performance.[7] So the second thing that a successful ergogenic supplement has to do is reduce ammonia accumulation.

Loss of Phosphate

Recent studies by Dr Richard Kreider at Old Dominion University, Virginia, show that whenever you exercise, either anaerobically with weights or aerobically with endurance sports, phosphate levels in the blood increase rapidly.[8] Studies in Britain by Dr G. Dale and colleagues at Newcastle General Hospital, show that this elevation of blood phosphate occurs because of loss of phosphate from muscle into the blood.[9] The muscle trauma that occurs in all heavy weight training also releases a lot of phosphate into the blood.[10]

Immediately after marathon races, triathlons, or other endurance events, some athletes have very low blood phosphate levels, low to the point of illness. Our findings agree with the British studies of Dr Dale, who has measured levels as low as 0.17 mmol/l in runners who collapsed after a half-marathon races.[9] Even athletes with high resting phosphate levels show marked reductions after endurance exercise.[11]

How does this loss of phosphate damage performance? First, there is a loss of acid buffering. Phosphate is a major alkaline buffer of muscle. Second, to make new muscle glycogen, your body has to use **pyridoxal phosphate**, a mix of phosphate and vitamin B_6. Also, before you can use glucose for fuel, it has to go through a chemical conversion called **phosphorylation**. Both these processes are partly dependent on the level of available phosphate.[11]

The third major effect of phosphate loss is to reduce delivery of oxygen to muscles. Phosphate forms part of a compound called **2,3-diphosphoglycerate (2,3-DPG)** which, in jargon terms, reduces your **hemoglobin/oxygen affinity**. That is, it helps red blood cells dump oxygen into muscle cells. As levels of 2,3-DPG decline, muscle oxygen, VO$_2$max, and performance decline also.[12] So, a third thing that a successful ergogenic supplement has to do is provide a source of bioavailable phosphate.

Oxygen Supply

The fourth factor that inhibits exercise is lack of oxygen supply to muscles and brain. Oxygen is not so important for short anaerobic *events*, but it is vital for *training* in all anaerobic sports. It is also vital for all endurance sports, where the goal is to exercise at as high an intensity as possible without going anaerobic. The more oxygen you can deliver to muscles, the higher your capacity to train for anaerobic events, and the higher your capacity to both train and compete in endurance events.

Some researchers claim that oxygen supply is not the limiting variable, but rather that muscles have a limited ability to use the oxygen. Even during maximal exercise, there is still a lot of oxygen left in the returning venous blood *after* delivery of oxygen to muscle by the arteries.[13] They claim that if the muscles could use more, they would extract it from the blood.

Wrong! A bit deeper into the biochemistry, we see that there is a whole unloading system that unlocks the oxygen from the hemoglobin of your red blood cells and delivers it to muscle cells. As we noted when discussing phosphate, this system is partly controlled by the enzyme 2,3-diphosphoglycerate (2,3-DPG). Under the stimulus of oxygen deprivation at high altitudes for example, 2,3-DPG increases, and a greater proportion of arterial oxygen is dumped into muscles.[14] So muscle capacity to take up oxygen can't be the limiting factor. And any successful ergogenic supplement should contain chemicals that will increase 2, 3-DPG.

Also, if you increase an athlete's **hemoglobin**, that is the amount of red pigment that carries the oxygen in blood cells, then oxygenation of muscle increases. And if you increase an athlete's **hematocrit,** that is the proportion of his blood that is composed of red blood cells, then oxygenation of muscle increases and performance improves.[15] That's the potent **blood doping** effect discussed later in the drug chapters. It is not the muscles that limit oxygen use, but rather the amount of oxygen that gets into them. So a successful ergogenic supplement should also contain chemicals that increase hemoglobin and hematocrit.

L-Carnitine Carries The Fat

During long endurance exercise, fats become a major energy source. You will not run out of fats, but you might run out of the chemicals that enable you to use them. One of the most studied is **l-carnitine**, a non-protein amino acid.

Transport of free fatty acids into the **mitochondria** (furnaces) of the cell for use as energy, requires l-carnitine-based enzymes as a transport system.[16] Endurance exercise rapidly depletes the pool of l-carnitine in muscle,[17] so the amount of carnitine available is a limiting factor on the energy supply of endurance athletes. Any successful ergogenic supplement for endurance, should contain chemicals that increase the free carnitine level in muscle.

Oxidation Hurts Muscle

Exercise increases the use of oxygen, so naturally increases the formation of **free radicals**, toxic wastes of oxygen metabolism that hurt every cell they touch. The effects of free radicals include damage to the muscle cells and a decline in mitochondrial metabolism.[18] Both these events reduce the production of energy.

Free radicals are neutralized by endogenous **antioxidants** including **superoxide dismutase, catalase,** and **glutathione.** They are also neutralized by nutritional antioxidants, such as vitamin A, vitamin C, vitamin E, coenzyme Q10, and the minerals selenium and zinc. See Chapter 20. A successful ergogenic supplement should include chemicals that increase the muscle supply of both endogenous and nutritional antioxidants.

There are over 100 other intermediate steps in the energy

chain that should be enhanced if you want optimum performance. But as yet, science has discovered few clues on how to do it. The items listed in Table 20, are the state of the art regarding nutritional ergogenics. The first two items are more concerned with building a better body. We covered them in earlier chapters. But the last five are purely ergogenic. Their pronounced effects on performance warrant a separate chapter for each.

Table 20. Real ergogenics: substances and mechanisms of action that improve performance. Each substance and action is covered in a separate chapter.*

Substance	Mechanism
Multiple antioxidants	Neutralize free radicals to maintain muscle integrity and mitochondrial metabolism. (Chapter 20)
Multiple	Increase hematocrit and hemoglobin to improve oxygen supply to muscle. (Chapter 21)
Bicarbonate, Phosphate	Reduce muscle and blood acidity. (Chapters 24 and 25)
Specific amino acids	Reduce ammonia levels. (Chapter 32)
Phosphate	Increases 2,3-DPG to improve oxygen delivery to muscle. (Chapter 25)
L-carnitine	Maintains free fatty acid oxidation for endurance exercise. (Chapter 26)
Caffeine	Stimulant: increases availability of free fatty acids for fuel. Multiple other actions. (Chapter 27)
Panax Ginseng	Stimulant: increases free fatty acid oxidation. Other actions. (Chapter 28)

*Source: Colgan Institute, San Diego, CA.

Chapter 24

Bicarbonate Buffers Acid

Do you know why your muscles fatigue and tie up when you do resistance exercises, such as a barbell curl or a bench press with heavy weights? Do you know what causes the burn that finally makes it impossible to complete another rep?

The biggest cause is lactic acid. Lactic acid and other acids and metabolic wastes build up in the muscles with repeated movements. The more anaerobic the exercise, the faster the build-up. Maximum strength output can tie up the muscles in just one rep.

Your muscles have a natural buffering system to prevent the tissue from becoming acid. But as reps continue, the level of acids rise beyond the capacity of the buffering system, the pH of your muscle tissue drops, acidity increases, and your muscle ties up. You have to rest until the lactic acid is cleared or chemically reconverted before you can continue.

Recent studies show that over 95% of the buffering muscle is done by three substances, carnosine which is the main buffer, phosphate which is the secondary buffer, and bicarbonate which does 5-10% of the buffering function.[1,2]

Improving Buffering Capacity

Acidity is not the only problem inside muscle cells. Continued exercise also acidifies your blood, mainly by release of some of the lactic acid build-up from muscles. Over the course of a workout, this acid build-up produces the feeling of overall fatigue we all know well. This fatigue occurs not only during anaerobic sports like weight training, shot putting or sprinting, but also during endurance sports like marathon running.

The main buffer in blood is sodium bicarbonate. Your body produces and uses plain old baking soda to protect its blood from acidity.[3] Armed with this knowledge, for more than 40 years, coaches have sought to use bicarbonate supplements to reduce muscle acidity and improve performance.[4]

Problems! Only a few top coaches know how much to use, when to use it, and what kinds of performance benefit. And they found the answer by trial-and-error and kept it to themselves. It has taken the last decade of intensive research to reveal the secrets of bicarbonate loading, and put the information into scientific journals.

The first problem is that sodium bicarbonate taken orally doesn't reach the muscle cells. It can't get through the cell membrane.[5] So how can it work at all, because the action you are trying to influence all goes on inside the cells? Dr GW Mainwood and colleagues solved this problem in 1980. They found that the less acid the blood becomes as you fill it with bicarbonate, the more it creates what is called a **pH gradient** between muscle and blood, which pulls acid out of the muscle.[6]

Subsequent muscle biopsy studies on athletes, show that the less acid your blood pH after bicarbonate supplementation, the less acid your muscle pH.[7] With this evidence bicarbonate was well on its way to creating the burp Olympics.

Bicarbonate and Performance

Once scientists were satisfied that increased bicarbonate in the blood could reduce muscle acidity, the race was on to see how it affects performance. In one of the well-controlled early studies, Dr D Wilkes and colleagues at York University, Toronto, gave 6 varsity track athletes 300 mg/kg bodyweight of sodium bicarbonate or a placebo. For a 70 kg (154 lb) athlete, that's a huge dose of 21 grams. Supplements were taken over a 2-hour period, up to 30 minutes before an 800 meter race.[8] Results showed that, in the bicarbonate trials, blood pH remained higher, meaning that acidity was reduced. Performance improved by an average of 2.9 seconds, which translates to a distance of 19 meters. In an 800 meter race, that's the difference between first and also ran.

After the success of Wilkes' study, Dr David Costill and his group, at the Human Performance Laboratory at Ball State University, Indiana, gave athletes a lower dose of bicarbonate (200 mg/kg bodyweight). That's 14 grams for a 70 kg (154 lb) athlete. Subjects then did five 1-minute sprints on the ergometer bicycle, with the last one to absolute exhaustion. The bicarbonate improved the time to exhaustion in the last sprint by a huge 42%.[9]

Other studies of maximal short-term exercise have also reported increased endurance after bicarbonate loading, and increased power output.[10-12] Some researchers have found no effects, but they have generally used lower doses of bicarbonate, or have used exercise bouts of longer than 5 minutes.[13-15] The evidence indicates that the dose and the duration of the exercise are critical. Bicarbonate works best as an ergogenic aid only at high doses (300 mg/kg bodyweight) and only for short, almost maximal exercise (2-6 minutes).

A new study by Drs Lars McNaughton and Rod Cedaro of the Tasmanian Institute of Technology, Australia, could be used as a model of the bicarbonate method.[16] They gave world-class rowers 300 mg/kg bodyweight of bicarbonate or a placebo. Ninety-five minutes later, subjects made a maximal effort for 6 minutes on a rowing ergometer. Compared with placebo trials, when receiving bicarbonate, subjects rowed almost 50 meters further in the same time. At the 1991 World Rowing Championships, that was more than the difference between first and last.

There is no longer any doubt that, in short events, bicarbonate can provide a winning edge. But there is one big problem -- explosive diarrhea. Because of biochemical individuality, different athletes react to bicarbonate very differently. About half the subjects we have tested at the Colgan Institute report no problems. The other half spend more time in the bathroom than on the track.

Two ways to combat the problem. First, take the bicarbonate in divided doses every 20 minutes, beginning three hours before the event, and ending one hour before the start. Second, drink very freely up to 30 minutes before the event. Practice it well in training before you ever do it in competition.

And remember, supplementation with 20 grams of sodium bicarbonate stuffs your body with 5 grams of sodium. That's very unhealthy nutrition, at least 10 times more sodium than you need.[17] It shoots some folk's blood pressure over the moon. So even if you get no gut problems, and have no trace of hypertension, reserve bicarbonate loading for the big one.

Chapter 25

Phosphate Loading

In both anaerobic and endurance exercise, you lose a lot of muscle phosphate into the blood.[1-3] Regular training also increases *resting* levels of blood phosphate, an indication that the body responds to training by increasing its overall level of phosphate, and that exercise increases phosphate needs.

Marathon runners, for example, have much higher resting blood phosphate levels than sedentary people. When we first measured them at the Colgan Institute in the early '80s, we thought some athletes had phosphate overload. Their blood levels were over 1.5 mmol/l, way above the normal range of 0.75-1.35 mmol/l. But other researchers have found the same,[4] and our athletes seemed to thrive on it. Also, whenever phosphate levels were low, performance usually bombed. So we came to the conclusion that elevated blood phosphate is a beneficial effect of training.

Your body can't make phosphorus. You have to get this mineral base of phosphate from your diet. Phosphates are added to numerous foods. The RDA is 800 mg, but the daily intake in America is over 1,500 mg in males, and almost 1,000 mg in females.[5] Because of these high levels in food, until recently supplement manufacturers have not followed the research on phosphate. But recent studies show pathologically low levels of blood phosphate in some athletes after endurance events.[2] So even our high food intake of phosphate may be insufficient to meet the demands of intense exercise.

Effects of Phosphate

Most athletes in good shape show resting phosphate levels at or near the top of the normal medical range. But does the normal range, conceived for sedentary folk, cover levels of phosphate required for optimal performance in athletes? What happens when you raise it even higher.

Successful ergogenic use of phosphate would have to do at least three things. First, it would have to buffer muscle acid. Dr Richard Kreider and his group at Old Dominion University, Virginia, the leading lights in this research, have recently shown exactly that effect in repeated studies of phosphate supplementation.[1,6]

Second, it would have to raise the level of 2,3-diphosphoglycerate (2,3-DPG), the enzyme that unloads oxygen into muscle. Studies from various laboratories have shown repeatedly that phosphate supplementation reliably raises blood levels of 2,3-DPG.[8,9,10]

Third, through its incorporation into numerous enzymes in energy production, it would have to improve the production and use of glycogen for fuel. There is some evidence that supplemental phosphate has this effect.[7]

Effects On Performance

The combined biochemical effects of phosphate supplements on performance are dramatic. Dr Robert Cade and his group at the Department of Medicine of the University of Florida, gave 10 well trained endurance runners either 1 gram of sodium phosphate four times daily or a placebo for three days. Then they ran them on the treadmill to exhaustion. During the phosphate loading trial, lactic acid levels were lower, 2,3-DPG levels were higher, VO_2max increased by 6-12%, and subjects ran 3-9 minutes longer.[9]

At the Tasmanian Institute of Technology in Australia, Dr Ian Stewart and his colleagues did a similar study of highly trained cyclists, giving them 3.6 grams of sodium phosphate a day or a placebo, for three days before a maximum effort on the ergometer bicycle. Results showed that phosphate loading reduced lactic acid accumulation, increased 2,3-DPG production during exercise, increased VO_2max by a whopping 11%, and increased time to exhaustion by an incredible 20%.[10]

One of the latest and best studies is from Dr Richard Kreider and his group at Old Dominion University. They gave trained cyclists 4 grams of sodium phosphate per day or a placebo, for 3 days prior to a maximal exercise test and a 40 km time trial on the ergometer bicycle. So they tested both anaerobic and endurance exercise.[11]

During the anaerobic phosphate trials, maximal power output increased by 17%. That's equivalent to adding 51 lbs to a 300 lb maximum bench press! During the aerobic phosphate trials, time for the 40 km ride was reduced by 3.5 minutes. That's the difference between winning and fell off the bicycle in cycling races. There is no doubt that phosphate works big time.

A dosage of 4 grams a day for three days seems adequate, which makes sodium phosphate a more healthy ergogenic than sodium bicarbonate. It also works in both anaerobic and endurance exercise, which makes it better all around. The sodium form has been used in most studies, but potassium phosphate might work too. With the high level of sodium added to our food and the big losses of potassium in food processing, potassium phosphate would be a lot healthier. But don't use calcium phosphate. Two studies that have tried calcium phosphate found no effect at all.[12,13]

There are two new controlled studies completed but not yet published, using the commercial phosphate/bicarbonate supplement Phos Fuel made by TwinLab. The first of these, done by Dr Richard Kreider's group was presented at the American College of Sports Medicine meeting in Dallas on May 27-30,

1992. It showed that Phos Fuel, at the recommended dose of 4 grams per day for 3 days prior to performance, significantly increased serum phosphate levels and reduced lactic acid accumulation in swimmers.[14]

The second study with Phosfuel has just been completed by Dr William Kramer, famous strength coach and Director of Research in Sports Medicine at Pennsylvania State University. Results were presented at the 1992 Annual Convention of the National Strength and Conditioning Association held in Philadelphia. Kramer and his group reported that Phos Fuel increased the athletes' levels of 2-3 DPG and increased power output in highly trained athletes. If anyone tells you that phosphate doesn't work, just smile, and keep your edge to yourself.

Chapter 26

Carnitine Moves More Than The Fat

Your muscles don't get much done without adequate carnitine. Throughout this book, I have stressed muscle glycogen as the most important fuel during exercise, because unless you supplement it, you run out very quickly, whereas you never run out of fats. Nevertheless, fats still provide about 50% of your energy during aerobic exercise and 80% of your energy towards the end of long endurance events.[1] So you have to be able to use them freely. Carnitine absolutely controls fat use because it forms the transport system that moves the fatty acid molecules into the **mitochondria** (furnaces) of the cell where they are burned for fuel.[2]

Carnitine also helps with the oxidation (burning) of **pyruvate** and **branched chain amino acids** in the energy cycle.[3] It also prevents the build-up of fatty complexes called **acyl-coenzyme A** that destabilize muscle membranes.[4]

Carnitine also operates to inhibit the build-up of **lactic acid** in muscle, one of the main causes of fatigue. In one recent study, patients with angina were supplemented with l-carnitine. The build-up of lactic acid during their moderate exercise routine was reduced by *half*, and exercise duration was significantly increased.[5] Because of all these functions, the amount of free carnitine in your muscles plays a major role in their efficiency, and places an absolute limit on the amount of energy they can supply.

The standard textbook answer to this problem is that the human body makes carnitine from the essential amino acids lysine and methionine (plus vitamin C, niacin, pyridoxine, and iron). So a sedentary person on a good diet does not need to take carnitine.

But athletes are different animals. During training they put their bodies into a state of stress that uses a ton of carnitine. Their demand for carnitine can easily exceed the body's ability to make it.[6] Even moderate exercise, such as cycling on an ergometer bicycle at only 55% of VO2max, causes a 20% drop in muscle carnitine.[6] Maximal exercise causes a much greater drop,[7] putting athletes into the same carnitine status as patients with carnitine deficiency diseases.

These patients can hardly use any fat for energy, they have high levels of blood lipids, they suffer extreme muscle weakness, they accumulate bodyfat from the *smell* of a bacon cheeseburger, and their heart function sounds like someone torturing a cat.[8,9] Every time you exercise to maximum without sufficient carnitine, you put your body into this detrimental condition.

Carnitine deficiency is easily corrected by oral l-carnitine. There is no doubt that increased carnitine intake increases the serum level of free carnitine.[10] Because of its involvement in normal heart function, oral l-carnitine has been used extensively to treat patients with angina. Because of its involvement with pyruvate metabolism, which regulates oxygen availability to muscle,[3] it has also been used to treat patients with respiratory insufficiency.

Oral l-carnitine is so successful in medicine that three US pharmaceutical companies now make prescription tablets.[11] Five well-controlled recent studies show that l-carnitine increases exercise tolerance and endurance performance in patients with angina and patients with respiratory disorders.[12-16]

L-carnitine Boosts Performance

What does carnitine do for athletes? Plenty! Physiological studies show that carnitine supplements inhibit the decline in free carnitine in muscle caused by maximal exercise, and completely prevent the decline in free carnitine during endurance exercise.[17]

Carnitine also increases maximum use of oxygen in athletes. This effect was first observed by Dr Brian Liebovitz at the University of California, Davis.[18] It has recently been confirmed by two Italian studies. Both gave athletes 4 grams of l-carnitine daily. The supplement significantly increased VO_2max.[19,20]

Supplementation also reduces the build-up of acids and metabolic wastes during maximal exercise. In a recent study, Dr Noris Siliprandi and colleagues at the University of Padua, Italy, gave athletes 2 grams of l-carnitine or a placebo, one hour before maximal exercise on the bicycle-ergometer. Carnitine reduced post-exercise levels of lactate and pyruvate, and significantly increased maximal work output.[7]

In another similar Italian study, normal subjects who were not athletes, were given l-carnitine supplements or placebo and tested for submaximal exercise on the ergometer bicycle. The carnitine trials showed a significant improvement in endurance.[14] So there is evidence that l-carnitine can boost both anaerobic and aerobic performance.

A dose of 2-4 grams taken for 2 weeks, one hour before exercise appears to be effective. That is many times the dietary intake in America, which runs about 100-300 mg per day.[21] But even at 4 grams daily, l-carnitine shows no toxicity.[20]

DL-Carnitine *IS* Toxic

Real l-carnitine costs an arm and a leg. That is why numerous sports supplements contain only a negligible few milligrams. Other supplements contain gram amounts, but it is cheap **dl-carnitine** or **racemic carnitine**, a very different compound than l-carnitine. Dl-carnitine contains about 50% of the **dextro,** or right-handed molecule of carnitine. This substance does not occur in normal foods, so during evolution the human body did not develop the mechanisms to deal with it. The body cannot use d-carnitine, and its presence inhibits use of l-carnitine, the **levo** or left-handed molecule. Dl-carnitine is therefore a toxin that causes carnitine deficiency and all its detrimental consequences.[22,23]

In 1984 the Food and Drug Administration issued a health warning about dl-carnitine,[24] but it still appears in the marketplace. Be especially wary of supplements labelled on the front, "L-carnitine" in big letters. On the back you may find in the tiniest print that is still legal, "in a base of racemic carnitine." They are all dl-carnitine. In one case reported by Dr Robert Keith of Auburn University, Alabama, a 35-year old runner took only 500 mg of dl-carnitine daily for two days before a race. His quadriceps became so weak, he had to miss the race and could not train for the next three weeks.[25]

So use only l-carnitine from a reputable company. At the Colgan Institute, we use the TwinLab brand of 250 mg capsules, which we have tested and have found true to label. That's about the most l-carnitine you can get into a pill and still keep it small enough to swallow.

Chapter 27

Caffeine: The Right Way

The word "coffee" comes from the ancient Arabic *qahweh*, meaning "gives strength". So the effects of caffeine, the main stimulant in coffee, have been known for thousands of years. The computer data-base at the Colgan Institute contains over 600 citations on caffeine, stretching back two centuries. But most of the work up to 1980 lacked the necessary controls to separate the effects of caffeine on sports performance from its effects in everyday life. The latest and best research shows they are quite different.

Numerous reviews on the use of caffeine in sports, lump together the many exercise studies of caffeine that have used sedentary people for subjects, with the few studies that have used athletes. So the usual advice you get in sports magazines comes to an aggregate conclusion that caffeine effects on performance are variable and inconclusive, and end with the vague conclusion that a couple of cups of coffee before competition might help, or might not.

The first error in these reviews is the assumption that a sedentary person who is coaxed to exercise, reacts to caffeine in the same way as an athlete. In a recent excellent review by Dr Luke Bucci, almost all the studies of sedentary subjects showed no effects of caffeine on performance, or on physiology. In contrast, 14 out of 16 studies with trained athletes showed significant benefits of caffeine, on performance or physiological responses or both.[1]

Caffeine Habituation

The second common error in much of the caffeine research lies in confusing subjects that habitually use coffee, tea, cocoa, caffeinated sodas, or chocolate, with those who have a low daily intake of caffeine. If you are a chocaholic, or it normally takes six cups of strong java to keep you perked throughout the day, then extra caffeine will not benefit your sport. Or if you use the herb **guarana**, the active constituent of which is caffeine, then no amount of extra caffeine will help you.

The only way round this problem is to ditch the caffeine from your everyday life. Three reliable studies have shown that it takes four days or more for caffeine tolerance to decline to the level where caffeine will start to influence performance.[2-4] Even then, effects are smaller than in people who normally avoid caffeine.

Many researchers continue to ignore this crucial variable. At least nine studies of caffeine and performance since 1980, failed to report on habitual caffeine use, or have required only 8-48 hours abstinence before studying the affects of caffeine supplementation on exercise.[3] No surprise then that results are variable and contradictory. Amounts of caffeine used in these studies varied from about 200 - 600 mg. That's about 2 - 5 cups of good coffee. To a habitual coffee drinker; that's his usual diet, so you would not expect it to have any special effect. Like giving an alcoholic a six-pack, and expecting him to keel over like a teenager losing his virginity to beer.

In the usual run of exposure to caffeine in the American diet, the amount of extra caffeine you have to use to get a significant effect on performance, seems to lie between the level used in most experimental studies and the level set by the US Olympic Committee for caffeine as a banned substance, (12 mcg/ml in urine). To reach this level, requires a dose of about 1,200 mg of pure caffeine. In pill form or as coffee, that's a great way to get an excruciating pain in the gut.

Dr Robert Voy relates one way athletes try to avoid this gastritis problem. At the 1984 Olympic Games, he intercepted a pile of pretty pink suppositories on their way to the US Cycling Team. Each one contained over 3000 mg of caffeine.[5] Next time someone flies by on the road when you are doing your best clip, look for the glazed eyes and strange movements of a man trying desperately to escape the nervous turmoil of an overstimulated rear end.

Excess caffeine can certainly screw you up. One study in the **American Journal of Psychiatry** reports anxiety, irritability, delirium and hallucinations, brought on by caffeine during exercise.[6] There does not appear to be a dose/response curve for caffeine benefits.[7] That is, above a certain amount, more caffeine does not produce better effects, probably because its toxic side-effects start to override the benefits. So there is no reason to take so much it sends you insane.

No one knows the right dose. A lot of good research from Dr David Costill's lab at Ball State University, Indiana, shows that there are large individual differences in responses to caffeine. He found performance improvements running from 0-80%.[8] From our 18 years of experience with athletes at the Colgan Institute, 1,000 mg is over the top for most athletes, especially if they abstain from caffeine in everyday life.

Caffeine Boosts Performance

Properly used, caffeine is a bonanza. Dr Melvin Williams and colleagues at Old Dominion University in Norfolk, Virginia have produced excellent reviews, showing that caffeine stimulates the central nervous system, increases the release of adrenalin, increases the use of bodyfat as fuel, and spares glycogen.[9,10]

There are also two *detrimental* effects of caffeine commonly cited by writers on sports nutrition: it is a well established diuretic (makes you lose water), and it is thermogenic (raises metabolic rate and body temperature).[11,12] Athletes are often warned that caffeine can make them dehydrate and overheat. But almost all the studies showing these effects were done with sedentary folk.

Recent research using athletes as subjects, found no diuresis or thermogenesis. Dr Baraket Falk and colleagues at McMaster University, Ontario, gave endurance runners caffeine at 7.5mg/kg body weight (560 mg for a 75 kg man). The dose had no effect on water loss, and did not raise temperature any higher than without it, in men running a treadmill to exhaustion at 70 - 75% of VO$_2$max.[13] That's about as fast as you can go in long endurance exercise. So forget those two old bogeys of sedentary caffeine use. Caffeine on the run is a different animal.

The most common beneficial finding of caffeine use is an increase in burning of bodyfat as fuel.[14,15] Compared with controls, up to 100% more bodyfat is used by subjects given caffeine. If your body is using more fat for energy, then it is sparing your muscle glycogen, and therefore will extend your time to exhaustion in long endurance events. One proviso: if you load carbohydrates, so that your muscles are filled with glycogen beyond their normal levels, then your body is more primed to use glycogen, and caffeine fails to increase the burning of fat.[16] Your body always takes the easiest of its many alternative routes. Supercharge one fuel source and it will use that first.

You also have to take the caffeine at the right time. Although many exercise studies have given caffeine one hour before exercise, studies focussing on measurement of free fatty acid metabolism, show that the fat-burning response to caffeine does not begin until 3 - 4 hours after ingestion.[16,17] Little use taking caffeine near the start of a race, as I watched some lively lads do at the last New York marathon, unless you are planning to be hyperkinetic *after* the race.

One of the latest studies controlled for all the above problems. At the Center for Physical Education at the Tasmanian Institute of Technology in Australia, Dr Lars McNaughton and colleagues selected cyclists whose diets had been analyzed to confirm their low habitual caffeine intake (less than 25 mg/day). They were tested against themselves as controls under double-blind conditions, pedalling a cycle ergometer to exhaustion under progressively increasing workload. Caffeine at 10 mg/kg bodyweight, or a placebo, were given as a flavored drink three hours prior to the test. That is a dose of 750 mg for a 75 kg (165 lb) man.

Results showed that the caffeine increased time to exhaustion by 18%, and exercise intensity by 24%. Caffeine allowed them to ride both longer and harder. It also increased use of free fatty acids for fuel, thereby sparing glycogen. It also raised the lactate threshold in relation to workload, suggesting that there was less build-up of lactic acid.[18] If you use caffeine correctly, that's the level of benefit you might expect.

A final tip. If you drink coffee to get your caffeine, which is a better way to do it than taking pills, avoid the cheap coffees made from *Coffea robusta* beans. They make a brown, sour brew that is hell on the gut. Go for *Coffea arabica* coffees, such as Gautamalan Antigua, 100% Columbian, or Kenyan AA. Grind the beans fresh and filter-brew a decent pot of maroon delight. Reserved for your hard training and competition days, it's ergogenic gold.

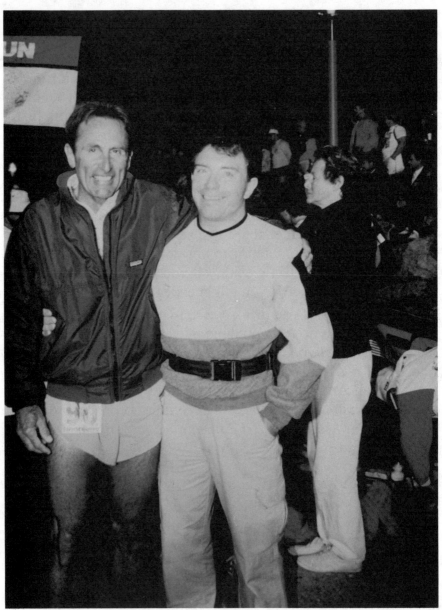

Michael Colgan with James Bond (the real one) at the start of the Western States 100 Mile Race. This running race over the Sierra Mountains, 100 miles non-stop is considered the most difficult endurance event in the world. James used a Colgan Institute nutrition and training program to help him win the coveted silver buckle in his first shot - at age 53!

Chapter 28

Real Ginseng Works

In 1985 I did a stint of lectures on sports nutrition to Chinese sports medicine specialists at Beijing Medical University, one of the largest medical schools and teaching hospitals in the world. It has a huge dispensary of herbal medicines. Not pills and potions, but the actual dried leaves, twigs and roots of the herbs, and a lot of stuff that looks like the dried remains of insects and animals. It also has a lot of ginsengs.

Following an ancient recipe, the Chinese pharmacists gleefully mixed several ginsengs and other herbs and pounded the lot to powder for me to use as a "sports tonic." The concoction didn't seem to improve my training, but I woke up every night with my heart pounding so hard it shook the bed.

Consulting their drug reference, the **Pen Tsao Kang Mu**, I found 42 formulas containing ginseng, many for relief of stress and fatigue. But they were all directed at sick people, not at athletes. The Chinese have concentrated on the medical effects of ginseng. They have not completed a single controlled trial on ginseng and sports performance.

Although Chinese physicians have been the authority on medical use of ginseng for over 4,000 years, they have never developed a methodology for its use with athletes. And nor has anyone else. Most of the research is new, and like any new development in science, fraught with error and ignorance.

First Find Your Ginseng

There are only three true ginseng plants (family: *Araliaceae*). **Panax** (*Panax ginseng*) is the original Chinese and Korean plant. **Sanchi** or **Tienchi** (*Panax notoginseng*) is the other ancient Eastern plant. **American ginseng** (*Panax quinquefolius*) is the modern American variant.

A fourth plant (*Eleutherococcus senticosus*), commonly called **Siberian** ginseng or **Wujia** ginseng is a member of the *Araliaceae* family, but sufficiently different to be considered a different species. It grows in wild profusion in Siberia, hence the name. Anecdotal tales of wonder from Russian athletes brought Siberian ginseng into the American sports market in the '70s. But there are no decent controlled studies showing beneficial effects on sports performance.

Even with the genuine ginsengs, the biggest problem is finding a potent source. The active chemicals in ginseng are 12 compounds (some researchers claim 13) popularly called ginsenosides.[1,2] In scientific gobbledegook they are, **triterpenoid saponin glycosides**. That's shorthand for, a fatty compound of hydrogen and oxygen that froths in solution, is derived from essential oils, and is usually linked to sugars. It is relatively simple to isolate.

Why am I laboring this point? Simply because many of the recent studies on ginseng and sports performance, especially American studies, have not analyzed the ginseng used, nor obtained any certification of its content of ginsenosides. A cardinal scientific sin: the researchers failed to determine whether the substance they were testing had any active ingredients.

The Colgan Institute has been testing ginseng since 1982. Almost two-thirds of the products we have analyzed are worthless. Ginseng teas are a good example. We have tested nine brands. All of them were over 95% plain table sugar. None of them showed any significant ginsenoside activity. Other experts have found the same. Dr Varro Tyler of Purdue University cites analyses of 54 ginseng products, 32 of which contained negligible amounts of ginsenosides.[3]

No active ingredients, no active effects. A typical example is the recent study on repeated, exhaustive exercise by Teves and colleagues.[4] They gave subjects 2 grams of ginseng per day. Sounds a lot until you realize that even top quality ginseng contains only 1-2% active ginsenosides. So, at best, these athletes were getting only 20-40 mg of active compounds, about one-tenth the amount needed to obtain significant changes.

Another negative study, published in America in **Federal Proceedings**, used even less ginseng. The researchers then panned the herb as ineffective when they found no evidence of its reputed anti-fatigue capacity.[5] But without a full analysis of the ginseng, they might as well have tested hedge clippings.

The problem is, the results of these easily accessible reports get repeated in American academic texts. But the harder to obtain European studies get left out. One example is the recent text, **Nutrition in Exercise and Sport**, edited by Drs James Hickson and Ira Wolinsky of the University of Texas.[6] It's review includes only a few studies that leave the reader with a false picture of ginseng research. It even states erroneously that there are no human studies with standardized ginseng extracts. I will give you more complete information.

The first step is to look for a standardized ginseng extract with a guaranteed percentage of ginsenosides. Today that is difficult. The recent explosive growth in US herb sales has caused a rapid revision of standards, as America tries to emulate sophisticated European herbal practices. "Standardized extract" has become a market buzzword, as new products seek to replace the uncontrolled and largely useless herbals made here from bulk powdered plants. So don't be fooled by shiny new labels.

Fortunately there is a Swiss standardized ginseng extract called G115, that has been used in many independent studies since 1971. It is sold in America under the trade name Ginsana.

Some of the recent research has focused on athletic performance.

Ginseng Improves Endurance

One way in which ginseng might boost endurance is by stimulating the brain and the adrenal/pituitary system to produce greater levels of excitatory hormones. In 1985, Dr M. Samura and colleagues showed with rabbits, that the G115 extract had pronounced stimulating effects on brain activity.[7] And Dr T. Kaku and colleagues showed in animals that ginsenosides produced significant resistance to fatigue.[8] In a recent study with human volunteers, Dr L. D'Angelo and colleagues showed that the G115 extract improved psychomotor performance on a series of tests, by maintaining alertness.[9] These studies suggest that ginseng could improve athletic performance by delaying fatigue.

There is also some research that measure energy use more directly. In a series of animal studies, Dr E.V. Avakian and colleagues have shown that standardized ginseng extract spares glycogen and increases oxidation of free fatty acids. That is, it reduces the body's use of its limited store of glycogen and increases use of the much larger store of bodyfat.[10,11]

Such effects should increase endurance. One study by Dr V.K. Singh and colleagues supports this view. In a nasty little procedure, rats were made to swim in a vat until they sank from exhaustion. After rescue from drowning, their diet was supplemented with ginsenosides for some weeks. Then they went in the vat again. Swimming time to exhaustion was extended by up to 40%.[12] That's a huge increase when you realize that both times they were swimming for their lives, so the first time was an all out effort, and the second time a big improvement on it.

Ginsenosides Lift Lungpower

Human subjects will not cooperate by swimming in vats until they sink. So measurements on men have to be a little more subtle. In a double-blind study with the G115 extract, Dr E. Dorling and colleagues gave subjects 200 mg per day for 12 weeks.

Then they measured lung functions that are reasonable predictors of athletic performance: vital capacity, forced expiratory volume, peak expiratory flow and maximum breathing capacity. After 12 weeks the supplemented group showed a 44% greater improvement than the placebo group.[13] A later study by Drs I. Forgo and G. Schimert in 1985 confirmed these findings.[14] G115 significantly enhanced vital capacity over nine weeks supplementation.

Another measure linked with capacity to use oxygen, is the level of serum lactic acid, which builds up in muscles during exercise and is a major cause of fatigue.[15] Drs I. Forgo and A.M. Kirchdorfer measured blood lactic acid levels at different workloads in 20 athletes. Then they supplemented subjects with G115 daily for nine weeks and measured them again. The supplement significantly reduced lactic acid levels.[16]

Ginsenosides & Performance

The above findings that ginsenosides increase brain activity, hormone activity, and lung power, and reduce lactic acid, fatigue, and glycogen use, are of great interest to scientists. But you as an athlete really want to know about improved sports performance. A representative study was completed recently at the Center for Physical Education of the Tasmanian Institute of Technology in Australia by Dr Lars McNaughton and colleagues. It was well controlled and ran double-blind for 12 weeks on experienced athletes. In addition to physiological measures, they measured direct effects on strength and on recovery time from exhaustive exercise.

Compared with a group given placebo pills, the group given ginsenosides showed significantly faster recovery. They also showed an average increase of 22% in pectoralis strength, and 18% in quadricep strength, above the increases achieved by the placebo group.[17] For trained athletes that's a great improvement.

The number of controlled studies is still small, but the consistent results do qualify ginseng as a legitimate ergogenic aid.

A dose of 200 mg/day of standardized ginseng extract appears to be effective. The G115 extract sold by Ginsana is the only product that has been tested in repeated studies. But, following these studies, there are now equivalent standarized ginsengs appearing on the market, including Sports Ginseng by Nature's Herbs.

Don't expect any overnight magic. If you examine the studies on physiological changes caused by ginseng, you will see that improvements are slow and steady, over months of daily ginseng use combined with continuous training. That's the way it should be. If we don't have to work to win, all the fun and pride of achievement go. Then we stop playing and do something else.

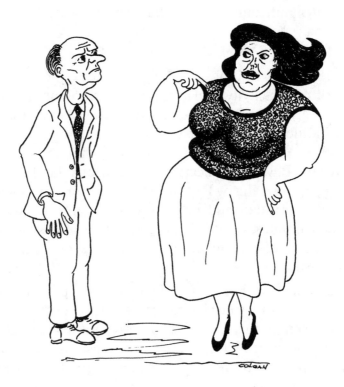

"You know how fat people all have a thin person inside them trying to get out.
I have three."

Part VI

Anabolics

If you continue to do what you've always done. You will continue to get what you've always got.

**Michael Colgan, Australian Institute of Sport
Lectures, 1987**

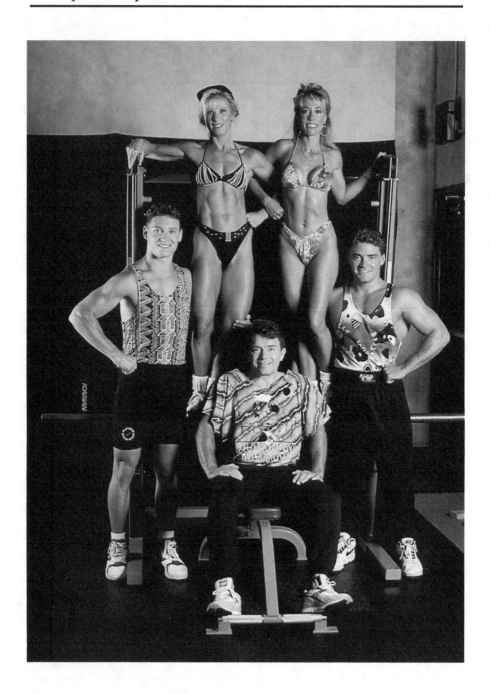

There is no better feeling . . . . . .

Chapter 29

Chromium Boosts Insulin Efficiency

Before the 1970s, chromium was considered great for car bumpers, but useless for human nutrition. In the 1968 handbook of the Recommended Dietary Allowances, chromium rated only two sentences of dismissal.[1] Then Dr Walter Mertz of the USDA showed that **trivalent chromium**, possibly containing an elusive compound that he dubbed **"glucose tolerance factor" (GTF)**, is essential for normal insulin metabolism.[2]

Because of the high incidence of diabetes in Western Society, most people know that insulin enables the body to deal with sugars and other carbohydrates. Not so well known is its equally important function in dealing with proteins. After protein is digested into its constituent amino acids, insulin facilitates entry of these amino acid building blocks into muscle cells. Once inside the cell, they are built into muscle proteins, again under the influence of insulin.[2] The more efficient your insulin metabolism, the more amino acids get inside the cells, and the more muscle you can make. Chromium enables the insulin to do its work.

Insulin also has complex roles in the control of bodyfat and in lipid metabolism. And it has a direct anabolic function in promoting the manufacture of **somatomedins** by the liver.[3]

These are the muscle growth factors produced under the influence of human growth hormone. Without somatomedins, also called **insulin-like growth factor**, you would grow very little muscle at all.[4] Chapter 32 gives you more details. Without adequate chromium to empower your insulin, manufacture of somatomedins is likely to slow down to a dribble.

These discoveries are hot off the press of today's science. Much of the work is not yet published, or even finished. But I am sketching the published studies here because of the great implications for athletes. We are coming to understand, that unless you have optimal chromium nutrition, your insulin metabolism, your muscle, your strength, your supply and use of glycogen and fats as fuel, your endurance, and your level of bodyfat, will all be sub-optimal.

Remember, I am talking about insulin *efficiency*, not insulin amount. Unless you have diabetes, you have all the insulin you need, because your body can make it instantly. To take extra insulin would be highly toxic to the non-diabetic. It would also cause a big rise in bodyfat, because the body protects itself from excess insulin by converting it into triglycerides (fats), which are then deposited into fat cells.[5] The effective supplement is not insulin but chromium.

Chromium Deficiency Widespread

What you are trying to do is make your own insulin work better. A giant step in that direction is adequate chromium in your diet. Unfortunately, the American diet is more deficient in chromium than in any other trace mineral. The 1989 RDA handbook recommends a daily intake of 50 - 200 mcg as safe and adequate (for sedentary folk).[6] Other studies show that some sedentary subjects require 290 mcg/day to remain in chromium balance.[7] Most people get nowhere near that amount.

Even a supposedly ideal American diet of 2,800 calories, carefully designed by dietitians to be complete in all nutrients, checked out at only 89 mcg of chromium.[8] Very few people get even that much. Drs Richard Anderson and Adriane Kozlovsky at the USDA Human Nutrition Research Center in Beltsville, MD, showed recently that 90% of the self-selected diets of a representative group of men and women contained less than 50 mcg of chromium a day.[9] The average chromium intake was only 29 mcg.

With that level of nutritional support, your insulin metabolism is barely limping along. We have measured the effects many times in athletes who are referred to the Colgan Institute with blood sugar problems. They cannot gain much muscle or strength. Their endurance is below par despite the best training. They are prone to infections and injuries. They have difficulty losing bodyfat. Their blood sugar is unstable, often swinging wildly between hypoglycemia (low blood sugar) and hyperglycemia (high blood sugar). But on all the usual medical tests for disease they appear perfectly normal. No disease: sound as a bell. In fact, they are a mess.

Does chromium help? Damn right! In more than 50% of these athletes, supplementary chromium significantly reduces symptoms. Our case findings agree with controlled studies throughout America. In more than half the patients treated with chromium, glucose tolerance improves dramatically.[10] Technically, a lot of the people in these studies are sick, and not comparable to healthy athletes. But chromium also works with healthy people who have no problem with glucose tolerance. In a well-controlled trial, normal men given supplementary chromium *all* showed improvements in insulin metabolism.[11]

Athletes Need Effective Chromium

But these men were not athletes. As I keep stressing throughout this book, athletes are a special case. Your body works differently to the bodies of sedentary people. Dr Richard Anderson and colleagues at the USDA, have shown repeatedly that the increase in insulin metabolism caused by exercise, increases the body's chromium requirement.[12-14] In one representative study, urinary loss of chromium increased almost five-fold after a six-mile run. Overall daily loss of chromium almost doubled on running days, compared with non-running days.[13] And the harder you train, the more you use.[14] Athletes may require twice as much chromium as couch potatoes to maintain efficient insulin metabolism.

As we saw above, you can't get the additional chromium from your food. It just isn't in there. It has to come from supplements. The best natural source is brewers yeast. But the best brewers yeast contains only a few micrograms of chromium per gram. If athletes in hard training need twice the chromium of sedentary people, then to get it from yeast means eating three or four ounces a day. We have tried it. You get the chromium O.K., but the yeast creates havoc in your gut.

Until recently, the other supplementary sources of chromium were inorganic chromiums, such as chromium chloride, and various inorganic chromiums mixed with yeast or chelated with proteins. There are two problems with these products. First, only one-half of one percent of inorganic chromium is absorbed, and there is little evidence that attaching it to other nutrients improves the situation.[15] Second, even if it is absorbed, the biological activity of inorganic chromium is very low.[16]

New Chromiums

Now there are two new forms of chromium with similar names, chromium polynicotinate, and chromium picolinate. Both are claimed to be highly biologically active. But, despite claims in articles in bodybuilding magazines, and in product literature from the manufacturer of chromium polynicotinate, there is only one published study in a reputable scientific journal showing that it has any effects. That study did report a reduction of cholesterol in some subjects.[17] It was only published in abstract, however, so there is no way to check the validity of the methods used.

In contrast, chromium picolinate was developed by Dr

Gary Evans at the USDA (Dr Evans is now Professor of Chemistry at Bemidgi State University, Minnesota). Chromium picolinate has since been patented and the patent is owned by the US Government, and is licensed exclusively to the Nutrition 21 company of San Diego, who are the sole supplier to the nutrition industry. I am spelling this out to indicate the legitimacy of this compound, because some magazine articles have accused Dr Evans of promoting chromium picolinate because he holds the patent. To clear up this matter, I wrote to the US Patent Office in 1989, and their reply is reproduced below.

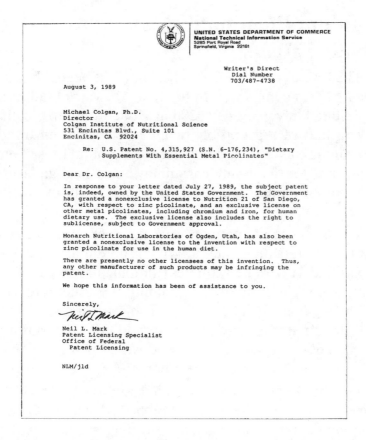

Figure 7. Letter from US Patent Office detailing ownership of chromium picolinate.

Chromium picolinate is five-fold better absorbed than inorganic chromiums. And it is very bioactive in improving insulin metabolism. Previous chromium compounds have improved glucose tolerance only in pre-diabetic conditions, but have failed most cases of overt diabetes.[18] Chromium picolinate is more powerful. In a controlled study at Mercy Hospital, San Diego, Dr Raymond Press found that chromium picolinate reduced fasting blood sugar by 18%, and significantly improved blood sugar stability in overt diabetics.[19] If it can do that with patients whose insulin system is shot, it may do even more for athletes.

Chromium Picolinate Has Anabolic Effects

The research with athletes has only just begun, but there are three studies completed. In the first, Dr Muriel Gillman at Bemidgi State University, gave 200 mcg of chromium picolinate per day to half of a group of freshmen who had enrolled in weight training classes. The study ran double-blind for six weeks. Freshmen not receiving any chromium made negligible gains. Those on the chromium gained an average of 3.5 lbs of lean body mass.[19]

That's a huge increase in six weeks, even for novices who have not exploited their muscle growth potential. So a larger study was done with trained athletes (football players) to validate it. Over six weeks intensive weight training, the athletes receiving chromium picolinate gained 5.7 lbs of lean body mass, compared with 4.0 lbs for the control group. In addition, the chromium group lost 3.6% of bodyfat, compared with 1% for the control group.[19] The chromium was a clear benefit.

Another independent controlled study was done in 1991 at Louisiana State University by Deborah Hasten and colleagues. They supplemented male and female college students with 200 mcg per day of TwinLab's Chromic Fuel brand of chromium picolinate, over a 12-week weight training program, in a double-blind trial. As we have found in case studies at the Colgan

Institute, 200 mcg of chromium picolinate made no difference in the male groups tested by Hasten. Probably because of their larger bodyweight, males over 165 lb may require 400-600 mcg per day to register a statistically significant difference in a short controlled trial. But for Hasten's female group, with their lower bodyweight, 200 mcg may have been sufficient. The females using chromium gained 2.7 kg of lean body mass, compared with 1.5 kg for the control group.[20]

New animal studies provide further evidence of muscle-enhancing and fat-reducing effects of chromium picolinate. In a series of studies at the Department of Animal Science at LSU Agricultural Center in Baton Rouge, pigs were fed chromium picolinate and compared with a control group. The chromium increased pig lean mass by an average of 7% and reduced what they term "tenth-rib fat" by 21%.[21] In three more studies at the same facility, chromium picolinate significantly reduced serum cholesterol levels in pigs.[22] As yet, these new studies are only published in abstract form. Nevertheless, there is no doubt that chromium picolinate is highly biologically active.

It certainly shows more biological activity than chromium nicotinate. In a study just gone to press in the **Journal of Inorganic Biochemistry,** chromium picolinate caused muscle cells to take up more than twice as much of the branched chain amino acid leucine, than chromium nicotinate or chromium chloride. It also showed about twice the affinity for insulin as the other two forms, and carried about three times as much insulin into the muscle cells.[23] All these effects indicate that chromium picolinate is the most active form of chromium on the market.

At the Colgan Institute, we have been using various forms of chromium with athletes for the past 18 years. Four years ago we began using chromium picolinate and chromium polynicotinate. Since then we have measured rates of growth of strength and muscle mass over periods of 1-2 years in individual athletes, and compared them with their rates of growth over the year before they began chromium supplementation. The anabolic effects we have found occur only with chromium picolinate. Based on our results with hundreds of athletes from club to Olympic status, three years ago we decided to switch entirely to chromium picolinate. The research published in the last two years supports that decision.

In our case studies, we use 200 - 800 mcg per day of chromium picolinate, depending on bodyweight and other factors. We compare the rate of muscle gain and the level of bodyfat with each athlete's records for the year prior to use of the supplement. Increases in muscle growth and strength, and reductions in bodyfat occur reliably, but more slowly than those reported in the controlled studies. Our results, however, which take 6-12 months to show, are more consistent with the chemistry of insulin metabolsim.[24]

Chromium picolinate will not build you up and slim you down overnight. But gradually, gradually, a little more muscle and a little less fat is what you might call "the picolinate advantage."

Chapter 30

Real Anabolics

Most young athletes who turn up at the Colgan Institute come seeking muscle and strength -- fast. They know from the TAC Track and Field Coaching Manual used in schools and colleges that strength is the key to greater speed and greater endurance.[1] In any sport, if you take two athletes of equal performance, and make one of them 10% stronger, he will start to beat the other every time. If you make him 100% stronger, it's no longer any contest.

With the right approach we can make many athletes more than 200% stronger. I'm talking 20 x 1-arm push-ups, one-arm pull-ups, double-bodyweight bench presses, 150 lb preacher curls, triple bodyweight squats - you name it. Don't believe me? Come on down, we'll be happy to demonstrate.

The four essentials for large and rapid gains in strength are, adequate sleep, complete nutrition, progressive intensity of training, and the anabolic drive. We covered sleep in Chapter 7. Suffice to say here, that 8 hours in bed per night is not enough. In agreement with the best coaches in the world, we advise all athletes to get 8 hours sleep (81/2-9 hours in bed), plus a 1/2-1 hour nap after each training session. Remember, you gain strength only during rest never during exercise. I was pleased to read the other day that the notorious, but very successful "Guru of Muscle," Dan Duchaine, is also recommending naps after training.[2]

The second essential for rapid strength gains, complete nutrition, we discuss repeatedly throughout this book. If even one essential nutrient is missing or insufficient, then growth is retarded. When training for strength, never allow your nutrition to falter, even for a few hours. Keep extra nutrient packs at work, at the gym, and in your bag. When you have to travel take all your nutrients with you, so all you have to find in the nutritional desert of American hotels is carbs and water.

The third essential for rapid strength gains is progressive intensity and variety of training. Once you are past the novice stage, your muscles quickly adapt to particular movements and to a given level of exercise. The sets, reps, weights, movements, and intensity that built them well two months ago, will not work today. That's the irony of the human machine. Exercise is stress that threatens the integrity of the muscle. The muscle responds to a given level of exercise by building just to the extent that the exercise no longer affects it.

In fact, muscles get ever more efficient at dealing with particular movements and levels of stress. Consequently, after about 8-12 weeks of doing any set of movements regularly, the muscles start to *lose* strength, if you continue the exercise that originally built them. Familiar problem? Should be. I watch it happening in gyms all across America. Unless you are committed to *progressive intensity and variety*, you haven't got a prayer.

A word of caution. Progressive intensity and variety doesn't mean that the best way for a novice to get strong is to increase weights every workout and make random changes to the exercises used. Unless you get strong in the basics first, which takes at least six months, you are simply setting up for injury. And unless you put all four essentials together you will make little progress. The *average* progress in strength gain in many gyms we have monitored is only a small notch above zero. Yet, if you put everything together right, you can more than double your strength in a year: which brings us to the most important principle of all.

The Anabolic Drive

The fourth essential for rapid strength gains is an ample anabolic stimulus. The most powerful anabolic substance made by the body is **human growth hormone.** Healthy adult males 20-40 years old, make 0.4 mg to 1.0 mg per day. Those who exercise intensely make the higher levels. You have a store of the stuff totalling 5.0 to 10.0 mg, in the pituitary gland, that pea-sized ball that hangs on a stalk off your brain about an inch behind your nose.[3]

Growth hormone is crucial to athletes. It is the primary stimulus to muscle growth *and strength,* bone growth *and strength*, tendon growth *and strength*, injury repair, and mobilization of bodyfat for use as energy. Low production of growth hormone and low release into the bloodstream place absolute limits on growth.[3]

It's a difficult job to increase your mean daily level of growth hormone release. So it is not surprising that many athletes take anabolic steroids in order to grow muscle. Steroids mimic natural testosterone function in the body, which itself is not half bad as an anabolic stimulus. But, as you will see in the drug chapters, steroids have a real unhealthy downside.

So what's to do? Unless you have a continuous, optimum supply of anabolic hormones, all the mega-nutrition programs, all the secret training systems, all the coaches, personal trainers, and chanting gurus in orange bedsheets, cannot make you achieve your athletic potential.

You read a lot about "good genetics" determining how one man can put on pounds of muscle and strength, while another on equal training and nutrition gains only ounces. And genetics has a lot to do with it. But measurements of case studies of hundreds of athletes at the Colgan Institute, indicate that insufficient anabolic stimulation is often the crucial problem. Genes can't be changed, but anabolic stimulation can. So we have spent a lot of years researching the best ways to do it with nutrition.

Human Growth Hormone

Recent studies with older men show unequivocally that injection of synthetic human growth hormone significantly increases muscle mass and bone strength, and reduces bodyfat in human subjects. Human growth hormone is the most powerful anabolic stimulus known to science. Its power is clear from these studies, because the subjects did not change their sedentary lifestyles, nor did they change their average American diets. So without any weight training, and without any proper nutrition, in six months they still gained a lot of muscle (8.8%), and lost a ton of fat (14.4%).[4]

Growth hormone also works with highly trained young athletes. In one recent study, Dr D.M. Crist and colleagues gave low doses of recombinant biosynthetic growth hormone to athletes doing intense training. Results showed very similar increases in muscle growth and reductions in bodyfat as those found in the studies of aging men.[5]

Since this research was publicized through television and other media in July 1990, we have received thousands of calls, including calls from physicians, scientists, and hospitals asking, - what's the real score? As I first warned in a popular article in 1988,[6] the real score is that these discoveries about growth hormone are one of the most important advances in medicine in the last fifty years.

The understanding we have gained about the hormonal control of human growth will revolutionize the way we think about athletic potential. But like every great advance, it will be abused to hell. Instead of using the knowledge to grow improved human bodies naturally, people will mistakenly scramble to use the drug itself. By the turn of the century, human growth hormone will be one of the most misused drugs in the history of science.

Already, thousands of athletes are *illegally* obtaining human growth hormone for their own use.[7] Don't be one of them! As we will see in the drug chapters, the downside is worse than for steroids. The real answer is to stimulate your own production of growth hormone. Adults have a fair store of the stuff in the pituitary gland, up to about 10 mg in males aged 25 to 45. The trick for those who want new muscle fast, is to get your body to release it into the bloodstream.

Once in the bloodstream, growth hormone goes to the liver, where it is destroyed within a couple of hours. But in the process it stimulates production of **insulin-like growth factors,** also called **somatomedins**. The somatomedins made by the liver are then used to control the steady growth of muscle during rest and sleep. This connection to insulin and the liver are crucial. We will return to them later, after I lay out the picture.

The best nutritional method to stimulate release of growth hormone is still to use certain amino acids. In this chapter, we cover the most effective: tryptophan, glycine, ornithine, and arginine. But you can't just pop a few pills like some of the supplement ads suggest. To do it right you have to know a bit about the link between aminos and the brain.

To release growth hormone you have to stimulate the pituitary gland in the right way. Because of its master role in controlling all your bodily hormones, the pituitary is well protected, hanging on an isolated stalk from the middle of your brain. Not many external substances can get at it, certainly not dietary amino acids. You have to hit it indirectly.

Getting Aminos Into the Brain

The pituitary is stimulated to release growth hormone by another hormone circulating in the brain, called **somatocrinin.**[8] Levels of somatocrinin can be increased by increasing levels of brain **neurotransmitters**. Neurotransmitters are the chemicals that carry information from one nerve to another. Their activity constitutes your mind, your consciousness, all your schemes and dreams. So before you mess with them you better know what you are doing.

To increase neurotransmitters, you have to get the amino

acids that influence them past what is called **the blood-brain barrier**. That is a system designed by evolution to protect the brain. To cross the barrier, amino acids have to be carried by specific transport molecules. The transport capacity is very limited and once it is full, no more aminos can get across for some time.

There are four different types of transporter. Each will carry only one specific class of amino acids. The four main classes are illustrated in Figure 8 below.

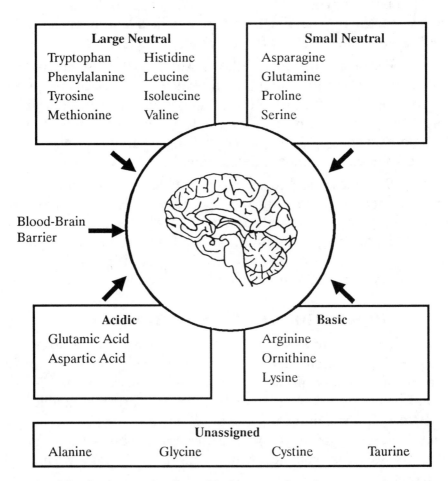

Figure 8. Main classes of amino acids, in terms of carrier systems that transport them across the blood-brain barrier.

To succeed in releasing growth hormone you need this chart, because even if you use two effective aminos from the same class, they compete with each other and less of each gets across. If you mix effective and ineffective aminos of the same class, then very little of the effective amino gets through.

Tryptophan Releases Growth Hormone

Tryptophan is a member of the **large neutral** class of aminos. It is a precursor of the neurotransmitter **serotonin,** a compound that slows down brain activity during rest and sleep. A short while after you fall asleep, your pituitary gland releases a burst of growth hormone. Recent research by Dr Richard Wurtman and colleagues at MIT, links the size of this burst to the amount of serotonin released from the brainstem.[9,10]

To get enough tryptophan into the brain to raise serotonin levels and increase growth hormone release, you have to take it in the absence of any other large neutral amino acid. So if you take it after a chicken dinner, or any other protein, it can't work. Or if you take it with a branched chain amino acid supplement (leucine, isoleucine, valine) it can't work. They are also large neutrals, and will compete with the tryptophan for blood-brain transport.

But on an empty stomach, oral tryptophan is a potent growth hormone releaser. A dose of 5 - 10 grams will cause a large rise in serum growth hormone, even when taken during the day.[9,11,12] Daytime use is not advisable though, unless you take it an hour before you plan to nap. Tryptophan has sedative action in the majority of subjects,[13] and may reduce performance. At night tryptophan does double duty for athletes, many of whom have mild insomnia. It helps put you to sleep, and also increases the release of growth hormone.

The only problem in using tryptophan, is that it is currently banned for US sale by the FDA. It was sold freely for the last 50 years, with great human benefit until 1989. Then a contaminated batch from Japan was widely distributed in many different products, and caused some 1,500 cases of **eosinophilia-myalgia syndrome (EMS)**, which is gobbledegook for high eosinophils (a type of cell in the immune system), with muscle pain. No joke: it is implicated in more than a dozen deaths.

The contaminated tryptophan has now been traced to a Japanese company,[14] and the contaminant identified by Dr Kasunori Sakimoto. Amino acids are made by bacterial fermentation. Use of a new strain of bacteria the fermentation, produced along with the tryptophan, the compound **1-methyl-1,2,3,4-tetrahydro-beta-carboline-3-carboxylic acid.**[15] It is toxic to everyone, but in sensitive individuals causes the serious disease EMS.

I am spelling out this incident to demonstrate how easy it is for chemical pollution to spread anywhere in the world, even from a chemical plant in Japan to the heartland of America. There is plenty of cheap and nasty stuff out there. Your sole defense in using amino acids, or any other supplements, is to buy only from reputable, long established companies.

Now that the tryptophan mystery is solved, the FDA could let it back on the market, but I doubt they will. If you can get pure l-tryptophan (it is freely available in Europe), then this inexpensive nutrient is a proven way to release growth hormone. Studies show that doses of 5-10 grams are effective.[9,11] Nevertheless, it is a banned nutrient in America, so I am **not** recommending that you use it.

Glycine Releases Growth Hormone

Glycine has had intermittent popularity as an ergogenic aid since the 1940s when Chaikelis first showed that 6 grams of glycine per day for 10 weeks caused large increases in strength of trained athletes.[16] But, until recently, it was thought that glycine worked because it is the precursor of **creatine,** which is needed for normal muscle contractions. Shortage of creatine causes muscle weakness. Now we know that glycine increases strength probably because it causes growth hormone release and consequent muscle growth.

Glycine has not been used much as a growth hormone releaser until recently, because medical research suggested that it functions only as an *inhibitory* neurotransmitter.[17] Recent research, however, shows that glycine potentiates the action of excitatory amino acids at important receptor sites on brain neurons called the **N-methyl-D-aspartate receptors.**[18] But don't, repeat don't, take glycine in conjunction with tryptophan. A derivative of tryptophan called **kynurenate** competes with glycine for space on the neuron receptors.[18]

Injection of as little as 4 grams of glycine can cause growth hormone release [19] a surprising finding because the body *makes* up to 20 grams of glycine a day. Effects of oral doses are equally surprising. In one study, 6.75 grams of oral glycine, raised growth hormone levels almost four-fold.[20] In another recent study reported by the late Dr Carl Pfeiffer, of the Princeton Brain Bio Center, an oral dose of 30 grams of glycine raised growth hormone levels *ten-fold!*[19]

Unlike most other amino acids that taste like the droppings of a moribund horse, even in high doses, glycine is pleasant to take, and has no reported side-effects in the controlled studies. One caution: at the Colgan Institute we have had several reports from athletes, that glycine doses above 15 grams can cause a doozy of a headache, especially if taken before a hard workout.

There are also reports that abnormalities of glycine metabolism are linked with Lou Gehrig's disease.[22] But, in healthy people, glycine metabolism is tightly controlled by multiple mechanisms. Nevertheless, the long-term safety of glycine use in humans is not known. As with any other nutrient in this book, I advise you to read the research studies given. Use of any nutrient is always at your own choice and risk.

Arginine/Ornithine Bonanza

The darling of free-form amino acids is still arginine, and research continues to pile up supporting its use by athletes. There are now more than 50 positive studies. Arginine is so reliable at releasing growth hormone, that it is used as a test of pituitary function in undersized children.[23-25] It works equally well on adults.[26-29]

Some skeptical folk, including some sports medicine professionals, who cannot have read the studies, still insist that arginine is at best a weak and variable stimulus to growth hormone release, or that the response is very small in adults, and non-existent in older people. There is a pile of new studies that prove these skeptics wrong. I can't review them all here, but will give some details from two of the latest that are representative of the evidence.

The first is in the medical journal **Regulatory Peptides,** by Dr Akitsugu Masuda and colleagues at the Institute of Clinical Endocrinology of Tokyo Women's Medical College, and Dr Nicholas Ling at the Department of Molecular Endocrinology of the prestigious Whittier Institute in San Diego. I'm spelling this out to show that it is not some rinkydink study in an obscure journal of irreproducible results, published in Outer Mongolia. This is as mainstream science as you get.

They gave arginine hydrochloride to 12 healthy men, in a study comparing the effects of arginine against the prescription drug l-dopa. L-dopa is a powerful growth hormone releaser. More important, they also compared arginine against injections of somatocrinin, the hormone used by the body itself to release growth hormone.

Peak growth hormone release to l-dopa was 14.6 mcg/l, a large amount. Peak growth hormone release to arginine was 15.4 mcg/l, even larger. Total growth hormone release to somatocrinin was 891.7 mcg.min/l, a very large amount. Total growth hormone release to arginine was 898.2 mcg.min/l, larger again. So arginine causes at least as big a boost to growth hormone release as the hormone naturally used by the body to do the same job.[30]

It still works even on people in their '70s. In a study just published, researchers from the Division of Endocrinology at the

University of Turin, gave 30 grams of arginine to eight normal but short children, eight normal adults aged 20 - 30, and eight normal adults aged 66 - 82.[31]

Results showed mean levels of growth hormone release of 12.6 mcg/l for the children, 14.3 mcg/l for the young adults, and 9.8 mcg/l for the older adults. Though the older subjects showed a lower response, it is still a highly significant release of growth hormone, about triple the average level found in the blood. From these and similar recent studies, there is no longer any doubt that arginine is a powerful growth hormone releaser, and that it works in adults of all ages.

Growth Hormone Released Is Active

All the above studies were with *injected* arginine. Further objections to arginine use by athletes concern whether it will work by mouth, and whether the growth hormone released is active, that is, will work as an anabolic. There is one report showing that external stimulation of the pituitary by chemical means, some-times produces growth hormone that is biologically inactive.[32]

Some researchers have also extrapolated from the studies of injected arginine, which usually use 15 - 30 grams, to suggest that oral doses would have to be massive, 40 - 60 grams, to have any effects. Considering the vomit-triggering taste of arginine powder, or the alternative of 100 or more arginine pills a day, and its tendency to upset the gut in large doses, that would be too tough for most athletes to swallow.

There are only two studies indicating that oral arginine can be effective in smaller amounts. At the University of Rome, Italy, Dr A. Isidori and colleagues found that 1,200 mg of l-arginine-2-pyrrolidone-5-carboxylate, plus 1,200 mg of l-lysine hydrochloride, given to healthy males aged 15 - 20, caused a *seven-fold* increase in serum growth hormone.[33]

These results are way out of line with the rest of the literature, and are the source of many exaggerated sales claims for arginine/lysine supplements. The form of arginine may have been important, because you will see from the illustration of the blood-brain barrier in Figure 12, that both arginine and lysine are **basic** amino acids. So the lysine would compete with the arginine for transport, thereby reducing the amount of arginine reaching the brain. In America this arginine is readily available as **l-arginine pyroglutamate**, but no studies have used it here with athletes.

The Isidori study also showed that the growth hormone released was biologically active. They found increased somatomedin activity, indicating that the growth hormone was initiating the sequence of chemical events necessary for the increased growth of muscle and other lean tissue.

Ornithine May Be Effective

The second positive study with small amounts of arginine also used ornithine. It did not measure growth hormone or somatomedins directly, but looked for effects of increased growth hormone activity. Researchers at the University of Texas, El Paso, gave 18 men 1 gram of arginine plus 1 gram of ornithine over a 5-week weight training program. (For many purposes arginine and ornithine act interchangeably, or are converted to each other in the human body). Compared with a control group, supplemented subjects lost more body fat, and made bigger improvements in their muscle to fat ratios. These effects provide *some* evidence that the oral supplements acted as an anabolic.[34]

We don't know whether it was the arginine or the ornithine or both that did the trick. *Injected* ornithine is effective at releasing growth hormone in animals.[35] But human subjects given oral ornithine show only minor effects.[36]

In the latest study, Dr Luke Bucci and colleagues at Biotics Research Corporation and the University of Texas in Houston, gave male and female bodybuilders either 40, 100, or 170 mg ornithine *hydrochloride* per kilogram bodyweight. Serum growth hormone levels tended to rise with all doses, but rose significantly only with the highest dose. The peak growth hormone level 90 minutes after taking the ornithine was four times the baseline. For a 75 kg man to copy this study, he would need to take a dose of 12.75 grams.[39]

It may be the form of ornithine that has been at fault. New studies on burn patients and on patients undergoing surgery show clearly that ornithine in the alpha-ketoglutarate form maintains muscle during severe trauma.[37,38] Patients given oral **ornithine alpha-ketoglutarate** after surgery reduced muscle loss and increased synthesis of muscle protein.

Alpha-ketoglutarate is what is called the **carbon skeleton** of the amino acid glutamine. It was developed during the '60s to treat liver disease by reducing ammonia build-up. But when combined with ornithine (2 molecules ornithine to 1 molecule alpha-ketoglutarate), it produces a release of growth hormone much larger than with either compound used alone.[39] Given orally, it also spares muscle nitrogen, that is, reduces the break-down of muscle and loss of muscle amino acids.[40] If you are using ornithine to grow muscle, make it alpha-ketoglutarate.

How Much Arginine/Ornithine?

No studies are completed yet on similar doses of arginine. Preliminary results from a study now ongoing at the Colgan Institute, suggest that 200 mg arginine hydrochloride, or 100 mg ornithine alpha-ketoglutarate per kilogram bodyweight per day, may be an effective level. That is 15 grams or 7.5 grams per day for a 75 kg athlete. Although arginine and ornithine seem to be non-toxic at this level, it's still a helluva lot.

Especially on an empty stomach. To avoid cancelling the arginine/ornithine effect, they have to be taken three hours distant from other amino acids of the same class, and from any protein food. That's a difficult condition to fulfill for athletes, who know that the best eating regimen is 5-6 small meals a day. We teach athletes to get up in the middle of the night to take growth hormone releasing amino acids.

The main variables we use to calculate arginine use at the

Colgan Institute are given in Table 21. For ornithine alpha-ketoglutarate, we use half the values given. We use these aminos in cycles of not more than 12 weeks, with a 6-8 week rest between cycles, and *strictly*, only in conjunction with training. No training on a particular day, no aminos that day.

Use of arginine at these levels causes stomach upsets, diarrhea, or headaches in some athletes. Arginine also tends to promote herpes outbreaks in athletes who have either oral or genital herpes.[40] When any of these conditions occur, the athletes cut back on use and symptoms disappear. To combat any herpes outbreaks we use 1 gram l-lysine three times daily, which has proved effective in some controlled trials.[36] But don't take lysine along with arginine. You will lose the arginine effect.

As with all amino acids, entering the brain in more than usual physiological amounts, the long-term safety is unknown. Read the scientific studies and decide for yourself at your own choice and risk, whether you want to use them. If you do, you also need to fulfill other conditions for maximum muscle growth. All the details are given in Chapter 32.

Table 21. Daily amounts of l-arginine hydrochloride used with athletes to stimulate anabolic processes. For l-ornithine alpha-ketoglutarate, use only half these figures. For a combination of the two compounds, use two parts l-arginine hydrochloride to one part l-ornithine alpha-ketoglutarate to total three-quarters of the figures shown.

Training hrs/week	Bodyweight (lbs) 80-130	131-170	171-220	Above 220
4-10	3 gm	6 gm	9 gm	12 gm
11-17	4 gm	8 gm	12 gm	16 gm
18-24	5 gm	10 gm	15 gm	20 gm
Above 24	6 gm	12 gm	18 gm	24 gm

Chapter 31

Anabolics/ Ergogenics and Snake Oil

Ancient Greek athletes used the seeds of *Areca catechu* (Betel nut) and the leaves of *Catha edulis* (Khat) arduously shipped in sailing scows from the shores of North Africa. Both plants contain stimulants with effects like amphetamines. The Greeks also used hallucinatory mushrooms and the entrails of poisonous fish, mixed by witches into brews that sent men mad with excitation, but didn't kill them if their heart and lungs were strong enough to stand the strain. Such is the legacy of ergogenics in sport.

It has gone on that way ever since. History contradicts sports officials such as Dr Robert Voy, former chief medical officer of the US Olympic Committee, who claim that athletes today are under greater pressure to win.[1] It has always been so. Ancient athletes were under the most extreme pressure: they were often competing for their lives.

The difference today is that modern performance enhancing drugs work so well we have to ban them to give everyone a fair chance. And we have convoluted testing systems to try to keep people honest. So the race is on like never before to find ergogenics that will not show on the tests. From sprays you squirt up your nose, to pellets you push up your rectum, to the foulest glop you can force down your throat, athletes have become prey to the weirdest collection of snake oil concoctions that ever came down the pike. The first one we tackle is glandulars.

Glandular Gobbledegook

The Greek poet Homer tells us that Achilles ate the organs of lions to increase his strength in battle. Masai hunters eat the lion's heart in the belief that they will gain its courage. Testicles of bull and bear have been consumed by numerous cultures in attempts to boost virility. These old traditions have spawned a lucrative modern market for the ground up glands of various unfortunate beasts.

The growth of the glandular industry stemmed first from the use of thyroid hormones extracted from animal thyroid glands in the 1920s to treat thyroid insufficiency, and the successful use of synthetic thyroid ever since. But unfortunately, there is no comparison between thyroid medication and glandulars. It takes many pounds of thyroid gland to produce one tiny bottle of thyroid, whereas glandulars are simply the ground up glands, freeze dried and made into a pill. The amount of gland you get is minuscule and the amount of active hormones it contains is negligible.

In a recent test at the Colgan Institute, we made a concentrated extract of a whole 100-pill bottle of orchic glandular in a search for its content of testosterone. Result: the content profile on our super sensitive instrument showed only a couple of milligrams. The usual dose of prescription testosterone is 100-200 mg.[2] Claims that glandulars contain effective amounts of hormones are plain fraud.

Nevertheless, booklets have flooded the health market, mainly by a Dr Alan Nittler, reporting that a German researcher, Kment, had found that radioactively tagged glandulars travel in the bloodstream directly to the "target organ".[3] Adrenal glandulars go to the adrenals, orchic glandulars go to the testicles, and pituitary glandulars go to the pituitary. All these remotely guided substances were claimed to carry genetic information that stimulated the respective glands. No one has been able to repeat these experiments.

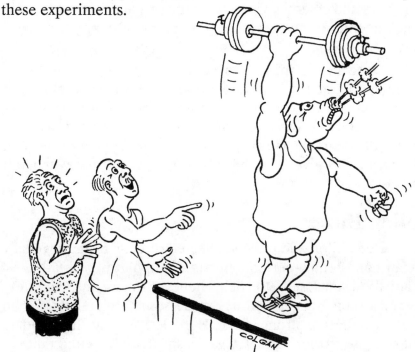

"Don's been great since he took those glandulars from bull's testicles."

The notion that oral glandulars carry genetic information which can strengthen the "target organ" is just plain stupid. The reported work of Kment was all done with *injected* glandular extracts. It had to be that way for any genetic information to get through. Genetic information is coded in DNA as a specific protein. Oral glandulars, like all proteins, are broken down during digestion. All genetic information is destroyed. Even if any did manage to squeak through, your immune system would immediately recognize it, and attack and destroy it. Just as well, unless you want to sprout horns and tail.

There is not a single study showing any effect of glandular supplements on sports performance. Yet the hottest protein supplement of the moment, displays glandulars prominently on the label, under its claim that the product boosts natural testosterone. On phoning the manufacturer, I was told that the glandulars add essential vitamins to the product. They do, but in minute quantities. You get more vitamins by chewing your finger-nails.

Despite all these problems, the glandular industry continues to trade on the myth, that swallowing the glands of spunky young bulls will make you an animal. Scientifically, it's nonsense. But to keep an open mind, if you do find such an effect, and you also start chewing your cud and snorting at open pasture, call me and I'll give up science, and we can go into witchcraft together.

Pollen Buzz

Bee pollen and pollen collected directly from flowers by human hands enjoy periodic bursts of popularity with athletes. Health food stores sell a ton of it whenever a new concocted story hits the streets, that pollen has made some athlete faster than speeding bullets or stronger than Hercules. We have followed up a lot of these stories at the Colgan Institute only to find that the athlete involved doesn't exist, or that he took a large wad of the folding green to let his name be used, or that the story came from the Soviet Bloc and is unverifiable.

Dr Melvin Williams of Old Dominion University in Virginia, reports a typical vague study by Korchemny, showing improved recovery of runners given "pollen".[4] But what pollen? There are hundreds of different types, each with a distinct chemical structure. One reason researchers have been unable to repeat these studies is because they have been unable to repeat the pollen.

In a representative American study, Dr Joe Chandler of Lander College, South Carolina, gave runners 400 mg of "bee pollen" per day for 75 days and found no effects at all.[5] In eight years of trying, the Colgan Institute has been unable to obtain even one sample of any American pollen product that is stable enough to provide a repeatable chemical profile, so that we can give athletes a standardized daily dose.

There is one pollen product that some researchers consider similar enough, batch to batch, to be used in controlled studies, Pollitabs by Cernelle. But results have all been negative. Pollitabs failed to improve running performance of cross-country runners, or swimming performance, or VO_2 max, or strength, or endurance of swimmers. And neither runners nor swimmers showed any beneficial changes in blood variables.[6,7]

In 1984, I tried repeatedly to get copies of research that distributors of cernitins (plant growth factors from pollen) claimed had been done. But all we received from them were useless anecdotes and promotional brochures. (I have just tried again in September, 1992 with the same result.)

Some other countries may have a better handle on pollen. In 1985, while lecturing to sports medicine groups in China, I visited a large Chinese study of bee pollen with athletes at their National Sports Center in Beijing. In contrast to American studies, which have used less than one gram of pollen a day, the Chinese were using 20-40 grams per athlete per day. The pollen came from special hives in special fields, and was made into government manufactured pollen wafers. They used huge ranks of treadmills going all day long with successive groups of athletes. Even with these large amounts of very controlled pollen, effects on performance were insignificant.

Returning to the States with cartons of these Chinese pollen wafers, we tested them on runners and weightlifters at 20 grams per subject per day for six weeks. These were pilot studies to determine whether it was worth doing controlled trials. Effects on performance compared with a control group given a fructose placebo -- a fat zero.

The pollen groups, however, did show increased resting heart rate and increased blood pressure, and reported that they felt an effect like strong coffee. They also reported sleeping problems. So there may be some yet unknown stimulant in pollen.

This stimulant action would explain why athletes keep buying it. It doesn't improve performance but it does provide a bit of a buzz.

Gamma Oryzanol, Ferulic Acid, FRAC

Japan and the rest of the Orient eat rice in the billions of tons, much of it refined with the bran removed. That leaves mountains of rice bran waste to dispose of. Waste products provide a very cheap source of base material, if you can find a use for them. So when gamma oryzanol was isolated from rice bran oil in the 1950s, manufacturers hustled to sell it for everything from fattening cattle to fortifying athletes.

Chemically, gamma oryzanol is a mixture of plant sterols and ferulic acid. It contains campesterol, cycloartenol, stigmasterol and beta sitosterol. The latter two especially, are often touted as "steroid alternatives", though there is no scientific evidence that they increase muscle growth. I cover plant sterols later. In any case, sterol levels in gamma oryzanol are way too low to have any physiological effect.

The ferulic acid fraction does have an effect, at least in animals. It reduces sexual hormone function. Ferulic acid (4-hydroxy-3-methoxycinnamic acid) is one of a group of plant cinnamic acids known to inhibit sexual and reproductive behavior in animals that feed the plants that contain it.[8]

Ferulic acid injected into heifers also causes a significant increase in prolactin, the milk stimulating hormone, which also has some small anabolic effects. There was also a minute increase in bovine growth hormone.[9] The results have been exaggerated by promoters of gamma oryzanol, ferulic acid, and its derivative FRAC, to claim anabolic effects in athletes. The animal evidence suggests the opposite. Athletes may do well to avoid any substance that promotes milk production and reduces copulation.

The only study on athletes using gamma oryzanol, also used glandulars, chlorophyll and other tomfoolery, as well as vitamins and amino acids. It did find beneficial effects on muscle size and a reduction of bodyfat, but there is no way to determine what caused them. The study was not even a double-blind, so the effect could have been pure placebo.[10] Even hedge clippings presented with enough hype and flapdoodle can improve sports performance, because the athlete will try harder under the belief he is being artificially enhanced.

Other studies with athletes, that you see in promotional literature, all come from a booklet sold in health food stores, of unpublished research by Joseph Bruni MD.[11] None of these studies employed even the minimum of scientific controls. So they cannot provide any reliable information. Rice bran is definitely a good source of fiber that can help to keep an athlete regular. But the ergogenic effects of the gamma oryzanol and ferulic acid it contains are pure hokum and flapdoodle.

Yohimbe Is Not Anabolic

Yohimbe is being widely sold in health food stores as an anabolic agent. But the evidence indicates it is something else entirely. The bark of the yohimbe tree (*Pausinystalia johimbe*) has been used as an aphrodisiac for centuries. And it works. The active ingredient is yohimbine, an alkaloid extract from yohimbe bark. After a long fight, it was approved recently by the Food and Drug Administration as a treatment for male impotence. In 1990, there were two drugs available, Yohimex, made by Kramer Laboratories of Miami, Florida, and Yocon, made by Palisades Pharmaceuticals of Tenafly, New Jersey. Both are used to treat males who have physical or psychological problems in achieving and maintaining erections.[12] They must be sought after because in 1992, six US pharmaceutical companies are offering to supply the world with yohimbine.[13]

It is certainly not a placebo. Male rats given yohimbine remain in a state of sexual arousal for extended periods.[14] And in a human study, Dr Alvaro Morales and colleagues of Queens University, Ontario, gave yohimbine daily to severely impotent men. After 8 to 10 weeks, half the men showed measurable improvement, and a quarter of them had their sexual potency fully restored.[15]

   Yocon is cautiously described in the 1990 Physicians Desk Reference (PDR) as "may have activity as an aphrodisiac".[12] First time I have ever seen "aphrodisiac" used in reference to a prescription drug. Sounds decidedly pleasurable, an emotion I thought was forbidden in American medicine.

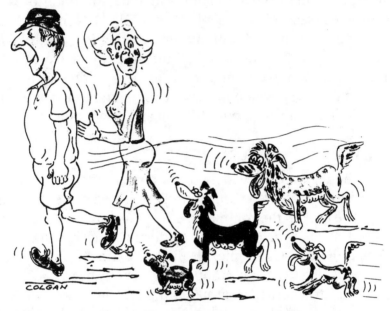

"You've been taking those aphrodisiacs again!"

   The authors of PDR may have been swayed from their usual strict scientific descriptions of drugs, by the startling effects of yohimbine on the brain and heart, as well as the genitals. In doses above the therapeutic range it causes a general excitation, including flushing, intoxication, shaking, mild hallucinations, elevated heart and blood pressure, and increased motor activity.[12,16]

   Perhaps it is the general excitation that huxters rely on when they tout yohimbe bark as an ergogenic aid for athletes that enhances both energy and strength. There are no studies at all on athletes to prove it. Nevertheless, excitation and euphoria are powerful motivators. Cocaine is the drug of choice among professional athletes, because of the euphoric, aggressive "rush" it produces. The modern trend to subvert sexual stimulants to athletic use, may have its roots in the ancient Greek belief that excitation to the point of madness improves sports performance. Don't discount it altogether; science just hasn't been able to measure it.

Although yohimbine is not anabolic, and there is no evidence that it enhances sports performance, new evidence shows that this complex drug has other roles in the human body that might be useful to athletes. It belongs to a class of compounds called **alpha-2-receptor antagonists**. Some of these drugs cause a large increase in the release of noradrenalin from nerve endings. This action stimulates the nervous system, raises core temperature, and causes the body to mobilize bodyfat or fuel. Yohimbine could prove effective in all these areas.

The latest study is reported by Dr C. Kucio and colleagues in the **Israel Journal of Medical Science**.[17] Weight-loss patients were given 15 mg per day of yohimbine hydrochloride and kept on a low-calorie diet (1,000 cal/day). A control group of weight-loss patients was given only the diet. Compared with the control group, Yohimbine increased noradrenalin output and energy expenditure. More important, the yohimbine group lost an average of 7.8 lbs in the three weeks of the study. The control group lost 4.8 lbs. Yohimbine may offer a new aid to dieting.

Unfortunately, yohimbe bark supplements sold on the health food market are far too weak to have any effect. Even the most potent contain only a few micrograms of yohimbine, whereas the dosage required for effective use of the prescription drugs is 8-16 mg, more than a thousand times greater.

Dibencoside Don't Do Diddley

Dibencoside (5,6, dimethyl-benzimidazolecobamide) is a coenzyme of vitamin B_{12}. In the 1960s it was confirmed that after vitamin B_{12} is absorbed through the intestines, it is converted into dibencoside. The body then uses debencoside rather than vitamin

B12 itself.[18] One of its functions is to assist protein synthesis. Another function is to promote hematopoiesis (formation of red blood cells).[19]

Because of these functions, some researchers thought that supplementation with dibencoside might assist sick children who were subnormal in height and weight and who might have difficulty absorbing and using vitamin B12. It was a wild thought and no controlled studies were done in America to examine the possibility. The only data of note are from a small Soviet study of 35 children, aged 1-13.[20] This study was done in 1969. The date is significant.

Average weight gain of the children was about 1 lb on the dibencoside, compared with 2 lb on the steroid stanozolol. Average height gain was 1.0 cm, compared with 0.5 cm on stanozolol. With this sort of result, researchers lost interest in dibencoside. Our computer database lists no controlled studies since.

But the flim-flam men saw a potential profit even in this old and shaky work. Since 1987, dibencosode has been widely marketed as an athletic supplement. Some advertisements claim it is "twice as effective as many prescription steroids." Almost all these ads depict a graph showing that dibencoside has a larger effect on height and weight than three anabolic steroids. All the claims infer that the graph refers to athletes. It doesn't. The graph is a hyped-up version of one that appears in the Soviet study of sick children.

Even if it did represent results found with athletes, you would still have to find real dibencoside. This compound is extremely light, oxygen and temperature sensitive, and degrades into plain old vitamin B12 in a heartbeat. Real dibencoside is difficult to make, and requires special laboratory conditions almost like a photographic darkroom. Then it has to be sealed in light-protected capsules and stored in a light-protected, airtight bottle in the refrigerator. Dibencoside that you see listed on labels of regular pills and powdered supplements, just isn't in there.

Gamma-hydroxybutarate Dreams

To read the ads selling gamma-hydroxybutarate (GHB) as a growth hormone releaser and anabolic agent, you would think it had received rave reviews from the scientific community. Not so. GHB was researched by pharmaceutical companies in the '70s as a possible sleep aid, and canned when it proved to be unpredictable and dangerous.

GHB was first identified in France in 1960 as a naturally occurring substance in the human brain.[21] Later it was shown to be an intermediate metabolite in the production of sleep.[22] Oral GHB supplements do produce sleep. The 5-gram doses being touted for muscle building will knock most people out cold.

There is also some evidence that GHB causes the pituitary to release growth hormone in healthy men.[23] This study, however, used intravenous injections of GHB. There are no studies of oral use of GHB to release growth hormone. But the strong effects of oral GHB on brain function, show that it does get to the brain via the oral route, and would probably work.

It is those strong effects that also cause the trouble. From June to November 1990, the Centers for Disease Control recorded 57 cases of GHB poisoning.[24] One of the worst problems is its unpredictability. People using GHB successfully for insomnia, may suddenly start getting headaches, vertigo and tremors during the day and disturbances of the heart. The worst cases show full blown epileptic seizures and comas.

The Food and Drug Administration issued a public warning against GHB in November 1990, and it has since been banned in most states. There is still a lot of it floating around though. If you value your body, leave it to float.

Inosine Aches

Athletes often show elevated levels of uric acid, especially in strength and explosive power sports. The body disposes of some of the excess uric acid by depositing it in joints, frequently causing chronic arthritis-like pain. The well-known high uric acid disorder is gout.

One thing we get athletes to do in cases of high uric acid is to avoid purines in the diet, because waste products of purine metabolism create a lot of uric acid. Combined with adjustments to the type and amount of protein they are eating, this simple strategy can move serum uric acid levels down below 5.0 mg/dl, where we like to see it stay.

But it is more difficult if they are hitting the inosine. Inosine is composed of the purine hypoxanthine and the sugar ribose. Excess inosine can send uric acid levels into orbit.[31]

Athletes continue to risk the uric acid problem because of evidence that inosine can increase the force of heart muscle contraction, thereby increasing blood flow and oxygen to the muscles.[25] Inosine has been used successfully for this purpose in coronary heart disease [26] and in transplant surgery.[27]

Inosine also increases oxygen/hemoglobin affinity. A large proportion of any inosine introduced into the bloodstream goes directly into red blood cells. Those cells then pick up increased amounts of oxygen when they pass through the lungs, and deliver it to the muscles.[28] The effect can last 1 - 2 hours.[25] This evidence, all from reputable research with **injected** inosine, has been used to sell many millions of inosine pills and tons of inosine powder for **oral use** by athletes.

I am partly responsible. In popular articles in 1987 and 1988, I reviewed this information and reported a study that we did with athletes at the Colgan Institute.[29] Weightlifters given inosine in a double-blind crossover trial, increased their strength more rapidly than without the supplement. I did report at the time that the study was preliminary, and that we were designing a larger trial with Dr Richard Telford, Head of Sports Science at the Australian Institute of Sport in Canberra, the Aussie equivalent of the US Olympic Training Center. But the preliminary results were widely quoted, and even reviewed in academic texts on sports nutrition.[30]

I also reported at the time, that continued use of inosine appeared to exhaust the weightlifters and **reduced performance** after a few weeks. But those data got lost in the selling shuffle. Since then new research has been published indicating that excess inosine can reduce performance because of its involvement in the uric acid cycle.[31] Also since then, the Australian trial we did has proved disappointing. Oral inosine does not appear to have any consistent beneficial effect. Ditch it before your big toe starts to ache.

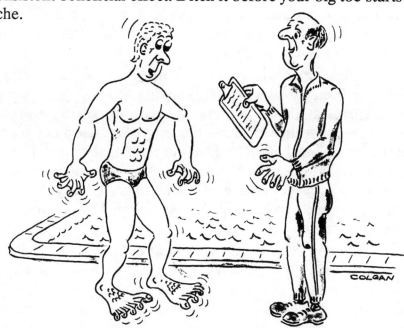

"The fish oil supplements work great coach!"

Dimethylglycine and Pangamic Acid

My last book warned athletes against so-called "pangamic acid", also called "vitamin B15".[32] Products sold under these names are neither a legitimate vitamin nor a legitimate acid. They are just another profitable flapdoodle.

Following reports that use of pangamic acid reduced lactic

acid accumulation in Soviet athletes,[33] the Colgan Institute bought samples of the Russian product and samples of eight different American and European products. No two of them had the same chemical profile. Mostly they were harmless but fraudulent mixtures of plain calcium gluconate and the amino acid glycine or dimethylglycine (DMG).

Despite a ban by the Food and Drug Administration, most of these mixtures are still out there, sold under rapidly changing names and formulas to dodge the law. There is no way that the tiny amounts of calcium or glycine in these concoctions could affect the performance of anything larger than my pet cockroach, who, I must admit, runs towards the pills at an accelerated clip and eats them avidly.

Only dimethylglycine mixtures are worth testing, under the faint possibility that boosting the body's supply of this naturally occurring methyl donor could improve transmethylation and hence the efficiency of muscle metabolism. But it is crude biochemistry indeed to think that all you need to do is dump a little extra methyl source into the system to boost the whole chemical cascade of events involved in lactic acid clearance. Research on rats injected with DMG shows no increase in transmethylation.[34]

The only study to report beneficial results with athletes was published in 1980 and only in abstract,[35] so there is no way to evaluate it. But it claimed a 28% increase in VO2max, which is enormous. Most researchers would give their eyeteeth for such a find, and would want to publish it widely. So it is mighty suspicious that it has never been confirmed in the last 12 years. But the VO2max effect has been hyped so well by the "pangamate" promoters, that a fair number of athletes still believe it.

The truth is more this way. Michael Gray and Larry Titlow at Northern Kentucky University, gave 16 track athletes 300 mg per day of the "Russian Formula" (61.5% calcium gluconate, 38.5% N, N-dimethylglycine). This is the expensive one you see for sale, sporting a US patent (#3.907.869). The study was run double-blind with a placebo control for three weeks, testing the athletes on a treadmill. Results showed **no effect** on a variety of exercise variables, including time to exhaustion, recovery, or lactic acid levels.[36] More recent studies confirm these findings.[37,38]

The same negative findings hold for VO2max. Three careful blinded experiments, using 115 - 200 mg of DMG per day, found no effect at all.[39,40,41] These studies, all in reputable, peer-reviewed journals, are not referred to by the makers of DMG, who continue to cite anecdotal reports or the unvalidated abstract noted above. DMG may be a breakthrough for boosting the performance of my pet cockroach, but for athletes it's no use at all.

Lactate: Subtle Shuttle Shuffle

A recent article in a popular sports magazine claimed that "lactic acid may well be one of the bodybuilder's most useful substances".[42] The author was extolling the ergogenic virtues of the recently introduced lactate supplements. Lactic acid, however, is no help at all in sports. Just the opposite. Excess production of lactic acid is one of the biggest causes of muscle fatigue.[43,44] Athletes are only too familiar with the acid burn of intense muscle contraction that crucifies performance.

Why then are lactates being touted as energy boosters? One reason offered by supplement sellers is that about 75% of the lactic acid formed during exercise is converted back to its former step in energy metabolism, pyruvic acid, and can therefore be used again as fuel. The other 25% is turned back into glucose by the liver, which also provides an extra source of fuel.[45,46] This **lactate shuttle** suggests that adding more lactates to the mix might increase the energy supply, help maintain blood glucose and spare muscle glycogen. Don't think, however, that you can drive yourself through the burn and suddenly perk up on your own lactate. No way!

There is a ton of evidence that muscles quickly produce

far more lactic acid than can be reconverted to pyruvate and glucose. In one representative study, Pendergast et al used anaerobic exercise to raise blood lactate to very high levels (12 - 14 mM), about three times the level usually found after moderate exercise. Then subjects were tested in both aerobic and anaerobic exercise. Far from improving exercise performance, the high lactate levels were followed by **reduced** endurance in both aerobic and anaerobic work.[47] Any athlete who has run a hard set of intervals, already has intimate knowledge of this problem.

Nevertheless, to be fair, lactic acid caused by exercise is not exactly the same as lactate, although the terms are often used interchangeably in biochemistry.[48] Lactate lacks one hydrogen, so it does not acidify the blood like lactic acid, which releases the hydrogen ion (H +) to lower blood pH and interfere with muscle contraction. So lactate supplements might be converted to glucose in the liver without affecting muscle pH, all clean and dandy. The extra glucose could then boost your glycogen supply and enhance performance.

The only study to date on athletes is by Dr Thomas Fahey and colleagues at California State University, Chico. They tested five elite cyclists for three-hour rides at 50% VO_2max.[49] For different rides they received either a 7% polylactate solution, a 7% glucose polymer solution, or water flavored with aspartame as a control.

Blood glucose at the end of the rides was similar for both polylactates and glucose polymers but, as expected, blood glucose dropped significantly with the aspartame flavored water. These results seem to suggest that the polylactate supplement was acting as an energy supply equivalent to the glucose polymer. And there are plenty of studies showing that glucose polymer is an effective ergogenic aid to endurance.[50,51,52]

So far so good. If polylactate works as well as glucose polymers, it could provide a new and powerful aid to endurance performance. The effect would also be likely to be additive with glucose polymers, because the lactate acts by conversion to glucose in the liver. This is a different metabolic pathway to glucose polymer carbohydrate, which acts by absorption of glucose directly into the bloodstream. A combination of the two is dynamic according to the sellers of polylactate.

But the only study that they rely on has just too many problems. I'll skip the complex biochemical problems and focus on the obvious. First, the polylactate did not raise blood lactate levels in the athletes, so it is doubtful that much of it was even reaching the liver. The researchers had no data on what happened to the polylactate once it hit the gut.

Second, the athlete did the rides at only 50% VO_2max, that is, very moderate exercise. That's no way to test performance. All sorts of supplements have apparently beneficial biochemical effects on endurance when you are just idling along. But when you start pushing your muscles and cardiovascular system, biochemistry changes radically. Wonderful sounding benefits disappear like smoke. So the Fahey study, which only raised heart rate into the 130s, provides no evidence that polylactate has any effect on performance.

Third, heart rate and perceived effort proved to be the same whether the athletes received polylactate or flavored water. You might fool an athlete about how hard he is trying, but you can't fool his ticker. The heart is a very good measure of exercise load. If it says the polylactate supplement was doing diddly, then it very likely was doing diddly. So if anyone claims there is evidence that polylactate supplements improve athletic performance -- don't believe them.

Tanking Up on Oxygen

You see a lot of ball players sucking on oxygen tanks to speed recovery from the anaerobic effects of an exhausting bit of play. The theory is that extra oxygen in the blood helps remove the lactic acid and carbon dioxide caused by anaerobic exercise from the muscle tissues and bloodstream. The theory is sound but the method doesn't work.

Olympian Dr Peter Snell and Dr James Stray-Gunderson at the University of Texas Medical School in Dallas did a double-blind trial that is representative of the research. They took 12 members of the Dallas Sidekicks soccer team and ran them to exhaustion on a treadmill. The subjects then rested, during which time they breathed either from an oxygen tank or a similar looking tank filled with regular room air. They didn't know which tank contained the pure oxygen. Levels of lactic acid in the blood were measured after 4 minutes of breathing either oxygen or air. Then they ran again to exhaustion on the treadmill.

The whole procedure was repeated three hours later with the subjects who had first breathed air being given oxygen and vice versa. Results showed no difference in time to exhaustion on the treadmill, and no difference in the blood lactic acid levels, whether the subjects breathed pure oxygen or regular air.[53]

The main reason oxygen tanks don't work, is that simply providing oxygen to the lungs does nothing to improve the oxygen transport system necessary to get it to the tissues. With exhaustive anaerobic exercise, your oxygen transport system is working at maximum capacity. Providing more oxygen than it can carry, does no good at all.

To take up additional oxygen you have to improve the oxygen transport system. You can do this two ways. First, you can increase what is called oxygen/hemoglobin affinity. That is, you can make the hemoglobin in each cell pick up more oxygen. The only known way to do that for athletes is to train at altitude.

Second, you can increase the number and the size of your oxygen transporters. You can increase the number of red blood cells, the proportion of the blood that is composed of red blood cells, and the amount of oxygen carrying substance in each cell. In blood analysis these are called the RBC count, the hematocrit, and the hemoglobin. Nutritional ways to increase these counts are discussed in the Chapter 21, Good Red Blood.

Although oxygen tanks may help the sick, they do nothing to increase the blood oxygen of a healthy athlete, or oxygen delivering to his tissues. They are just expensive toys, part of the razz-ma-tazz of clowns in fuzzy animal suits and angora goat mascots, that pump up the athletes and the fans in the arena of professional sports.

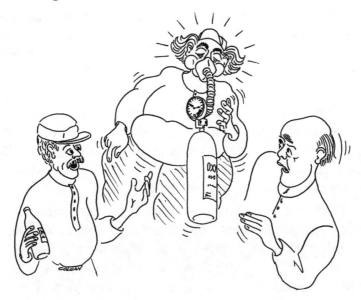

"Hank pumps in the oxygen till he gets liftoff."

Excitable Herbs

Hundreds of products claiming anabolic and ergogenic effects load their formulas with plant sterols, mainly beta-sitosterol, stigmasterol and campesterol, and the herbs that contain them, in the hope that the combination may somehow overcome the ornery resistance of the human system. Vain hope!

Smilax is perennially popular. *Smilax officianalis* and *Smilax aristolochifolia* are both forms of the old sarsaparilla plant that used to be popular in sodas. The notion that smilax might be anabolic arises from its traditional use as an aphrodisiac. There is a small amount of evidence that a properly made extract of smilax provides a stimulant effect, including a stimulation of the male genitalia.[54,55] Perhaps that is where it gets the mistaken reputation for raising testosterone levels. There is no evidence whatever that smilax is anabolic. It is used freely in America to flavor baked goods and candy but you don't see any couch potatoes suddenly sprouting muscle.

Saw Palmetto is another favorite of the steroid replacement brigade. *Serenoa repens* and *Serenoa ferrulata* have spiced the food of countless lovers, and have been used fervently by countless damsels seeking larger breasts. There is no scientific evidence showing growth of either muscles or mammary glands. Like smilax, the reputation of saw palmetto has grown from people confusing sensation with physiology. Studies show that a strong extract of saw palmetto causes feelings of stimulation and euphoria in both male and female reproductive systems.[56] But there is no evidence of an anabolic effect.

Damiana, gotu kola, fo-ti, Mexican yam, even innocuous aloe vera, spirulina, wheat grass and barley grass, and a variety of algaes enjoy periodic popularity as "anabolic alternatives." The basic error in trying to use these plants as anabolics, is equating the sterols they contain with anabolic steroids. Most plant sterols have very different chemical structures to human steroids. So there is little chance that they can function anabolically in the human body.

They can act as stimulants, however, and have been shown to do so. The euphoria they produce is probably the reason behind their continued use. We use a herbal mixture with athletes for exactly that purpose. Foremost herb authority, Dr Jim Duke of the USDA, suggests his "Root Buster Tea" composed of ginger, ginseng, smilax, and sassafras. Smart supplement manufacturers include herbs in their supplements, not only for buzz-word value, but also for the buzz that keeps them selling.

To claim the above herbs are anabolic or ergogenic is hokum. As I write this, I am pleased to read that the hottest selling of these products at the moment, has just been served with a cease and desist order by the FDA for making unsubstantiated claims.[57] This dubious stuff not only contains three of the above plants, plus an unidentified "sterol complex", but also five of the other bogus "anabolics" reviewed in this chapter. Save your money for real nutrition.

There are some exceptional sterols and steroids from plants, invertebrates, and insects that have sexual steroid activity in mammals. The prothoracic gland hormone **ecdysone** of some insects, and estrogens from some starfish are close enough in chemical structure to animal sex hormones to have a weak effect on steroid receptors in mammals.[58] But despite the ads for supplements supposedly made from insect or invertebrate steroids, there is no evidence at all that they are anabolic.

The plant sterol genistein from a type of Australian clover causes cattle to go into continual estrus (become continually sexually receptive).[58] Similar phytoestrogens (plant estrogens), **equol, diadzein,** and **coumestrol** occur in soybeans and other legumes, and cause disturbances in the sexual behavior of sheep[59] and in the sexual development of mice.[60]

Coumestrol has the strongest effects because its chemical structure is the most similar to the female hormone **estradiol.** Coumestrol causes uterine growth in rats and probably in humans.[61] So it is anabolic to female sexual organs, but there is no evidence it is anabolic to muscle. With the distinct possibility of femininization from their use both male and female athletes should avoid estrogens, plant or human, like the plague.

The latest plant sterol to hit the market is ecdisterone extracted from the rare herbs *Pfaffia paniculata* and *Leuzea carthemoides.* There is one sketchy Russian study reporting that ecdisterone has a weak anabolic effect on muscle in animals.[62] As usual, it is being hyped to the skies in the sports supplement marketplace, as if there is all sorts of evidence on athletes. No evidence at all folks. Scam city!

Vanadyl Sulfate/Vanadium

Since 1973, research has shown consistently that vanadium is essential for normal growth in animals and probably in man.[63]

Daily requirements for this mineral, however, are easily met by the amounts normally occurring in a wide variety of foods.[64] Why then is it being marketed in the vanadyl sulfate form as a hot anabolic that will increase muscle growth and reduce bodyfat?

The notion that vanadium might be anabolic arose from a series of reports showing that supplements of this mineral improve glucose tolerance and reduce muscle loss in animal studies of diabetes.[65] Vanadium appears to improve the efficiency of insulin action inside the cell.[66]

Insulin efficiency is intimately connected with protein synthesis and use of bodyfat as fuel. But the vanadium effect has been shown only in diabetic animals whose insulin metabolism is disordered to the point of producing disease, and then only in some of them. Just as in many other diseases that can be treated with high levels of particular nutrients, it is likely that the disease state of these animals can be treated with high levels of vanadium.

Such studies provide no logical reason to use vanadium with healthy athletes, and no evidence at all that vanadium is anabolic. It is about the same level of silliness, as saying that because a splint can help a broken bone to heal, then athletes should all wear splints to strengthen their bones. The effect would be just the opposite. Splinting a healthy bone weakens it, because it deprives the bone of the applied forces that keep its matrix strong. The same may well apply to vanadium, because repeated animal studies show that an excess of this mineral *reduces* muscle growth in healthy animals.[67]

The other big problem with vanadium is that it is highly toxic. Studies of mineral toxicity on animals show vanadium to be about as toxic as arsenic.[68] How then did it get onto the supplement market?

In 1985, a report by Heyliger and colleagues in the prestigious journal **Science** showed that vanadium in the drinking water of rats that had been made diabetic, controlled their high blood glucose.[69] Diabetes researchers were excited because vanadium is effective by mouth, whereas insulin has to be injected. Maybe vanadium offered a new, more convenient medicine for diabetes.

Other reports confirming the action of vanadium on diabetic rats quickly followed in 1987.[70,71] To their shame, however, these researches did not report, or detail, the toxic effects of the vanadium, only the positive effects. Seeing a possible positive effect on the glucose metabolism of athletes, supplement manufacturers ignorant of nutritional toxicology jumped in and began making vanadium supplements.

Unfortunately, by 1989, reports of vanadium toxicity were pouring in. In the original 1985 paper the Heyliger group reported no evidence of toxicity. But in a 1989 paper they admitted:

the concentration of vanadate used in the drinking water was toxic to some animals, resulting in severe diarrhea and death because of dehydration.[72]

Of course by then there were at least six other studies showing severe vanadium toxicity, so the original group had to 'fess up to cover their butts.

So by January, 1990, you have a group of supplement makers out big bucks on vanadium supplies, bottles, labels, literature, and ego, with a potentially toxic product on their hands. Well, no one had called in sick from the supplements because mild vanadium poisoning is difficult to distinguish from flu and other illnesses that inflame your liver and kidneys. So why not sell the hell out of it before someone calls the bluff.

Think that I am overstating the case? The latest joint study, by Dr Jose Domingo and colleagues at the University of Barcelona Medical School, and the University of California, Davis, indicates just how toxic vanadium can be.[73] They compared three forms of vanadium, **metavanadate**, **orthovanadate**, and **vanadyl sulphate**. All three improved glucose metabolism in diabetic rats. But the survival rates were horrific. A control group of normal rats given no vanadium remained 100% in good health. A control group of rats made diabetic but given no vanadium, lost 20% of their subjects to the complications of diabetes. The three groups given vanadium all became very unhappy campers. In the orthovanadate group, 40% died. In the metavanadate group and the vanadyl sulphate group (the form usually used for supplements) half the rats died!

Deceptive supplement literature has now appeared in the marketplace trying to con you by claiming that those poor rats got far more vanadium than they put in supplements. So what! The experimental rats were given the amount of vanadium necessary to improve glucose tolerance. In every case where sufficient vanadium was given to improve glucose tolerance, it also caused toxic side effects. That's the chemistry! You can't get the improvement without the toxicity. Thousands of promising drugs are dumped because of that problem.

So if you claim a vanadium supplement is not toxic, you can't expect it to do anything beneficial either. And if you take enough of the pills to produce a gain in glucose metabolism, then you can also expect it to beat the hell out of your liver and kidneys.

I would love to be able to tell you that vanadium supplements work. And if the science supported it, I would sing praises for a new advance in sports nutrition. But vanadium doesn't work, it can't work and its presence in the sports market is, like so many other scams, a result of ignorance and greed.

Colostrum Capers

In the first few days of an infant's life, mothers milk contains colostrum a yellowish fluid that conveys a host of nutritional goodies to the babe. These goodies include insulin-like growth factors I and II (IGF), the major promotor of protein synthesis in muscle, that we cover in detail in Chapter 32. The IGF in colostrum causes rapid infant growth, especially of the visceral organs.

Colostrum containing IGF can also be collected from cows. In newborn infant cows it causes rapid growth of lean mass. Some supplement hustlers have twisted these facts to conclude that bovine colostrum will act as an anabolic for athletes. Articles acclaiming this hokum have recently appeared in bodybuilding magazines. Probably the biggest reason for the hype is that some makers of colostrum are offering to provide pre-written pieces and to obtain advertising for the magazines in return for running the articles.[74]

Oral bovine colostrum cannot work in adults for two reasons. First a polypeptide such as IGF, which consists of a 67-amino acid chain, is slaughtered by adult digestion. It is broken into dipeptides (two amino acids), tripeptides (three amino acids) and single amino acids. The information only gets through in newborn infants because their digestive systems have not yet kicked in. The newborn gut has a neutral ph of around 7.0. It can't split polypeptides into their constituent amino acids. But after a day or two, the infant gut changes to a harsh acidity of 1.0, same as an adult. That's why colostrum stops flowing from the mother around Day 2. After that the IGF and other important peptides are no further use, because they can't survive the stomach acid.

Second, bovine IGF is chemically different from human IGF. Even if it got past digestion, your immune system would recognise it as foreign immediately, and attack and destroy it before a molecule of new muscle could be formed. Even if by some miracle your immune system left bovine IGF to run free, its chemical structure will not fit with the IGF carrier proteins that are essential to move IGF around your body and enable it to attach to muscle cells.[75]

Finally, the meat industry spends millions on anabolic steroids and other synthetic drugs to promote lean mass in cattle. If the IGF in bovine colostrum grew muscle in cows don't you think they would use it. They don't because it doesn't work. Selling bovine colostrum as an oral anabolic agent for athletes is the type of scrape-the-bottom-of-the-barrel scam that drags the whole nutrition industry down in the dirt.

Diosgenin: Yam Yam Scam

Disgenin is a compound derived from various species of

yam, especially *Dioscorea composita*. How it comes to be offered to athletes as a steroid alternative is a typical example of ignorance and perfidy. Some species of toxic yams (and other plants) contain up to 13% diosgenin. In this concentration it is used by natives as a fish poison. but it also contains the chemical building blocks of steroid hormones. Following the lead of an eccentric chemist named RE Marker, by the 1960's diosgenin was being fermented with bacteria that contain exactly the right enzymes to convert it to human steroid hormones, including estrogens, testosterone and cortisones.[76] That's how these hormones became cheap enough tomake oral contraceptives, cortisone creams and testosterone affordable for general public use.[77]

Twenty years later this science finally penetrated the layers of sedimentary misconception that cake the bottom end of sports nutrition. Low-life denizens of the pseudonutrition swamplands briefly turned their thoughts from gluttony to profit. If diosgenin contains all the building blocks of steroids, then let's feed it to athletes. Their bodies will convert it to testosterone and they'll grow like the Jolly Green Giant.

Hogwash! First, the human body doesn't contain the necessary enzymes to make the conversion. Second, the human system makes all its steroid hormones from cholesterol, under the strict control of specific hormonal signals from the hypothalamus and pituitary centers in the brain. Diosgenin as a sports supplement is 100% flim-flam. Suspect any supplement that contains it, and suspect the company too. If they will scam you for one thing . . . .

Octacosanol: Marginal Effects?

Professor Thomas Cureton at the University of Illinois began research on wheat germ oil and sports performance in the '50s. After 20 years of studies on more than 900 swimmers, weightlifters, wrestlers, track and field athletes and military personnel he reported that wheat germ oil improves strength, reaction time and endurance.[78] He concluded also that the active compound in the oil is **octacosanol**, a peculiar solid, white alcohol.

In a typical study, matched groups of Navy SEALS were fed either 3.85 mg of octacosanol daily or a placebo for six weeks. All subjects followed the same training schedule of 5 hours exercise per day, lived in the same barracks, and ate at the same cafeteria. Results showed that the octacosanol group improved their mile run time by 46 seconds more than the placebo group. They also made larger gains in strength.[78]

Sounds terrific. Problem is, most researchers have been unable to replicate Cureton's work. In 1982, the Colgan Institute set up a tightly controlled experiment to replicate and extend the above study. Result: a fat zero! Even at doses of 10 mg per day we found no difference in strength or endurance.

One recent report, however, does show an increase in strength with octacosanol, but no increase in endurance.[79] There is also one study showing an anabolic effect of octacosanol on comb growth in chicks.[80] So it is not an inert substance.

No one knows how octacosanol may work in the body. Cureton explained it in vague terms as a catalyst, a chemical that speeds up existing functions. Medical studies suggest a different idea. Recent trials of octacosanol with Lou Gehrigs disease and Parkinsons disease reported some gradual improvements in neuro-muscular coordination.[81,82]

Octacosanol may act to improve the efficiency of transmission of nerve impulses. These effects, however, are with patients. Until there are independent studies that clearly confirm Cureton's work, it remains a question mark. The most we can say is that octacosanol might "steady your nerves."

Placebo Effects Are Real

Whenever I lecture on anabolics and ergogenics, there is always the guy who comes up to me afterwards and swears he got great results with one or other of the bogus mixtures. I don't doubt that he did. It was not the mixture that did it though. It was the placebo effect, which is real and measurable, and often extremely powerful.

In my medical school teaching days, I used to do a class demonstration on how the stress of fear raises heart rate and blood pressure, causes a burst of adrenalin, and a dozen other measurable physiological changes. My problem was to get these responses on the lab instruments from a volunteer out of a bunch of smart, cynical, medical students.

I used a light and the threat of an electric shock. I couldn't actually shock the student, because then his body would be reacting to the shock, and not to the fear. Many of the students had figured that out, and used to set me up by not responding at all.

Then I found an old Edwardian chair in the laboratory basement that solved my problem. It was dark oak with big square legs, heavy arms, and a solid back. It looked a ringer for the electric chair. Fitted with straps to buckle in the students, and a sinister black shock electrode the size of a dinner plate, I never had any more trouble. Physiological fear responses to the wink of the light went right off the chart. Once you set the scene up right, placebos work a treat.

The same real placebo changes are found in all sports. In one well known study, weightlifters were given chalk pills and told they were the latest and best anabolic steroids. They all made large and measurable gains in strength, significantly greater than the gains they were making before getting the pills.[83]

If you believe, truly believe, that a supplement is helping, because it is endorsed by a top athlete, or because it comes from Russia, or because of the pseudo-scientific hype that litters promotional brochures, then it is likely that you will make real, measurable gains while using it. That's the placebo effect. All the better if the supplement also contains a stimulant that gives you the additional feeling that something good is happening to your body. It's the power of placebos that keeps bogus supplements on the market.

Conclusion

We have covered the worst offenders amongst the fake anabolics and ergogenics. There are plenty more waiting in the wings. Every one of the thousands of intermediate chemicals in human metabolism is fair game.

To have any possibility of an effect with any metabolic intermediate of steroids, you would first have to boost your supply of adrenocorticotrophic hormone (ACTH), which directs the body to make steroids. Then you would have to boost a dozen other biochemicals. But I am not going to name them, because some clown is sure to make a supplement to suit, and claim I said it works.

So that you will know to avoid them, there is also no evidence to support "ergogenic" supplements of cyclofenil, succinic acid, lipoic acid, creatine, betaine, choline, cytochrome C, pyroloquinolone, wheat grass, barley grass, spirulena, propolis, royal jelly, aloe vera, yucca, devils claw, dong quai, ho shou wu, oxygen drinks, and the encapsulated slime of warty green toads. Some of these things are very useful for other purposes, but ergogenics they are not.

When you paid your dollar for a snake oil remedy on the boardwalk at Coney Island, you knew it was really a fee to watch the old barkers perform. And you threw the bottle away or gave it to someone you wanted to torment. Today the snake oil comes in shinier packages, surrounded by pseudoscience, touted by hired champions, and sold with the best of Madison Avenue flim-flam. This chapter saves you from much of this sham and mendacity.

Table 22. Substances that have no anabolic or ergogenic effects.

Bogus Ergogenics	
Glandulars	Pangamic acid
Orchic	Dimethylglycine
Pituitary	Lactate,
Adrenal	Oxygen tanks
Pancreas	Oxygen cocktails
Heart	Vanadyl sulfate
Bee pollen	Smilax
Flower pollen	Saw Palmetto
Cernitins	Damiana
Gamma oryzanol	Gotu kola
Ferrulic acid	Fo-ti
FRAC	Mexican yam
Yohimbe	Cayenne
Dibencoside	Capsicum
Gamma hydroxybutarate	Beta sitosterol
Inosine	Campesterol
Vitamin B15	Stigmasterol
Diosgenin	Fucosterol
Muira puama	Plant sterol complex
Ammi majus	Colostrum

Chapter 32

The Anabolic Drive and Anti-Catabolism

The **anabolic drive** is a precise synergy of nutritional, hormonal, and metabolic activities that completely control growth. In the last five years, science has finally made some sense of how it works. Unless every link in the chain of growth is complete, not a molecule of new muscle will form in your body. This chapter covers the guts of it, the information that turns donkeys into stallions, also-rans into champions. If you really want the gold, you better know it good.

Many athletes and trainers do not appreciate that the mechanisms controlling growth are a prime illustration of the principle of **synergy**. Growth hormone, for example, cannot work alone. It is useless to take arginine and ornithine alpha-ketoglutarate to increase the release of growth hormone (see Chapter 30), unless you also fulfill a host of other conditions that set your body up for growth.

Failure to fulfill these conditions is the reason athletes who use growth hormone injections, and even some experimental studies of growth hormone, get only marginal results. Simply pumping growth hormone into the system, is like maximizing the pedal power of a bike with no wheels.

Even when you do fulfill many conditions, you may still

make meagre gains. Net growth is the quantity of new proteins formed in muscle, minus the quantity of proteins lost by muscle breakdown. A marathon runner may have new proteins forming at a very high rate. But, because of the extreme endurance exercise of his sport, muscle protein breakdown for use as energy can equal or even exceed new muscle growth. So marathoners generally remain skinny and physically weak.

And don't believe that weak doesn't matter in endurance running. From 18 years of working with athletes, I'm here to tell you it matters in every sport. Give me two equal marathoners. If I make one of them 20% stronger he will become the superior runner - period!

Because strength is so crucial to sports performance, smart coaches are very interested in the new research on **anti-catabolic** nutrients. These are compounds that inhibit muscle breakdown. Combining them in the right sequence with anabolic nutrients is a potent strategy to increase net growth of muscle and strength.

The biochemistry of anabolic and anti-catabolic processes is so complex that no one has yet made complete sense of it. Nevertheless, science has uncovered enough of the system to form a concise plan to optimize your anabolic drive. In explaining this plan, we have to throw in a bit of biochemistry here and there. Stick with me. If you follow each step precisely, you will gain more strength than you ever dreamed possible. Healthy strength, without drugs, strength that needs no chemical crutches to support it, strength that will stay with you for the rest of your life.

Figure 9 shows a bare-bones schematic of the anabolic drive that we have developed at the Colgan Institute since the research began to look promising in 1982. The biochemistry is a lot more involved than the figure suggests, I have left out the whole adrenal-pituitary axis for example. Nevertheless, the components shown are all you need to maximize anabolism. Complicated? Nah! Apple-pie simple when we take it step-by-step.

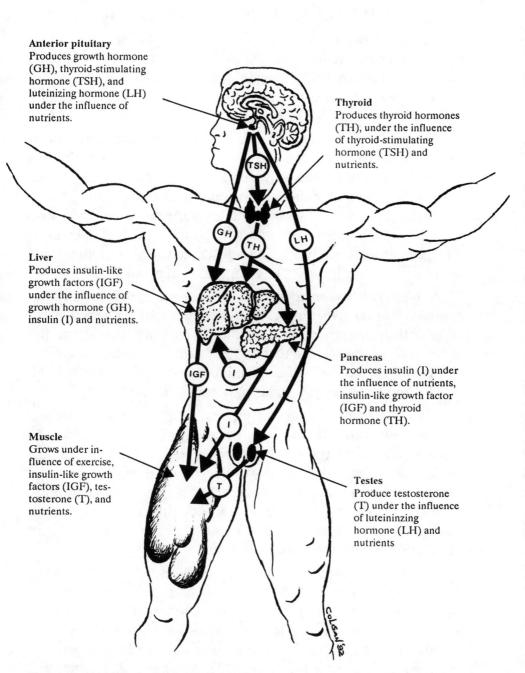

Anterior pituitary
Produces growth hormone
(GH), thyroid-stimulating
hormone (TSH), and
luteinizing hormone (LH)
under the influence of
nutrients.

Thyroid
Produces thyroid hormones
(TH), under the influence
of thyroid-stimulating
hormone (TSH) and
nutrients.

Liver
Produces insulin-like
growth factors (IGF)
under the influence of
growth hormone (GH),
insulin (I) and nutrients.

Pancreas
Produces insulin (I) under
the influence of nutrients,
insulin-like growth factor
(IGF) and thyroid
hormone (TH).

Muscle
Grows under in-
fluence of exercise,
insulin-like growth
factors (IGF), tes-
tosterone (T), and
nutrients.

Testes
Produce testosterone
(T) under the influence
of luteininzing
hormone (LH) and
nutrients

Figure 9. Simplified schematic of the Anabolic Drive.

Step 1: Releasing Growth Hormone.

To promote anabolism, first you have to increase output of growth hormone from the anterior lobe of the pituitary gland. We covered the basics of using amino acids to do that in Chapter 30. Here we look at some more details of nutrient synergy that will help you maximize results.

Growth hormone is released into the bloodstream in bursts. Some of each burst goes directly to bone and muscle cells where it initiates a little growth.[1] The rest is neutralized by the liver within 60-90 minutes. Before it is neutralized, the growth hormone causes the liver to manufacture **somatomedins** also called insulin-like growth factors.[1] The most studied is **insulin-like growth factor I (IGF)**. This substance travels to muscle and other cells where it causes large amounts of growth.

You can maximize this sequence of events only by fulfilling numerous other conditions. Animal studies indicate that the size of growth hormone bursts, and their frequency, determine the amount of muscle growth that occurs.[2] But you can't force growth hormone release just by taking amino acids any time you feel like it. The bursts occur only under particular circumstances.

In humans the largest growth hormone release occurs 30-60 minutes after falling asleep, and during heavy exercise.[3] To take advantage of these normal physiological functions, smart athletes increase the frequency of sleep and exercise periods and make their use of amino acids coincide. Arginine and ornithine alpha-ketoglutarate, taken in the absence of competing amino acids, one hour before exercise or sleep, reach the blood-brain circulation at just about the right time.

A practical scheme is to train twice daily, mid-morning and early afternoon, take the aminos an hour before training, and take a 30-60 minute nap immediately after training. In addition split your night sleep into two periods with a short waking period between them. Take the aminos an hour before bed and immediately you wake for the split. That way you can get four hits with aminos to increase growth hormone release in each 24 hours. How to work out the amounts of arginine and ornithine alpha-ketoglutarate to suit your biochemical individuality and lifestyle dynamics is explained in Chapter 30. Rule 1 for maximum anabolism: **Train twice, sleep twice, take aminos an hour before each**.

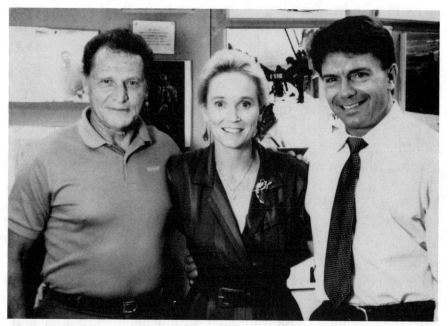

Michael and Lesley Colgan with renowned Olympic coach Arthur Lydiard whose work guides our training of runners.

An additional amino acid that causes some release of growth hormone in studies of catabolic patients is leucine.[3] Like the other two branched-chain amino acids isoleucine and valine, leucine is a **large neutral** amino acid. So inclusion of leucine in the mix that you take before sleep and exercise, does not compete with arginine and ornithine for transport across the blood-brain barrier, because they are **basic** amino acids. As explained in Chapter 30, they use a different transport system to get into the brain. So, although the evidence is scanty, leucine may add to arginine and ornithine in promoting release of growth hormone.

At the Colgan Institute we add 2-4 grams of leucine to the mix taken before sleep and exercise.

Other nutrients also boost the system. Release of growth hormone from the anterior pituitary depends on stimulation by another hormone in the brain called **growth hormone-releasing hormone** or **somatocrinin**. As we saw in Chapter 30, arginine and ornithine activate somatocrinin very nicely. So do glycine and tryptophan, except that tryptophan is currently banned by the FDA for sale in America. But before any of these amino acids will work, you have to fulfill another essential condition. The brain must have an adequate supply of vitamin C.

Research has recently established that activation of the growth hormone-releasing hormone, somatocrinin, requires another enzyme called **alpha-amidating monooxygenase**, which is absolutely limited by the amount of vitamin C available for use as a co-factor.[4] So you better have plenty around if you want to maximize growth hormone output. Linus Pauling guessed this connection many years ago, long before there were any scientific data about it. The link between vitamin C and growth hormone is one reason that his mega-intake of ascorbate has enabled him to retain his hormones, and thus his vigor, into extreme old age.

Another condition for growth hormone release is adequate supplies of phosphatidyl choline and pantothenic acid. These are the main constituents of the brain neurotransmitter **acetylcholine,** and we know that eating more of them increases brain acetylcholine levels.[5] One job of acetylcholine is to *reduce* production of another brain hormone called **somatostatin,** the hormone that *inhibits* release of growth hormone. And vitamin C helps acetylcholine do the job.[6]

A final but vital wrinkle for release of growth hormone is the essential mineral potassium. Most sports medicine folk seem unaware of the recent research showing that even marginal potasium deficiency causes profound inhibition of growth.[7,8] The accepted belief is still that potassium deficiency inhibits growth because it is required for development of muscle cells themselves. It is indeed, but that's not the only level of action. New work done by Dr Inge Dorup and colleagues, at the University of Aarhus in Denmark, shows that growth inhibition occurs after only a few days of reduced potassium intake, long before there is any significant decline in muscle potassium.[7]

In the latest series of studies, animals made potassium deficient showed large reductions in levels of growth hormone, and IGF, and strong inhibition of lean tissue growth. Injections of the growth-hormone-releasing hormone, somatocrinin, did not correct the problem, indicating that inhibition was occurring at the level of the anterior pituitary, not at the level of muscle. Simple oral supplementation with potassium promptly restored growth hormone levels and IGF levels.[9]

The synergy that controls all nutrient action provides a ready explanation. When serum levels of potassium decline, as they do almost immediately on a potassium-deficient diet, it is likely that the decline signals your brain to reduce growth hormone output and slow down muscle growth. That way your body avoids forming defective muscle cells because of an inadequate potassium supply.

I explained in Chapter 15 that much of the potassium is removed from American food by processing, and how athletes need more potassium than couch potatoes. Use this chapter to work out your individual need for potassium, and don't miss a day of it. Rule 2 for maximum anabolism: **Ensure adequate supplies of leucine, vitamin C, phosphatidyl choline, panthothenic acid and potassium**.

O.K. You have followed the rules, you are training like a madman, and enough growth hormone is coursing through your veins to grow a hippo. To read a lot of popular nutrition books, you might think that's all you need to grow muscle. I wish it was that easy! As many users of injectable growth hormone have found, pumping yourself up to the eyebrows with the drug doesn't grow much of anything in normal-sized adults, except a big jaw and a neanderthal shelf of bone above your eyes. Getting the growth hormone to produce IGF and to act on muscle depends on a host of other factors. The first of these is insulin.

Step 2: The Insulin Drive and IGF

As we saw earlier, the bulk of growth hormone goes to the liver where it is destroyed. Prior to destruction it stimulates the liver to produce insulin-like growth factor I (IGF). This is the real growth compound which travels to muscle cells and causes massive growth.[1] Recombinant DNA scientists have already produced some synthetic IGF. God help sport when that stuff hits the marketplace. To produce your own supply requires insulin, lots of insulin.

Drs DJ Millward and JP Rivers at the London School of Tropical Medicine in England are the leaders among researchers who have uncovered convincing evidence that your level of IGF and your rate of muscle growth are absolutely dependent on your insulin supply.[10] I can't cover the research here so will give only one example. Insulin dependent diabetics are the best model we have of people with inadequate insulin levels. They have great difficulty putting on muscle. Even if you inject them with growth hormone, their levels of IGF do not increase, and they make no muscle gains.[11] Throughout their lives they have very low levels of IGF simply because they do not have a steady level of insulin to help produce it.[12]

In addition to its effect on IGF, numerous researchers have shown that insulin also acts directly on muscle to drive amino acids into muscle cells for protein synthesis.[13] These are great finds for athletes, because evolution linked our insulin production directly to nutrient intake. So with a few simple principles we can manipulate the insulin drive at will.

The first principle is: keep it going. I have explained already why you should keep growth hormone release going 24 hours a day with amino acids taken before two exercise and two sleep periods. To keep the insulin drive going in a steady stream to combine with the growth hormone, you have to eat every few hours. It is useless to eat only three times a day. That causes a yo-yo rise and fall of insulin that disrupts the whole sequence. To keep insulin levels high and steady you have to eat at least six small meals each 24 hours.

A typical sequence to fit in with growth hormone release is given in Table 23. The post-exercise meals and night-time meal are best achieved by use of a pre-mixed protein/carb drink, mixed once a day in a large jug and used repeatedly. One drink that contains the right mix of amino acids, carbs and first-class protein sources is Lee Haney's Mass Fuel. Rule 3 for maximum anabolism: **Maintain insulin drive by eating six small meals a day**.

Table 23. A program for spacing of meals, growth-hormone releasing amino acids, exercise, and sleep to maximize growth hormone levels and insulin drive.

Time	Activity	
6 a.m.	Meal 1	
8 a.m.	Aminos 1	EXERCISE 1
10 a.m.	Post-exercise Meal 2 30 - 60 minute nap	
12 noon	Meal 3	
2 p.m.	Aminos 2	EXERCISE 2
4 p.m.	Post-exercise Meal 4 30 - 60 minute nap	
7 p.m.	Meal 5	
9 p.m.	Aminos 3	SLEEP
1 a.m.	Meal 6	SLEEP
4 a.m.	Aminos 4	SLEEP

Step 3: The Right Food

The composition of your meals is also critical in maintaining the insulin drive. As we saw in Chapter 9, during intense exercise your muscles lose glycogen fast. Whenever you finish a hard workout muscle glycogen levels, liver glycogen levels, and blood glucose levels are reduced. Consequently, insulin production is also reduced, and the insulin drive essential to anabolism cannot occur.

In this situation some athletes take only whole food proteins or amino acid mixes. Dead wrong on two counts! First, whole food protein is too hard to digest immediately after exercise. And, as we saw in Chapter 13, free amino acid mixes are very inefficient in building muscle. Second, by themselves proteins and free amino acids cause only a slight rise in insulin.[14] Consequently, muscle protein synthesis is inhibited, because the body has insufficient insulin drive to stimulate IGF synthesis, and to push amino acids into muscle cells.

Other athletes take only complex carbohydrates with low glycemic index scores after exercise, under the false belief that the only important job is to trickle glycogen back into their muscles. Big mistake! Complex carbs release sugar only slowly into the body, where it is immediately sucked up by muscles and liver to bring their glycogen levels up towards normal. Blood glucose cannot rise sufficiently to stimulate the insulin drive because there is insufficient sugar available. The first part of the mix you need immediately after a workout is some *quick* sugar. Sufficient must get into the body both to satisfy the increased muscle and liver demands for glycogen, and to raise blood sugar and stimulate the insulin drive.

To maintain the post-exercise insulin drive, first you should follow Chapter 9 and sip a 7-10% carbohydrate drink *during* training, such as Twinlab Hydra Fuel. That prevents your blood glucose and consequently your insulin being driven too low by the exercise. Second, you should include some glucose itself in your post-exercise meal.

Some athletes reject glucose because of the belief that simple sugars will disrupt insulin metabolism and also make them fat. They will if you take them into a system that is already full. But post-exercise sugar doesn't put on a molecule of bodyfat. Your body is far too busy using the glucose to replenish muscle glycogen and to assist protein synthesis.

But taking glucose alone as the first sugar source is not the best way. The body also responds to fructose by using it preferentially to replace liver glycogen. There is a ton of recent evidence that the combination of glucose and fructose stimulate much greater insulin production than glucose alone.[15]

The third part of the post-exercise meal is complex carbohydrates that digest slowly and continue to trickle sugar into the body for at least a couple of hours. The types and amounts of these carbs are explained in Chapter 9. For a 75 kg (165 lb) athlete in intense training, 200 grams of a maltodextrin based formula is about right. combine this with about 10 grams of glucose and 15 grams of fructose to yield 900 calories of carbohydrates.

The fourth part of the post-exercise meal is protein. As Chapter 13 explains, best is a whey or egg protein hydrolysate, the form of protein that yields the highest nitrogen retention. Together with carbohydrates, hydrolysates consisting of dipeptides (two amino acids), tripeptides (three amino acids) and single amino acids, stimulate far more insulin production than carbohydrates alone.[14] In some studies the addition of amino acids to glucose doubled insulin output.[14]

One further reason that a hydrolysate is the best post-exercise form of protein is digestibility. Because of the high amino acid flux in the body immediately after exercise, you should take about one-quarter of your total daily protein after each training session. As shown in Chapter 12, for some individuals protein intake needs to be 200 grams a day. For them a post-exercise meal would include 50 grams of protein. That's far too much to digest, unless you take a predigested hydrolysate that can be transported directly into the system without much modification by your intestines.

A final stimulus to the insulin drive is the mineral chromium, in the form of chromium picolinate. This compound is so important in increasing the efficiency of insulin that I gave it the whole of Chapter 29. Use that chapter to work out your individual chromium requirement, and take it every day.Rule 4 for maximum anabolism: **Each post-exercise meal should consist of glucose, fructose, complex carbohydrates, chromium picolinate and 25% of your total daily protein as a whey or egg protein hydrolysate.**

Step 4: Specific Amino Acids

Some amino acids also act independently to stimulate insulin release and should be included separately in the mix. In addition to their presence in the protein hydrolysate. Arginine is a potent stimulus to insulin and this action is specifically enhanced by a small amount of glucose.[16] In contrast, a study just completed by Dr Luke Bucci and colleagues at the University of Texas, Houston, found that ornithine has no effect on insulin levels.[17]

Ornithine combined with alpha-ketoglutarate is a whole different story. And you should know this story, because it explains a lot about the action of the essential branched-chain amino acids, and about the non-essential amino acids **glutamine** and **alanine** that are probably the keys to anti-catabolism.

Glutamine is the most abundant free amino acid in muscle, comprising over 50% of the free amino acids.[20] Alanine comprises about 10% of the free aminos in muscle.[18] The level of glutamine, but not alanine, is also highly correlated with muscle protein synthesis.[7] Because glutamine can carry two nitrogen molecules, it is also the main transporter of nitrogen waste.[20] So it is likely glutamine is the more important.

During and following exercise or trauma, large amounts of alanine and glutamine are released from muscle, much more than any other amino acids.[19,20] The loss of alanine and glutamine induced by exercise is way above the amounts available in muscle, and more than 50% of the total loss of muscle amino acids. So other muscle amino acids must be used to make them.[18]

Studies on the rapid uptake of branched-chain amino acids during and after exercise, indicate that they provide the building materials for alanine and glutamine.[10,15,19] These findings explain one major way that supplements of branched-chain amino acids support muscle growth. They prevent catabolism of muscle by serving as substrates for the large amounts of alanine and glutamine that are lost from the body during and after exercise.

Why Ornithine Alpha-Ketoglutarate?

Why should we go to the trouble of using ornithine alpha-ketoglutarate: why not use glutamine itself? Oral glutamine certainly maintains muscle in catabolic patients.[21] There are six reasons, all of them important to athletes. First, as we saw in Chapter 23, ammonia is toxic to the body in numerous ways. The most important finding for athletes is: the higher the ammonia level created by exercise, the poorer your performance.[29] If you use glutamine, you whack your body with ammonia.

Unless kept absolutely dry, glutamine powder degrades into ammonia and pyroglutamic acid. It degrades even if you put it in solution only a few minutes before you drink it, and even in the stomach if you take it dry. Consequently, glutamine is not used with catabolic patients because it adds to their ammonia burden and jeopardizes recovery.[20]

To overcome this problem researchers in France developed alpha-ketoglutarate, which has the same carbon skeleton as glutamine, that is, provides a substrate for glutamine, but contains virtually no ammonia. Far from adding to the ammonia burden, alpha-ketoglutarate acts in the body as an ammonia scavenger.[30] Ornithine also acts as an ammonia scavenger.[31] The combination of the two is a potent way to reduce your ammonia burden.

Second, as we saw in Chapter 30, ornithine alpha-ketoglutarate produces a much larger release of growth hormone in patients and in healthy subjects than either compound used alone.[22]

Third, the body can make glutamine from both ornithine and alpha-ketoglutarate. Animal studies show that oral ornithine alpha-ketoglutarate increases the muscle glutamine pool and reduces muscle catabolism.[23] Oral ornithine alpha-ketoglutarate also reduces muscle catabolism in burn and surgery patients.[24,25] So it is a strong anti-catabolic agent.

Fourth, ornithine alpha-ketoglutarate increases insulin secretion in patients[26] and in healthy subjects.[27] In a recent study, the pioneers in use of this compound, Dr Luc Cynobar and colleagues of the Laboratoire de Biochemie at the Hopital Saint Antoine in Paris, fed healthy males oral doses of 10 grams of ornithine alpha-ketoglutarate or a placebo. Ornithine alpha-ketoglutarate caused a marked increase in insulin levels.[28] So it is a potent stimulus to the insulin drive.

Fifth, arginine is the end product of ornithine in the body's **urea cycle**. So ornithine alpha-ketoglutarate can add to the arginine pool available for growth hormone release. In cases of severe muscle catabolism such as that caused by overtraining, arginine may become an essential amino acid. Available ornithine would then be used to create additional arginine in order to preserve muscle.[16]

Sixth, as we saw in Chapter 22, muscles provide a continuous supply of glutamine to the immune system. Proliferation of immune cells requires glutamine but they cannot make it. Studies show that the traumatic effects of intense training on the muscles and on the immune system easily overwhelm your body's ability to make glutamine. Without supplemental glutamine it is likely both muscle cells and immune cells will be poorly supplied.

This problem is likely whenever you step up your training.

It is most obvious in the overtraining syndrome. Without adequate glutamine, strength and immunity gradually decline, and health and performance go to hell in a handbasket. Ornithine alpha-ketoglutarate may be a key to prevention.

To sum up, ornithine alpha-ketoglutarate provides a strong releaser of growth hormone, a ready source of glutamine, an anti-catabolic, a big stimulus to the insulin drive, a source of arginine, a support for the immune system, and a great ammonia scavenger. Any athlete who doesn't use it is giving away a potent edge. Rule 5 for maximum anabolism: **Each meal should include 2-4 grams of ornithine alpha-ketoglutarate.**

Special Properties of Leucine

Leucine and probably the other two branched chain amino acids, isoleucine and valine, act to protect muscle in a variety of ways. We have already covered their action as substrates for alanine and glutamine. [10,15,19] They are also used directly for fuel, thereby sparing muscle amino acids. [32] Leucine especially, is burned in large quantities during long exercise, [33] and the better trained the athlete the more leucine he burns. [34]

Leucine also increases growth hormone release, [3] which is why we included 2-4 grams of leucine with each amino acid mix taken before sleep and exercise. But we do not use supplemental leucine with post-exercise meals, even though such use causes great improvements in protein synthesis in patients after surgery. [35] Leucine suffers from the same problem as glutamine. It increases the ammonia burden of catabolism. As chapter 23 explains, ammonia is serious nastiness for athletic performance. [29]

Very recent reasearch has solved this dilemma. We now know that the growth hormone releasing action of leucine depends on the amino acid itself, whereas its other anabolic and anti-catabolic actions depend on what is called its keto-acid derivative, **ketoisocaproate.** [36]

That's good news for athletes because ketoisocaproate contains no ammonia. Athletes on the high protein diets essential to fast increases in muscle and strength, produce scads of ammonia from protein metabolism as well as from training. Studies on patients who have been put into a high catabolic, high ammonia condition by surgery or disease, show that ketoisocaproate acts as a strong ammonia scavenger.[36,37] Any nutrient that will suck up ammonia is a big benefit for sports performance.

To cover all the other actions of branched-chain keto acids is way beyond the scope of this book. Suffice to say here that ketoisocaproate is the best form of leucine for post-exercise meals because, in addition to scavenging ammonia, it also stimulates insulin release, spares muscle protein and promotes protein synthesis.[32,37,38] Rule 6 for maximum anabolism: **Each post-exercise meal should include 2-4 grams of ketoisocaproate.**

Combination of the ketoisocaproate form of leucine with the ornithine alpha-ketoglutarate forms of ornithine and glutamine provides the most potent anabolic and anti-catabolic mix of these amino acids yet known to science. Unfortuantely, very few companies make it yet, except at highway robbery prices for use with patients after surgery. The only sports supplement I know that has these forms of the amino acids in the right concentration, in combination with some decent carbs and proteins, is Lee Haney's Mass Fuel made by Twinlab. Having won Mr Olympia 8 times, and having trained such champions as Evander Holyfield for strength, Lee has more of a handle than most on the stuff that works.

Step 5: Nitrogen Balance

Throughout this book I have emphasized the importance of a positive energy balance and a positive nitrogen balance *all the time*, if you want to grow an optimum body. But a lot of coaches still keep their athletes on mediocre calorie intake or mediocre protein intake. They do this in order to keep down bodyfat, or keep athletes in lower weight classes, or keep them looking sleek and cut for what you might call decorative sports. That way of

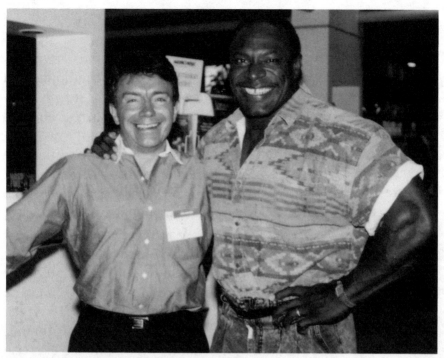

Dr Michael Colgan with Lee Haney in 1991.

doing it is crazy for all sorts of reasons that we covered in earlier chapters. But the main craziness is, it kills the anabolic drive.

At one of my recent lectures to sports medicine folk, some members of the audience objected that athletes need only the RDA for protein, and that low-calorie intakes **increase** growth hormone levels. So they do.[1] But remember the focus of this chapter. Growth hormone is only the first step towards muscle growth.

Growth hormone *levels* do little to determine growth hormone *action*. Undernourished children, for example, have very high levels of growth hormone. But they have very low levels of insulin-like growth factor (IGF), so no muscle growth takes place.[39] If you fast animals for 3 days, their IGF levels drop by a third.[40] If you fast human subjects for five days, IGF levels drop by two-thirds.[41] Without adequate IGF, you can't even grow a toenail.

The pioneering research on regulation of IGF by protein-calorie nutrition in humans is being done by Dr David Clemmons and Louis Underwood of the Department of Medicine and Pediatrics at the University of North Carolina. Recently they threw in the exercise variable. Normal subjects were exercised intensely for a week. They were fed a supposedly protein-adequate, calorie-adequate diet of 35 calories per kilogram bodyweight. That's 2625 calories a day for a 75kg (165 lb) athlete. The exercise used about 1000 calories per day. According to some coaches, that should have left plenty for vital functions and muscle maintenance.

The exercise also significantly increased growth hormone output. Uninformed folk might think that would yield increased muscle growth. No way! IGF levels declined by 40%, and the athletes were in *negative* nitrogen balance, that is *losing* muscle, throughout the test.[42] These are important findings for athletes. On a diet deemed adequate for sedentary folk, intense exercise kills the anabolic drive and decimates muscle.

But the key to this problem is not just calories. The answer comes from other studies in Clemmons' laboratory. Levels of IGF are directly correlated with nitrogen balance.[43] Rats put on a 5% protein diet instead of their usual 15%, but with as many calories as they want, show large reductions in IGF levels. And injections of growth hormone don't raise their IGF levels even a whisker.[44,45] Animal studies from other laboratories confirm that protein intake affects IGF production in a dose-dependent fashion.[46]

This need for protein to stimulate IGF is best illustrated by Clemmons' studies of sedentary human subjects. Subjects fasted for five days lose two-thirds of their IGF. If you then feed different groups varying levels of protein, all in calorie-adequate diets, the IGF response is proportional to the protein intake. Low protein diets (0.4 grams/kg bodyweight) do not restore IGF. Higher intakes (1.0 grams/kg bodyweight) quickly bring IGF levels back to normal.[41]

But remember, that is in sedentary folk. Athletes in intense training need a lot more protein than 1.0 grams/kg to remain in positive nitrogen balance. It is crucial to your anabolic drive, that you use Chapter 12 to work out your individual need for protein and then stick to it.

Protein quality is also crucial. Proteins high in all essential amino acids, in the correct ratios to each other, yield the highest levels of IGF. Clemmons has shown that adequate protein-calorie diets supplemented with essential amino acids cause a 20% greater increase in IGF levels in human subjects, than the same diets supplemented with non-essential amino acids.[47]

So make sure all your protein is top biological value. That's a difficult job in the sports marketplace where most protein powders use casein as their main source of protein. It bears repeating from Chapter 12 that the highest biological value proteins are whey protein concentrate (lactalbumin) and egg white protein (egg albumin). Note I said whey protein concentrate, not whey itself which is low in protein but cheap, and therefore much used.

Beef, poultry and fish proteins have a 20% lower biological value, followed by casein from milk, followed by soy protein. All other vegetable proteins have a much lower value, about half the value of whey protein. Buying low quality protein is a sure road to a low anabolic drive and poor muscle growth. Rule 7 for maximum anabolism: **Maintain nitrogen balance every day with top quality protein**.

Step 6: Thyroid Hormones

Look back at Figure 9. It illustrates how thyroid hormones (TH) are released from the thyroid gland at the base of your throat, under the influence of **thyroid-stimulating hormone** (TSH) and nutrients. An adequate supply of the thyroid hormone **T3** is essential for your anabolic drive, because it directly influences insulin secretion.[48] In animal studies, low levels of thyroid hormone T3 reduce the insulin response to food, and injections of T3 improve the response.[49] Thyroid is an essential component of the insulin drive.

Insulin also interacts in synergy with the thyroid hormone **T4** at the liver,[50] which may affect insulin's influence on production of IGF. No one has sorted that one out yet. But we do know that thyroid hormone T3 interacts with insulin to inhibit protein catabolism in muscle.[51] So, *at correct levels*, T3 is anti-catabolic.

Correct levels is the operative phrase. Any excess of thyroid hormones is big-time catabolic to all tissues.[51] Because it is easily available, some athletes use synthetic thyroid to reduce bodyfat. They don't realize it is also chewing away at their hard-earned muscle. High levels of thyroid are so catabolic that whenever the pituitary increases output of growth hormone, it automatically reduces output of thyroid-stimulating hormone.[52] So it is likely that certain amino acids can affect thyroid production through their influences on the pituitary. But no one has sorted that one out either.

The first thing you need to know about thyroid hormones is that your body needs **iodine** to produce them. With the supplementary iodine now added to salt and other foods, the level of iodine in the American diet is probably sufficient for sedentary folk. But athletes may need more iodine, because it is rapidly lost in sweat.[53] Use Chapter 20 to help you work out your iodine requirement: then don't mess with it.

Protein quality also affects thyroid levels. Recent research by Dr CA Barth and colleagues at the Institut fur Physiologie und Biochemie in Kiel, Germany compared milk protein and soy protein diets in a series of experiments with rats and pigs (whimsical choices as models for men). Soy protein caused a greater rise in both T3 and T4 hormones.[54] Other laboratories have recently reported similar evidence of a sharp rise in thyroid hormone levels after feedings of soy and gluten proteins.[55,56]

These important findings uncover a major reason why soy and other vegetable proteins are inferior for growth of muscle and strength. They raise thyroid hormone levels towards the catabolic zone. If you are one of those athletes who has been influenced by the "cult of the cuddley" (Oops! I mean ethics) not to eat milk, egg, or other high quality animal proteins, then give this book away to someone who will really benefit from it. Soy and other vegetable proteins will get you by, but you will *never, never* achieve your athletic potential.

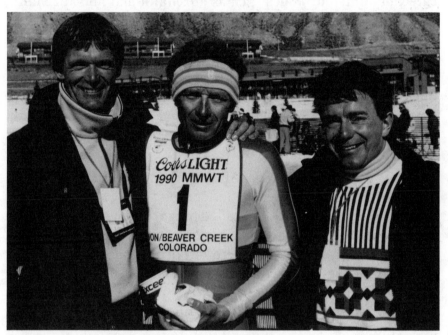

Michael Colgan with mountain sports athlete Rex Keep and champion triathlete Andre Boesel at the Winterman Triathlon, Vail.

And don't point to those champions who wear vegetarianism as a trademark. I have broken bread with some of them, watching as they inhaled huge bowls of egg whites and brown rice, or swallowed whey-based protein drinks by the quart. Without those first-class proteins their bodies would resemble Olive Oil not Popeye. Rule 8 for maximum anabolism: **Protect thyroid metabolism with iodine and first-class proteins**.

Step 7: Testosterone

Figure 13 shows that testosterone is produced in the testes under the influence of **luteinizing hormone** from the anterior pituitary, plus nutrients. That's correct as far as it goes, but it covers only a tiny piece of the testosterone story. I deliberately left out the **adrenal glands** and the whole collection of **catecholamine hormones** such as **adrenalin** and **nor-adrenalin**, because it would have made the picture much too complex. Suffice to say here that the catecholamine hormones are generally catabolic, that is, they break down glycogen, bodyfat and muscle proteins for fuel and also inhibit the insulin drive. But, and it's a big but, **adrenocorticotrophic hormone (ACTH)**, the main hormone released from the pituitary that stimulates production of catecholamine hormones by the adrenal glands, also increases production of testosterone.

It happens like this. All sex hormones are made from cholesterol. Greatly under the influence of ACTH, cholesterol is converted to an intermediary called **pregnenolone**. If ACTH goes up, so does pregnenolone, and so does testosterone. We know this happens because excessive secretion of ACTH by the anterior pituitary occurs in certain inherited diseases. This excess increases production of pregnenolone, which in turn increases production of testosterone. Growth of all lean tissues is thereby accelerated.[57]

But it doesn't produce giants, it produces muscular dwarfs, because excess testosterone causes early maturation of bone.[57] Disreputable coaches who supply teenage athletes with synthetic testosterone, take note. For a modicum of quick muscle, you are condemming these lads to never reach their true height.

The testosterone story would remain fairly simple if it was all made in the testes. But a good deal is also made in the adrenal glands under various influences of the catecholamine hormones, and, for women, also in the ovaries, and even in muscle.[58]

Males make up to 10 mg of testostrone a day: Females only

0.25 mg. Testosterone affects female cell growth just as it affects males. So the huge potential for growth of muscle and strength in adult women by increasing testosterone levels is obvious. Remember the giant East German female athletes. Ben Johnson's coach, Charlie Francis, underscored the anabolic power of excessive testosterone injections, when he likened two East German throwers in dresses and high heels to the dancing hippos from Disney's Fantasia.[59]

But as Chapter 33 shows, sports careers built on anabolic steroids often collapse into grim disease. Far better to go for the long haul and healthy life thereafter, by stimulating your own production of testosterone. That way the body can use all your individual genetic checks and balances to keep it within healthy bounds.

Stimulating testosterone production is a tough job. To show you how tough I will sketch the process as it happens in your body. After cholesterol is turned into pregnenolone under the influence of ACTH, it goes through a precise series of chemical steps outlined in Figure 10. I left out some of the steps, but you get the general idea. At the progesterone step, specific hormonal influences chop off most of that intermediary (indicated by the size of the arrow) and turn it into other essential hormones called **corticosteroids**. These are the **glucocorticoids** that increase catabolism of body proteins and fats, and the **mineralcorticoids** that control your water and electrolyte metabolism.[57]

The little that is left at the end of the chemical trail is then turned into androgens (male hormones) **androstenedione** and **testosterone** under the influence of luteininzing hormone. Genetic controls in males then turn a tiny fraction into the estrogens (female hormones) **estrone** and **estradiol**. Genetic controls in females turn most of the androgen production into estrogens.

I have tortured you with a sketch of the exquisite control of testosterone formation in the body to emphsize one thing. *None* of the so-called steroid alternatives sold in the sports supplement marketplace can increase testosterone production. The bodily controls are far too tight. As explained in Chapter 31, some plant sterols (**phytoestrogens**) do have estrogenic action in animals, but in a drug-like fashion, not by increasing estrogen production.[60] Certain other plant sterols and insect steroids possibly have a weak influence on human anabolism, but again in a drug-like fashion, not by increasing testosterone production.[61]

The element boron is another steroid alternative scam. As explained in Chapter 15, boron probably is an essential mineral for testosterone production. But it doesn't *cause* it. It's just one of the links in the chain of synergy. You should use Chapter 15 to ensure you have a sufficient intake of boron. Beyond that, extra

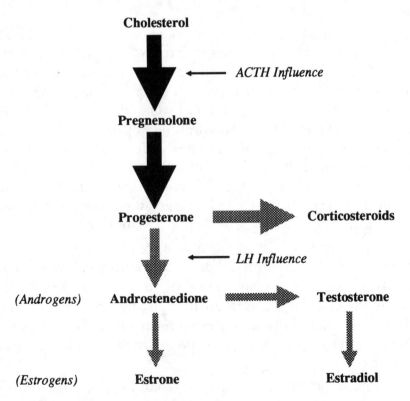

Figure 10. Bodily production of steroid hormones. Size of arrows illustrate progressive reductions in the amount of substrate available.

boron cannot raise your testosterone by a molecule.

The evidence is a lot stronger for vitamin C as a stimulus to testosterone production than for boron. One of the main jobs of testosterone is to maintain the structure of the testes. Vitamin C deficiency is notorious for destruction of testicular tissue through its effects on testosterone.[62] And large doses of ascorbic acid restore fertility in some impotent men through complex multi-hormonal influences on testicular tissue, sperm production, and sperm motility.[63]

But the strongest influence of vitamin C on testosterone takes place further up the chemical chain. Dr Abbas Kitabchi and colleagues at the University of Tennessee in Memphis, recently confirmed earlier research that high intakes of ascorbic acid partially inhibit the adrenal gland response to ACTH, so that it makes less of the catecholamine hormones. Consequently, more of the body's pregnenolone is available for conversion to testosterone. [64,65] Whether the conversion takes place has still to be proven. But it is likely, given the evidence discussed above that high pregnenolone levels produce high testosterone levels.[57] Use Chapter 20 to work out your individual requirement for vitamin C, and take it every day.

There is also a pile of evidence from animal and human studies that the essential mineral zinc dramatically influences testosterone production.[66,67] These effects occur because the **Leydig cells** in the testes that produce testosterone require continuous adequate supplies of zinc to maintain their function.[68]

In a representative study, experts in zinc metabolism, Dr Ananda Prasad and colleagues at Wayne State University School of Medicine, Detroit, made normal human subjects zinc deficient. Blood levels of testosterone promplty declined. Supplementary zinc just as promptly restored levels to normal.[68] So, for optimal testosterone, use Chapter 15 to assess your individual need for zinc, and include it faithfully in your daily nutrient mix.

The final nutrients that may improve testosterone levels are the branched-chain amino acids. New research indicates that supplements of leucine, isoleucine, and valine taken an hour before intense training can increase serum testosterone levels after training.[69,70] Directly after training is when you need the circulating testosterone most. That is when it has maximum effect in promoting new protein synthesis. We currently add only leucine to the pre-exercise mix. But the evidence is growing that isoleucine and valine may also be involved.[69,70] Chapter 13 gives a table that will help you work out daily amounts.

There is one other thing you can do to stimulate testosterone production. The brilliant work of Dr C H Li at the University of California, established over thirty years ago that growth hormone increases testosterone levels. It achieves this difficult task by enhancing the action of leuteinizing hormone, the direct influence on testosterone production.[69,70] So whenever you focus your efforts on secretion of growth hormone, you also get a bonus in testosterone. Rule 9 for maximum anabolism: **Maintain adequate boron, zinc, and vitamin C and branched-chain amino acid status, and increase growth hormone output to raise testosterone levels.**

Maximum Anabolic Drive

I have sketched the main influence of exercise and nutrients on the anabolic drive. Numerous other nutrients are involved, because all of them work in synergy with each other. We only separate them out in order to make the picture understandable. The picture I tried to draw here is a bare-bones sketch, citing only a tiny, but hopefully representative fraction of the evidence. Nevertheless, the rules summarized in Table 24 give you a pretty decent shot at maximizing anabolism. Go do it!

Table 24. A program to maximize the anabolic drive.

To increase release of growth hormone:

    1. Train twice, sleep twice daily. Take arginine, ornithine alpha-ketoglutarate and leucine before each.

    2. Ensure adequate daily supplies of leucine, vitamin C, phosphatidyl choline, panthothenic acid and potassium.

To maintain the insulin drive and IGF production:

    3. Eat six small meals a day.

    4. Each post-exercise meal should contain glucose, fructose, complex carbohydrates, chromium picolinate, and 25% of your total daily protein as a whey protein or egg protein hydrolysate.

    5. Each meal should include 2-4 grams of ornithine alpha-ketoglutarate.

    6. Each post-exercise meal should include 2-4 grams of ketoisocaproate.

    7. Maintain nitrogen balance every day with top quality protein.

To ensure correct levels of thyroid hormone:

    8. Protect thyroid metabolism with iodine and first-class proteins.

To stimulate testosterone production:

    9. Maintain adequate boron, zinc, vitamin C, and branched-chain amino acid status, and maximize release of growth hormone.

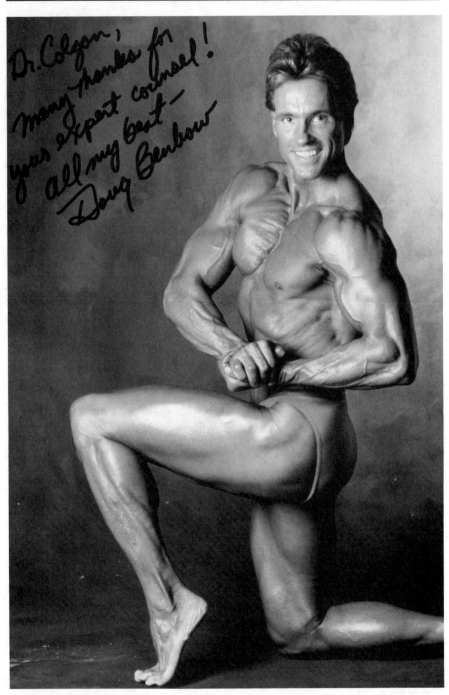

In his forties, athlete Doug Benbow shows the effects of nutritional stimulation of the anabolic drive by use of a Colgan Institute program.

Drugs work, no doubt about it. But optimum nutrition works equally as well and has no downside, neither for health nor for the human spirit.

Michael Colgan, Olympic Scientific Congress, 1984

Chapter 33

Steroids: The Real Story

"I lied, I lied, I lied." In July 1991, Lyle Alzedo admitted in **Sports Illustrated** that he had used massive doses of anabolic steroids since 1969, since he was 20 years old. And that he had lied through his teeth all those years to conceal it. Stricken with inoperable brain cancer, he had lost 60 lbs of his famous muscle and was, in his own words, "sick and scared."[1] A few months later he was dead at age 42.

Raiders' physician, Dr Robert Huizenga admits he warned Alzedo for years about the consequences of steroids. Alzedo himself was convinced that steroids caused his cancer, a virulent T-cell lymphoma. Huizenga believes he was probably right.

Ex-Pittsburgh Steeler and Tampa Bay Buccaneer offensive lineman, Steve Courson, was a regular steroid user since age 19. In 1988 at age 32, he was rushed to intensive care only to be told he needed a new ticker.[2] Today, he still awaits a suitable heart transplant that might allow him to limp along to age 50.

Steve Vallie, Connecticut bodybuilder and football standout, suffered a heart attack at the Phoenix Gym in New Haven, in March 1989. He died. An autopsy found that his heart was pathologically enlarged and thickened. He was a heavy steroid user -- dead at age 21.[3]

Nine-time American powerlifting champion Larry Pacifico also wrecked his cardiovascular system with steroids. He was rushed to the hospital for a quadruple coronary bypass at age 35.[3]

I have hundreds of these celebrity cases on computer. But I also have thousands of cases where steroids did no apparent damage. The most famous is Arnold Schwarzenegger. Now chairman of the President's Council on Physical Fitness and Sports, Arnold used steroids throughout his bodybuilding career.[4,5] Of course, at that time they were perfectly legal.

Another famous steroid user that apparently kept his health, is footballer Brian Bosworth,[3] the "Boz," with his abrasive demeanor and multi-colored haircut beloved of hordes of adoring fans. Another is Bill Toomey, Olympic gold medalist in the decathlon, and recipient of the AAU Sullivan Award as an outstanding American in every way.[6] His use of steroids was legal also.

Hulk Hogan, the world's best known wrestler, is widely reported as receiving steroids from ringside physician Dr George Zahorian. Hogan denies it. Zahorian was convicted of selling steroids to professional wrestlers in July 1991. Another well-known "steroid doctor," Dr Walter Jekot, has just been convicted of selling steroids to a reported list of Hollywood clients, whose names the attorneys warn me I better not mention.

And among the Eastern block athletes who were given steroids officially as part of their training, is the most beautiful woman ever to don a pair of skates, Olympic gold medalist and Diet Coke advocate, Katarina Witt.[3]

The problem in all these cases is not whether steroids cause illness, nor even whether steroids work, but that they have been used by the stars, the cream of the human crop, the models of greatness adored by our youth, and emulated minutely, even to the color of their socks.

Today, Arnold does a great job of warning young athletes that steroids are sick, and Hogan preaches a no-drugs litany to children. But the kids see only the Terminator and the Hulkster, and crave anything they think may have given them that power.

Recently, the National Youth Sports Coaches Association surveyed 2,700 young athletes in 17 states. Almost half the respondents believed that drugs will improve their sports performance, that steroids will improve muscle and strength, and that steroids will not harm a user who is careful.[7]

In fact, there is strong evidence that warning athletes about steroids by zealous campaigns to keep kids off drugs only further encourages their use.[8,9] When will authorities learn that educating athletes about the dangers of performance enhancing drugs does not change attitudes towards drugs. Experts in this field, Dr Linn Goldberg and colleagues at Oregon Health Sciences University, have shown repeatedly that threats or warnings about the dangers of drugs do not reduce their use, but rather increase it.[8-10]

The only way to eliminate steroids from sports is to give athletes an alternative program for growing an optimum body that works at least as well as the drugs, and that also leaves your health and longevity intact. That's what this book is all about.

Steroid Use

Whenever I read the official stance that only a tiny percentage of athletes use steroids, it smacks of hypocrisy by officialdom to protect their fat sinecures from public criticism. Official pronouncements are based on surveys and drug testing. They go this way. Surveys of football players in six high schools in Oregon reported only 1.1% steroid use.[11] (Official stance: "Praise the Lord, our kids are clean.").

In two recent national surveys of high school seniors, 3% reported steroid use.[12,13] And in the **1991 National Household Survey on Drug Abuse**, 2.5% of high schoolers reported steroid use.[14] (Official stance: "Well, the kids are almost clean.").

But the accuracy of surveys depends on who did them. Studies sponsored by the federal government get few truthful responses because of public suspicion of hidden agendas. More incisive studies in high schools in seven states got reports of 5% to 12% steroid use, up to *five times* the government figure.[21]

By college, students are even more suspicious. Surveys in 1991 report that 5% of college athletes admit steroid use.[15] (Official stance: "There is a bit of slippage in college."). But if you don't ask students to admit their own steroid use, but rather to say how many of their peers are using, they are less reticent. Using this technique with 1,600 NCAA Division I athletes, Dr Charles Yesalis and colleagues found 14.7% steroid use among males and 5.9% among females.[16]

Elite athletes are very closed-mouthed to any official inquiry about steroids. Even when asked to give use amongst their peers, they shy away. At the 1992 Winter Olympics, out of 155 Olympians, 53 athletes reported use of only 1-9%, and 35 athletes reported that there was *no steroid use at all* in their sports.[17] If you believe that I have some prime swampland in Florida that might interest you. Some 67 of the Winter Olympians worried officialdom by reporting steroid use of 10% plus. (Official stance: Finger to side of nose: "Bad foreign influences.").

But even these figures are a huge under-report of steroid use. You get the real position only from the inside. Olympic runner, now popular TV commentator, Marty Liquori, was asked before the Seoul Olympics. His reply, "I doubt whether you'll find many athletes on our '88 Olympic team who haven't had some steroid use."[18]

I promised you the truth in this book. The official stance on steroid use in America is patent garbage! In the '80s, drugs in sport became naughty-naughty. Athletes who valued their careers publicly distanced themselves from users. By 1988 it was an offense to prescribe steroids to healthy people. By November 1990, the Anabolic Steroids Control Act made it a felony to sell steroids, on penalty of 5 years jail, plus a $250,000 fine. It's as thick as two bricks dumb to believe that most steroid users are going to tell you about their little secret.

Take the National Football League, for example. Dr Charles Yesalis, world expert on drug use in sports at Penn State University, estimates that 75-90% of NFL players have used steroids.[19] From the inside, former New York Jets lineman Joe Klecko put use at 65-70% in 1987.[20] But they are too smart to admit it publicly. In 1990, the NFL did a league-wide anonymous survey of drug use among its 1,600 players. Only 7.5% of the players responded. The others refused or ignored the letters and reminders.[19,21]

Wouldn't you? If you have a $1 million a year contract with a no-drugs clause, how do you know any questionnaire sent to you doesn't identify you personally. It's pie simple to code the computer to rig any questionnaire. You simply put in an extra comma in a specific location to identify the questionnaire sent to say, NFL lineman Bill Fralic, and you leave out a comma in a specific location to identify say, the paper sent to Mike Keen. Then if the NFL wants to dump anyone who reports steroid use, they have them by the short and curlies on a downhill pull.

I'm sure all was kosher with the NFL survey, and Fralic and Keen are two of the strongest voices in the fight against steroids. But if you are in college or on an athletic scholarship, or have anything to lose, and you use steroids, keep it to yourself.

What about those deadly accurate drug tests? Don't they show how many athletes are users? Give me a break! There is nothing wrong with the chemistry of the tests, but any physician with a basic knowledge of biochemistry can teach athletes how to beat them in a day.

In 1984 and 1985, US Olympic Committee drug testing, always announced well beforehand, found less that 1% of athletes positive for steroids. But during the same years with the same athletes, the US Olympic Committee did a number of unannounced tests. For these the athletes were guaranteed that results would not be subject to sanctions, and would not go on the athlete's record. *One in every two* tested positive for steroids. Half of our finest athletes were on the juice![3] You have to conclude that drug testing is more a deterrent to public criticism of fat cat sports officials than to drug use.

Medical Profession Responsible

Most media reports today don't seem to realize that the witchhunt against steroids is very recent. They used to be lauded by some of the very people that now condemn them. They were legal, freely available, and prescribed in multi-millions of doses for athletes by thousands of physicians. The American medical profession popularized and promoted the use of steroids in sports for 20 years. **The Track and Field News**, official organ of The Athletes Congress (TAC), openly called steroids the "breakfast of champions."[22]

Here are the facts. In 1954, Dr John Ziegler was physician to the United States weightlifting team at the world championships in Vienna. He noticed that the superior Soviet team had very heavy body hair, and some team members had to have catheters inserted in order to be able to urinate, indicating enlarged prostate glands. On questioning a Soviet team physician, he learned that the athletes were using synthetic testosterone.

At that time in America, various anabolic/androgenic steroids were being developed from testosterone to treat muscle-wasting diseases, and to increase red blood cells in certain forms of anemia.[23] They were also being tried for hastening recovery from surgery or injury. Incidentally, we use the word "steroid" here to mean anabolic/androgenic types of steroid. These are all derivatives of testosterone. But there are many other steroids, such as cholesterol, that have no anabolic or androgenic activity.

When Ziegler returned to the US, he was concerned about the androgenic effects of testosterone derivatives and approached CIBA Pharmaceuticals to develop a drug that was less androgenic and more anabolic. Dianabol (methandrostenolone), was born, and the athletic world changed forever.

Ziegler took this fairly crude drug to the York Barbell Club in Pennsylvania where top weightlifters trained. Results were so spectacular that reports spread throughout America.

Within months thousands of physicians were prescribing anabolic steroids for athletes.

Footballer Steve Courson is a typical example. Like tens of thousands of college athletes, he was turned on to steroids by a college coach, when he was 19 at the University of South Carolina. He went to the team physician, got a prescription, and *the University paid his drug bill.* Now Steve needs a new heart.[24]

Ziegler, who used steroids himself, also wrecked his heart, and died of a heart attack on 18 November 1983. Before he died he warned everyone in a tape-recorded message:

I wish I had never heard the word steroid...All these young kids...they don't realize the terrible price they are going to pay.[25]

Meanwhile, American doctors were getting rich on steroids, pumping out prescriptions like pulp novel printing presses. Unlike some whitewash inquiries conducted in America, the Dubin Commission, set up by the Canadian Government in 1989 to investigate the Ben Johnson affair, got right to the guts of it. The testimony of Dr Robert Kerr, a sports medicine specialist in San Gabriel, California, gives you a handle on the extent of steroid prescription.

When my steroid practice peaked in 1983, I must have been seeing 2,000 patients for just steroids....There were seven physicians who prescribed steroids right here in San Gabriel, and at least 70 in the Los Angeles area. Nationwide, thousands of doctors were involved, and I knew hundreds of them (p.1703).[26]

Now that the American climate has gone cold on steroids, and rightly so, many former prescribers and users have turned violently against them, at least in public. As the old saying goes, there is no prude so zealous as the reformed prostitute.

I have laid out the facts because I want you to be clear about who is responsible for the steroid mess. I want you to know how two-faced it is. There are now no legal steroids, but according to the US Drug Enforcement Administration, the black market for steroids and similar drugs tops $400 million.[27]

And many of these street drugs include all sorts of fake compounds. Many are also laced with toxic stimulants such as strychnine, or a touch of amphetamines and heroin to give them an obvious kick and keep you coming back. Damn all you irresponsible medicine men. You knew what you were doing.

Are Steroids Effective?

In 1935, Dr David Laqueur and colleagues in Amsterdam, first isolated testosterone.[28] Chemists then busily developed hundreds of derivatives trying to separate testosterone's **androgenic** (masculinizing) effects from its **anabolic** (tissue building) effects. They also developed forms that work orally.[29] Testosterone itself is not active orally, because it degrades to neutral compounds in the first pass through the liver. No one achieved total separation of androgenic and anabolic actions, but by the 1950s oral compounds were developed that could increase nitrogen retention in rats up to *10-fold*.[30]

Researchers developed effective oral steroids by the chemical procedure of **alkylation of the 17-alpha position** of the testosterone molecule. These 17-alpha alkylated steroids dodge destruction by the liver, but are more toxic than injected steroids causing much liver inflammation and misery.

Despite the toxicity, human studies show that provided subjects eat sufficient protein, nitrogen retention can be enhanced up to *30-fold* in convalescent patients.[31] Some of the most successful oral steroids in human trials were **oxandrolone** (Anavar), **methandrostenolone** (Dianabol), and **stanozolol** (Winstrol). All became very popular with athletes.

Injectable steroids are much less toxic to the liver. They are made by the chemical procedure of **esterification of the 17-beta hydroxyl group** of the testosterone molecule. The injectable veterniary form of stanozolol was the steroid used by Ben Johnson.[26]

As we might expect in the climate of hypocrisy that surrounds anabolic steroids, the 40 or so controlled studies on strength, lean body mass, and endurance in athletes are a mass of contradictions. Only by applying the principles in this book can we make any sense of the mess.

The first problem is physiological dynamics. Nature needs time to grow new tissue no matter how much you stimulate that growth. Three months, one blood turnover, might be a reasonable minimum. Most of the studies, however, have tested steroids for only a few weeks. Research by Dr D.M. Crist and colleagues, for example, tested experienced weightlifters for strength increases for 3 weeks with 100 mg of **nandrolone decanoate** (Deca-durabolin) per week.[30] As we have seen throughout this book, 3 weeks is not long enough to test physical changes in anyone.

The second problem is building materials. Steroids provide a stimulus to growth, but they don't provide the additional proteins, vitamins, and minerals required for the new tissue. More than half the controlled studies on steroids failed to provide any increased building materials, or even to control subjects' diets.[33] How naive can you be, to give athletes a powerful drug, and expect it to grow new body parts out of thin air! Sorry guys, I can only conclude that many of these studies were designed to demonstrate that steroids don't work.

Training intensity and duration is also critical. Most studies have failed to control for the weight training program. Unless it is *individually* designed to suit the level of the athlete and his previous training, it will not work. Many studies have also used non-weight trainers who have no idea how to train at all. They have also used low-intensity, short-duration exercise. If you want a study on strength to fail, that's just the way to set it up.

There are so many other laughable things wrong with most steroid studies, including incorrect drug dosages, no measurements of prior steroid use, measuring body composition with *skinfold calipers*, that it's a miracle they found any changes at all. Nevertheless, there are at least seven studies that found significant increases in strength and lean body mass that put the question beyond reasonable doubt.[34-39]

A representative study is that of Dr G.R. Hervey and colleagues in 1981. They gave experienced weightlifters either 100 mg per day of **methandionone** (another name for Dianabol), or a placebo for six weeks. They found substantial increases in bodyweight, lean mass, and strength.[35]

Studies on steroids died in America about 1985 when public opinion turned against them. But they continued in Europe. One of the most recent good studies, representative of the gains that can be made with steroids, is by Dr H. Kuipers and colleagues at the University of Limburg in Holland. They selected 26 male bodybuilders of average age 30, with at least 3 years strength training. They controlled the training, giving the athletes a regimen in which major bodyparts, back, buttocks, arms, thighs, calves, and abs were each trained 3-4 times a week for 4-6 sets of 10-12 reps. The subjects also kept diet diaries. Average intake was 4,200 calories per day. Mean daily protein intake was 2.4 grams/kg bodyweight. Subjects refrained from taking steroids for 15 weeks before the study began. Urine was sampled for drug testing to ensure compliance.[39]

Fourteen of the subjects were given intramuscular injections of nandrolone decanoate (Deca-durabolin), or a placebo for eight weeks. Starting dose was 200 mg, followed by 7 doses of 100 mg in the next seven weeks. On the placebo, subjects gained only 0.7 kg (1.5 lbs) of lean body mass. But on the steroid they gained a highly significant 2.7 kg (6 lbs). Another group of subjects who self-administered higher doses of nandrolone decanoate (200 mg a week), or who self-administered stanozolol (200 mg/week) or testosterone (2,000 mg/week), made even greater gains in lean mass, 3.6 kg (8 lbs).

In both groups, tissue water content remained unchanged, so the additional lean mass was not water weight. The most significant finding was that 12 weeks after ceasing steroid use, but continuing to train, most of the increase in lean body mass was still there.[39]

This study is representative of many similar findings. Given the right steroid, the right dose, the right training, and the right diet, anabolic steroids can stimulate growth of about 1 lb of lean mass per week for 8-10 weeks. And if you continue to train like hell, you keep most of it.

That's the max. Higher doses do not yield much greater gains, because the limiting factor on muscle growth is the number of specific steroid hormone receptors in the cytoplasm and neucleus of skeletal muscle cells. Once these are saturated with steroids, higher doses have no further effect.[40-43] All they do is make guys froth at the mouth (you've seen them), and act like rabid dogs.

The Beast From the East

The most telling evidence that steroids work comes from East German athletes. Since the fall of the Berlin Wall all sorts of skullduggery has been coming out of the rubble. West German molecular biologist Dr Werner Franke, has uncovered a huge scientific program on steroid use in the former East Germany involving top research institutions. This **State Plan 14.25** was a well-funded, government-backed, comprehensive effort to improve methods of using steroids with athletes while avoiding detection on international drug tests.[44]

Franke uncovered charts showing the effects on athletic performance of different steroids, different dosages, and different cycles of the drugs, for more than 200 top East German athletes. According to one of the scientists involved, who is now confessing all, the program involved over 1,000 scientists, physicians, and trainers. It covered top athletes in almost every sport.

The most sinister evidence uncovered, proves that some athletes continued to be given steroids even though they showed liver damage and other pathological side-effects. This practice is the long suspected reason why many East German athletes emerged from nowhere, became world dominant for a couple of years, and then disappeared into oblivion. As soon as their bodies sickened, they were cast off by the State like worn out shoes.

But while the athletes remained healthy, there is no doubt the drugs worked. Let's take East German female swimmers as a potent example. There are no Western studies on female athletes because of the ethical problems (and potential lawsuits) of the irreversible masculinization caused by steroids. But because women have lower testosterone levels than men, effects of steroids are likely to be even greater than on males. Animal studies show very large effects of steroids on female rats.[45] They create huge, muscular females that literally kill and eat untreated males.

Does that scenario remind you of the era of the huge, unbeatable East German swimmers such as, Petra Schneider, Ulrike Richter, Kornelia Ender, and Barbara Krause. While American athletes were being given steroids arbitrarily by chump physicians, with no knowledge and no science, East German and Soviet use was backed by a top level scientific effort since the '60s. Twenty former East German coaches have just testified that by the mid '70s, they had developed a tremendous drug program with female swimmers.[46]

At the 1972 Olympics, East Germany won zero gold medals in women's swimming. At the 1976 Olympics, out of nowhere, they won 10 of the 12 gold medals for individual events. When Western coaches remarked on their huge musculature and deep voices, the East German swim coach snapped, "Ve came here to svim, not to sing."

In 1980, America boycotted, East German women swimmers won 10 golds and 9 silvers, and a look at their times indicates we wouldn't have had a chance. When East Germany was dismantled in 1991, and its steroid program diminished, by the '92 Games in Barcelona, America was back in the medals.

Now we have to contend with the East German steroid

doctors who fled to China, where the huge, muscular female syndrome is rearing its ugly head again. For the record, no East German or Chinese swimmer has ever tested positive for steroids. Yeah, they really know how to do the drugs, and, as their coaches used to say, "bodies are expendible."[46] So it did not restrict their use if the individual athletes were crippled or dead after a couple of years of glory.

The East German and Soviet steroid program for men started earlier and was well in place by 1968. Let's look at the shot put. American *owned* the men's shot put until 1968, taking the gold and silver in every Olympics since 1900 (excepting a bronze in 1920 and a 4th in 1936). From an 11th place in 1964, East German jumped to 4th in 68, and 3rd and 4th in '72. By 1976, East Germany took the gold, and the Soviets the silver and bronze. At the boycotted 1980 Games, East Germany and the Soviets again swept the medals.

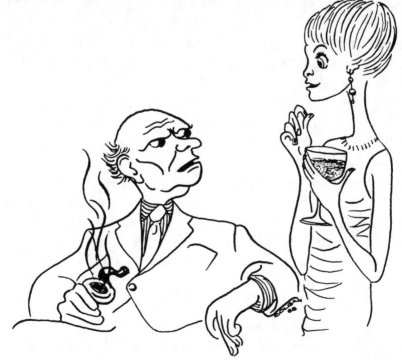

"That was wicked of you to tell your grandma I lost my hair from using steroids."

In '92 after the collapse of the Soviet Union and its drug programs, American shot putters Mike Stulce and Jim Doehring put us back in the gold and silver again.

The evidence that steroids work is now so solid that, after decades of denial, even the most conservative American scientists have to agree. The most extensive analysis of anabolic steroids ever is the new text edited by Dr Charles Yesalis of Penn State University, and written by him and other leading experts on drug use in sports. After analyzing all the studies from 1930 to 1992 they conclude:

> Anabolic steroids are associated with increases in strength and lean body mass in subjects - especially experienced weight lifters - who perform high intensity work and consume adequate diets.[21]

Perhaps the last word on the subject should come from the American College of Sports Medicine, the premier repository of scientific expertise in sport:

> Anabolic-androgenic steroids in the presence of an adequate diet, can contribute to increases in bodyweight, often in the lean mass compartment (p.13).[47]

> The gains in muscular strength achieved through high-intensity exercise and proper diet can be increased by the use of anabolic-androgenic steroids in some individuals (p.1).[48]

So, if anyone tells you steroids don't work, *don't believe them!* But don't use steroids either. In Chapter 41, I outline a strength program that can at least equal steroid effects. Follow this book precisely and you will perform better without steroids. You will also have a much healthier, longer, and prouder life.

Why Drug Tests Don't Work

Ben Johnson was caught in Seoul because he was being advised by a bunch of chumps. The Canadian team was all serviced by Dr George ("Jaime") Astaphan. The worthy doctor cloaked himself in mystery, and parlayed a little knowledge he got from a poorly documented booklet, **The Practical Use of Anabolic Steroids With Athletes**, by another steroid doctor, Robert Kerr, into a wealthy practice as the "steroid maestro." He gave athletes his special expensive mixture "estragol," which turned out to be plain old Winstrol V - a horse steroid he bought in bulk for pennies.[26] With that sort of backing no wonder Ben was caught.

The people who know their business never get caught. Drug testing is kindergarten for any competent biochemist. And there are experts, such as Dr Mauro Di Pasquale, editor of the scientific journal, **Drugs In Sports**, and Dan Duchaine, the Los Angeles steroid guru, who can tell you how to beat any drug test that can ever be devised.

Some pompous sports officials are going to disagree with me, so I better document why drug tests don't work. Briefly, the modern era of drug testing began with the 1983 Pan American Games in Caracas. Dr Manfred Donike of West Germany developed a new testing system using sophisticated gas chromatography and mass spectrometry that is almost 100% accurate. You have any of the drugs they are looking for in your urine, the tests are going to find them.

A few drops of urine are dispersed through a long tube by a stream of helium gas. Detectors spot molecules containing nitrogen and phosphorus present in almost all banned drugs, and plot them as peaks on a graph. Each drug has characteristic peaks. Any suspect pattern is then retested by mass spectrometry which breaks the molecules into their components, and positively identifies the drug from which they came by reference to its known spectrum profile.[49]

Officials in 1983 knew this system would catch most athletes using drugs, so they warned them and let them take anonymous tests in Caracas before the Pan Am Games began. On getting their results, athletes withdrew from the Games in droves including at least 10 Americans, and all but one of the Australian team. Dr Robert Voy, former Chief Medical Officer of the US Olympic Committee, reveals that there was also a secret agreement only to test medal winners.[3] So other athletes did compete, but didn't go for the win, enabling them to save face and not be counted with the obvious druggies who fled for home.

Even so, US heavyweight weightlifter Jeff Michels was caught and stripped of his gold medals. So were 20 other athletes, from Canada, Nicaragua, Venezuela, Chile, Cuba, and the Dominican Republic. The media trumpeted a new era of fairness and justice in sports.

But there are two big problems. First, it's one thing having a system that can detect drugs: it's another finding people with the integrity to use it. Most people don't realize that the Donike system was first used one month *before* the Pan Am Games, at the World Track and Field Championships in Helsinki. No athletes tested positive in Helsinki, not one! Yet droves of the same athletes who competed in Helsinki fled from the Pan Am Games a month later.

The International Amateur Athletics Federation (IAAF) concealed the positive tests in Helsinki, and let the athletes compete anyway! Here were the very officials who scream loudest against drugs condoning their use! How do we know this? Because Professor Donike himself appeared before the Canadian Dubin Commission on the Ben Johnson fiasco, and admitted that there were positives in Helsinki.[50] The fox is watching the henhouse again; business as usual.

The second big problem with drug tests is they are time specific and drug specific. If the athlete stops using the drug so that it clears from his body before the test, then he tests clean. Or if the drug he uses is not one of those tested for, he tests clean. Some athletes were caught using the beta-agonist anabolic drug **clenbuterol** at the Barcelona Games, for example, because they didn't know that the IOC instituted specific testing for clenbuterol just before the Games began. Before then many athletes used clenbuterol freely and were never caught. If athletes, such as hammer thrower Jud Logan, had stopped using clenbuterol 10 days before the test, it would have cleared their bodies and they wouldn't have been caught either. By the way, you have to use pretty big doses of clenbuterol before it is detectable at all.

Many water-based **oral** steroids such as stanozolol (Winstrol) and oxandrolone (Anavar) are undetectable if athletes stop using them 5-10 days before the tests. In contrast, oil-based injectables, such as nandrolone decanoate (Deca-durabolin) can be detected up to *a year* or more after use. So drug testing has pushed athletes into using the more dangerous orals, the **17-alpha alkylated steroids**, that are strongly linked to steroid caused cancer.

But this is all kid's stuff to biochemists. It's a piece of chemical cake to take any anabolic steroid and change its spectrum signature so that it can no longer be recognized by the computer analyzing the gas chromatograph in a test. Computers are swift idiots. Change a comma and they become blind. And don't think the biochemist doing the test can eyeball the printout to spot a designer drug. Guys that good you can count on one hand, and they are not wasting their time drug-testing athletes.

To show you how easy it is to create designer steroids, Dr Mauro Di Pasquale gives the example of methandrostenolone (Dianabol). The chemical structure of this steroid has what is called a **methyl group in the C 17 position**, part of its signature, which helps identify it and its metabolites. By removing the methyl group you change the signature and make it invisible to the computers.[51]

If athletes can't afford the thousands of $$ per month for designer drugs, then their physicians can send urine monthly for private testing, and titrate the steroid dose a week or two before drug tested competition, so that it is no longer detectable. They can also use cattle or poultry steroids that are not usually tested for. More risky is the common use of masking or diluting agents, or drugs that reduce the excretion of steroids such as the

norethindrone in some oral contraceptives, or the product "Defend," which is both diuretic and inhibits excretion.

Just drinking a gallon of water during the day of testing to dilute the urine will beat a lot of tests. Then there is the use of natural forms of testosterone and human growth hormone that can't be detected at all, as we see in following chapters. The procedures are endless and mostly effective.[51] For anyone with a modicum of brains, drug testing just can't catch them. I wish to hell the biochemists would put the same time and effort into improving human nutrition to grow better bodies, instead of into drugs to destroy them. But, that's the way it is.

The Dark Side of Steroids

For the last decade the medical media have damned steroids for producing disease with the same enthusiasm they once used to praise them for producing strength. And with the same degree of hot air and lack of science. Steroids have been cited recently for prostate cancer, kidney cancer, heart disease, liver disease, impotence, tendon damage, and mental disorder. Let's get to the truth of the matter.

I will only mention the cosmetic side-effects because they are more comical than life threatening. There is good evidence that steroids cause rapid hair loss in some individuals.[52] Of course all the young athletes we see shaving their heads is probably just high fashion, and nothing to do with concealing sudden baldness.

Increased testosterone or testosterone derivatives in the blood also frequently cause acne on face and trunk.[53] They also increase facial hair in women. But what's a few zits or a mustachioed girl or two between friends.

Gynecomastia (bitch tits) is a well-known effect of high androgenic steroids such as methandrostenolone (Dianabol). We have seen this problem in very young athletes after reportedly only one use of steroids. Some folk use anti-estrogenic drugs to block the effect, but they are usually unsuccessful. One judge at the last Mr Olympia bodybuilding championship, was heard to remark that the progression of gynocomastia in some contenders was a better indication of their continued steroid use than drug testing. Cosmetic surgery is the only real answer.[54]

Prostate Cancer

To get down to the nitty-gritty, steroids all attack the prostate gland, because it is an androgen target tissue just like the breast. Prostate inflammation caused by steroids is so reliable, researchers use it in animal studies as a measure of the degree of androgenicity of different steroids.[55]

Long-term steroid use leads to irreversible prostate enlargement, and prostatic enlargement is a risk factor for prostate cancer. In rat studies, steroids readily produce prostate cancer.[56] But the problem in trying to connect human prostate cancer to steroids, is the time it takes the cancer to develop, a latency period of up to 40 years.

Nevertheless, there are some cases of early onset prostate cancer in bodybuilders.[57,58] The latest report is from Dr Luke Larkin of West Virginia University. Two retired bodybuilders both in their early 50s, both have malignant prostate cancer. The only identifiable risk factor: prior steroid use. Combined with the animal evidence, these cases indicate that steroids increase your risk of this cancer, well recognized as one of the more agonizing ways to die. Worst part: it will come home to roost when you are 50 or 60, when the few pounds of extra muscle you got from the steroids are long gone and forgotten.

Kidney Cancer

I hear medicos echoing each other in speeches against steroids, citing their use as a cause of kidney cancer. Puzzles me? Our database tracks every case of steroid induced disease. There is only one case of a steroid user developing kidney cancer, and that is a strange one. This guy got a rare cancer called **Wilms' tumor**, that almost never affects adults.[60] With that little evidence you could equally claim that steroids cause big ears or flat feet.

Safe to say that the risk of kidney cancer from steroids is virtually non-existent.

Heart Disease

Steroids do affect the heart and cardiovascular system -- big time! I gave some of the celebrity cases at the beginning of this chapter, Steve Courson, Larry Pacifico, Steve Vallie, and Dr John Ziegler, the man who started the steroid mess in America.

Steroids cause a severe decline in HDL cholesterol, the "good" cholesterol that "scrubs" your arteries clean. With only mild steroid use this effect appears to be reversible.[39] But don't push your luck; low HDL level is a major risk for heart attack.

Steroids can also raise blood pressure.[64] As with HDL cholesterol, this effect is reversible with mild steroid use.[39,64] Even in heavy users it has been exaggerated by uninformed physicians who seem to read the abstracts of research rather than the studies themselves. In one often quoted study, for example, systolic blood pressure rose from 118 mm/Hg to 121 mm/Hg after 8 weeks of steroids.[65] Big deal! Systolic pressure can rise 10 points watching a pretty girl titupping down the street. Steroids may raise blood pressure in a few sensitive individuals, but as a general rule -- not a problem.

Steroids can pathologically enlarge the heart. There is strong evidence that they thicken the left ventricle and change the function of the heart to predispose you to heart attack.[66-68] I am citing the recent studies because some people have suggested that weight training itself thickens the heart. So it does, but *not* in a pathological way in which the left ventricle grows bigger and thicker, and can no longer function in proper rhythm with the right ventricle.[69] That's purely a steroid effect.

Adding to the heart attack risk are steroid effects on **platelets** in the blood. These little discs are vital for blood-clotting after injury, and have just the right amount of stickiness to clump together and seal off broken blood vessels. Steroids cause them to become too sticky, thereby increasing the risk of forming clots in arteries.[70]

In the latest study, Dr Gary Ferenchick and colleagues at Michigan State University tested the platelet aggregation of experienced weightlifters. All were drug tested. Although many initially denied using steroids, 24 of 28 volunteers tested positive. The risk of thrombus formation was significantly higher in users, and the older the user the worse the risk.[71] Because steroids are not usually tested for on autopsy, some researchers now believe that a lot of unexplained fatal heart attacks may be linked to concealed steroid use. Don't become one of them.

Liver Disease

Steroids definitely damage the liver. At the Colgan Institute, we use elevated liver enzyme counts to identify covert users. Elevated **serum glutamic oxaloacetic transaminase (SGOT)** and **serum glutamic pyruvic transaminase (SGPT)** in a SMAC 26 blood screen indicate liver inflammation. If the subject is not sick and seems in top shape, suspect steroid use. If you state straight out "Your blood tests show you are using steroids," most guys 'fess up immediately. Sneaky? No. Steroids drastically affect nutritional needs, so we need to know.

Oral steroids are especially hard on the liver. Heavy users often get jaundice.[72] Yellow skin is easily hidden by a tan, but a yellow cast to the eyes is a dead giveaway.

The next step for repeat oral steroid users is growth of liver cysts.[73] Whether these cysts turn cancerous is unknown, but anabolic steroids readily produce liver cancer tumors in animals.[73] And there are almost a hundred cases of liver cancer in steroid users.[73] In fact, they are now so well recognized in oncology, they have their own diagnostic category. Ugly stuff! Some of these cancers regress when patients stop using steroids, but others progress remorselessly to the grave. If you value your liver and your life, leave the juice alone.

Impotence

Beside cancer, impotence might seem a minor inconvenience of steroid use. But there are a lot of lads out there spending big bucks on hormone treatment to get back their manhood. Average sperm count of bodybuilders during steroid use and for many months after is about 25% of normal levels.[74] The effect is so reliable that the World Health Organization is conducting trials of steroid as a male contraceptive to reduce the overpopulation in Third World countries.[75] Now you know why many heavy steroid users seem to be sexual neuters.

Tendon Damage

Beside cancer and chemical castration, steroid induced tendon damage seems a nothing. Don't believe it. Injured tendons are one of the most frequent problems we see with steroids. They are serious, not because of the injury itself, but because they immediately ruin your training.

Athletes often deny that the injury has anything to do with steroid use. But animal studies show clear and consistent damage to the muscle-tendon junction when steroid treated animals are made to exercise.[76] The problem occurs because steroids cause the body to make abnormal **collagen**.[77] Collagen is the white gelatinous substance that forms the tendon fibers. Steroids reduce the tensile strength of new collagen until much of the tendon is weakened.[78] One big lift and, bingo! A rupture that permanently creases your potential.

I say permanently because you can't afford three months off while a tendon heals. The secret to achieving an optimum body is consistency. We've watched many athletes who went big on steroids. As tendons get sore, first it's knee and wrist wraps. Then it's big doses of anti-inflammatories, elbow wraps, ankle wraps, elephant size wraps up the thighs, and good-bye Charlie.

Yet if you search the literature, there are only a handful of case studies linking steroids to tendon rupture in athletes.[79]

That's because most tendon injuries go unreported, or are reported while steroid use is concealed. We've seen it many times in 18 years of work with athletes. Steroids are a no-no for tendons in anyone making maximal muscular efforts.

Mental Disorder

You can find "roid rage" in most serious gyms. And it's a real effect. East German athletes were given steroid nasal sprays designed to promote aggressiveness. And testosterone levels are a good predictor of aggressiveness in healthy lads,[80] violent rapists,[81] and prison inmates.[82] And hockey players known for whacking the opposing team rather than the puck, have testosterone levels almost off the scale.[83]

There is a world of difference, however, between increased aggressiveness and mental disorder. Most reports of violence by athletes on steroids are anecdotes, usually from friends and family members.[84] Because such reports have been widely publicised, it's likely many athletes act aggressively while on the drugs, because that is what people expect. Such acting out bears little relation to mental disorder, in which you are totally incapable of controlling your behavior.

So it's not surprising when you search the scientific literature for evidence of madness in steroid using athletes, that all you come up with is anecdotal reports. A recent review of the controlled studies concluded only that, "irritability is slightly increased in many users."[84]

That sure doesn't look like those guys I see in Venice Beach biting corners off the floor mats and bowling 45 lb plates. But their behavior is more likely a performance than madness. Pretty convincing act. Sure scares the hell out of me.

The problem expressed by many researchers trying to settle this question, is that athletes in a steroid aggressive state will not enroll for the studies, even for pay. Anyone red-eyed with steroids doesn't want to be put under a microscope about it, especially by some pencil neck bureaucrat in a polyester suit.

The scientific view and we have to bow to the science, is that uncontrollable "roid rages" don't exist. So next time you see a hulk in the corner of the gym snorting like a bull, and staring you down through a bloodshot haze, don't give it a thought. He's probably just allergic to gym chalk.

Chapter 34

Testosterone Tales

Why do athletes bother with synthetic anabolic steroids when they could use the natural anabolic steroid testosterone to produce muscle? Testosterone works at least as well. In the latest study by Dr Gilbert Forbes and colleagues at the University of Rochester, New York, normal subjects gained an average of 16.5 lbs of lean body mass in 12 weeks.[1] Testosterone is also widely available, legal by prescription, much cheaper than steroids, and very difficult to detect in drug tests.

Seems ideal, but the problem lies in the androgenic action of testosterone that produces maleness in the first place. Like the synthetic anabolic steroids developed from it, testosterone, has two distinct modes of action, **androgenic** (masculinizing) and **anabolic** (tissue building). Up to a certain level of testosterone in your body, a level that varies widely with biochemical individuality, the androgenic action produces more maleness, broader features, more hair, deeper voice, and larger sex organs. Along with it, the anabolic action produces larger muscles and greater strength.

But if you take more than that level of testosterone in an attempt to stack on the muscle, the androgenic action turns nasty. Normal male fearlessness becomes aggression, violent anxiety, paranoia, and manic-depressive reactions. East German athletes were given testosterone sprays exactly for this purpose. That's why so many of them have such sweet personalities.

Excess testosterone also deposits in the scalp as dihydrotestosterone that causes irreversible baldness. Excess testosterone in the genitals causes overgrowth of the prostate, which chokes the bladder, leaving the athlete dependent on a forcefully inserted catheter in order to urinate.

Also, just like synthetic anabolic steroids, there is the acne as the blood fails to contain the excess hormone and overloads the sebaceous glands. There is the impotence and shrinkage of testicles. There is the increased risk of cardiovascular disease and cancer, especially prostate cancer. All these risks are higher with testosterone than with man-made steroids.[2]

Testosterone injections also quickly shut down the body's own production. Athletes who use testosterone either give up sex entirely or are always running to physicians for shots of **human chorionic gonadotropin (HCG)**, because they have "lost their balls". HCG helps because it mimics the pituitary signal to the testes to increase testosterone production.[3] It even helps the testicles to grow back a bit -- but only temporarily. I've seen a sad parade of athletes over the years who have become permanently neutered as a result of testosterone use.

Some of them tell me it's not so bad because another side-effect of excess use of synthetic testosterone is a permanent loss of libido. Sex is no longer an option, but they no longer want it. Women, who needs them? Then why do some of the biggest names in bodybuilding and professional wrestling spend tens of thousands of $$ on specialist hormone treatment trying to regain their virility?

Testosterone Use

Despite these risks, many athletes continue to use testosterone. Weightlifters, powerlifters, football players, especially like this drug because it is cheap and effective in building size. Other competitive athletes, including Olympians, like testosterone because they will not get caught.

The most popular form is **testosterone cypionate**

(depo-testosterone) which is quickly in and out of the body, so it can be used within days before a drug-tested competition. **Testosterone propionate** is slower, staying in the body a week or so, and is probably the least effective form. **Testosterone enanthate** is slower still, staying in the body about two weeks. And you can spot many users easily because they hold more water than a sponge, and puff up to beat the Michelin Man.

The quickest and most dangerous testosterone is a simple suspension of the actual hormone in water. It has become popular with Olympic athletes because it is in and out of the body in a day. Because of this quick processing, it is highly toxic to the liver. In his book, **Drugs, Sport and Politics**, Dr Robert Voy, former Chief Medical Officer of the US Olympic Committee, blames the Olympic drug testing program for pushing athletes away from easily detectable but relatively safe steroids, such as nandrolone decanoate (Deca-Durabolin), and towards toxic drugs like testosterone.[4]

Testing for Testosterone

If you call the Olympic Training Center in Colorado Springs, they will deny pushing athletes towards testosterone. They will tell you that the IOC has a very effective screen to detect testosterone that is helping to stop the use of testosterone worldwide. Don't believe them!

Let's get at the facts. Along with testosterone, the testicles also secrete an inactive form of the hormone called **epitestosterone**. Usually the ratio between testosterone and epitestosterone in urine is 1:1. If you inject testosterone, then obviously the testosterone:epitestosterone ratio will increase. This occurs for two reasons. First, there is now more testosterone in the system. Second, the extra testosterone signals the brain which reduces its own production, both of testosterone and epitestosterone. So total testosterone goes up and epitestosterone goes down.

Seems simple to detect. If an athlete's testosterone:

epitestosterone ratio is markedly above 1:1 then he is a drug user -- right? Wrong! Some individuals have a natural ratio of 4:1. So the test cutoff has to be set higher than that. Otherwise, the test would falsely select some drug-free athletes as users. The current Olympic drug test cutoff is a testosterone/epitestosterone ratio of 6:1.[5] As Dr Robert Voy points out, that cutoff allows any athlete with a usual 1:1 ratio, to load up with injected testosterone until he reaches 5.9:1, and still test drug-free. But you can't lower the test ratio or you will unfairly catch some athletes who are really drug-free. So right off the bat the test is a bummer.

Even if the test worked perfectly, it is still useless. All the Eastern bloc coaches and sports physicians, and any Western sports medicine professional who reads the scientific literature, knows that you can normalize a high testosterone:epitestosterone ratio with a single injection of HCG.[6] Better still, you can inject epitestosterone along with the testosterone in a ratio of 1:30.[7] Then the ratio in urine remains within the normal range.[8] This strategy has been known and practiced ever since drug-testing began.

Dihydrotestosterone

Then there is **dihydrotestosterone**, a natural, highly androgenic hormone produced by the body. Its main functions are to grow facial hair (but not head hair), male genitalia, and the prostate gland. Inject dihydrotestosterone and you get all these effects -- guaranteed.

Seems a dopey way to go, because there is no scientific evidence at all that dihydrotestosterone is an effective anabolic. Even so, it has become popular among Olympic and other drug-tested athletes, because *it is completely undetectable*.

Some researchers might object that measures of the ratios of excretion of various different hormones have been proposed to detect dihydrotestosterone use.[9] Injections of dihydrotestosterone inhibits bodily production of testosterone itself, and production of another compound called **luteinizing**

hormone, explained in Chapter 32. Injected dihydrotestosterone also changes the ratios of excretion of other hormones. So the simplest method involves testing for a low testosterone level and low levels of luteinizing hormone, plus high levels of **dihydrotestosterone glucuronide**, a metabolite of the hormone.

Sounds like sophisticated biochemistry doesn't it. Gimme a break! These guys seem to think no one else understands the metabolism of anabolic hormones. Even a mediocre chemist could counter all these measures by using a combination injection of dihydrotestosterone, epitestosterone, and testosterone. If he even had to bother. Because of biochemical individuality, the range of individual differences in normal levels of these hormones is so broad, that any cut-off points that would register users as positive on the test, would probably register half the Olympic Committee as positive too.

Transdermal Testosterone

The latest development is testosterone patches. These were first made by Alza Pharmaceuticals of Palo Alto, California in 1985 as an experimental treatment for aging men with low testosterone levels, and for men who had lost their testicles by accident or surgery. The 2" square patch is stuck on the scrotum, or anywhere on the body, and releases testosterone slowly, evenly, and painlessly through the skin. They are not officially on the medical market yet, but plenty of athletes seem to have acquired them.

Transdermal delivery of testosterone to the scrotum is far superior to testosterone injections. First, in six years of testing, the patches have shown much less prostate enlargement and no increase in prostate cancer.[10] Second, serum levels of testosterone remain level, with none of the wild swings and side-effects caused by testosterone injections. Third, patients can use them anywhere without the risks of pills or injections.

These are all medical indications, and bode well for the use of the patches in treating the elderly. But they also make them very popular with athletes. Serum levels do not increase wildly because a lot of the testosterone is converted to dihydrotestosterone in the scrotum.[11] So athletes can use them right up to a drug-tested meet.

Testosterone patches still carry all the risks of introducing excess testosterone into the body. They are meant for guys who don't have sufficient. They can elevate the blood level of dihydrotestosterone by 10 times. In someone who has had testicular surgery, that might bring behavior up to normal. There are no reports of violence or paranoia in treated patients.[10,11] But if you see a bald, bearded athlete in the shower with sticking plaster on his scrotum, and a sour demeanour, don't make any sudden moves in his direction.

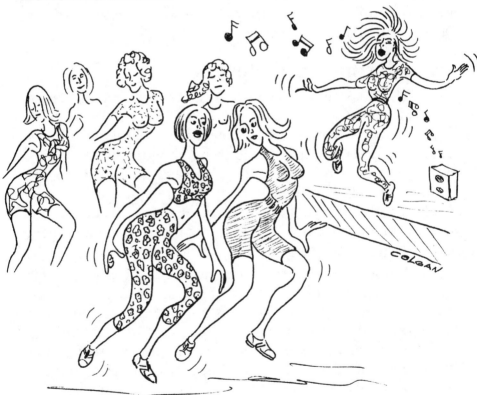

"I had to quit jogging. My thighs rubbed rogether so hard they caught my underpants on fire."

Chapter 35

Human Growth Hormone

"The drug of choice." In 1985, drug guru Robert Kerr MD, who boasted a steroid clientele of over 2,000 athletes, predicted that synthetic human growth hormone would become the elite sports drug throughout the world. Available since 1986, there are two FDA approved brands of this genetically engineered drug in America, Protropin (**somatrem**) produced by Genentech, San Francisco, and Humatrope (**somatropin rDNA origin**) produced by Eli Lilly, Indianapolis. There are three other growth hormone drugs almost on the market as pharmaceutical companies race to cash in. They are all made by growing the hormone in a special strain of *Escherichia coli* bacteria that have been genetically modified by inserting the gene for human growth hormone. Drugs from bugs, the wave of the future.

Humatrope is an exact copy of the 191 amino acid sequence of human growth hormone. Consequently, the human body accepts it as self and does not develop antibodies to the drugs except in about 2% of unexplained cases.[1] Protropin, however, is not exactly human growth hormone because it contains 192 amino acids. It has an extra methionine which enables the immune systems of many people to attack the drug as foreign to the body. Between 30% and 40% of people treated with Protropin develop antibodies to it,[1] which helps explain the frequent reports from athletes that growth hormone makes them sick.

You don't want antibodies to growth hormone in your body. The evidence is not in yet because abundant supplies of growth hormone only became available in 1986, but with these antibodies, the immune system could begin to attack its own growth hormone. Without continued injections for life, that would quickly and permanently shrink you down to a Pee Wee Herman.

Growth Hormone Use

Synthetic growth hormone is approved only for the treatment of pituitary dwarfism, that is children who fail to grow because of an inadequate supply of their own growth hormone. One medical journal, **The Medical Letter**, states that there are about 4,000 legitimate cases in America.[2] Deborah Swansburg, Director of the Human Growth Foundation, puts the figure at 10,000 to 12,000, depending on what individual physicians judge is pathologically short for a child. But there are tens of thousands of parents who think that bigger is better for their normal height kids, and zillions of athletes who think that humungous is better for everything.

Both Lilly and Genentech swore to the Colgan Institute that synthetic growth hormone is kept under super tight controls, drug registers, multiple licenses, triple IDs, mother's deathbeds, cross your heart and hope to die. And they are sincere. But that's not the way it is. Industry watchdog, the Smith Barney Company, reports that Genentech's Protropin grossed $185 million in sales in 1991.[3] And Eli Lilly refused to tell the Colgan Institute their sales figure for Humatrope.[4] Judicious analysis by our own staff suggests it's at least $50 million. That's a total of $235 million in growth hormone, all to treat a small number of short kids.

Either the stuff costs over $20,000 per child or a lot of it is being diverted to unapproved uses. The bottom line is that many elite athletes are now using synthetic growth hormone. Top bodybuilders reported to us that there is no difficulty buying it, provided you have five figure wads of the folding green. Dr

Robert Voy, former chief medical officer of the US Olympic Committee agrees.[5]

There is also some foreign natural growth hormone floating around. Brands are Crescormon (Pharmacia Labs) and Assellacrin (Serano Labs). But you have to be seriously out of your mind to use either. They are made from the pituitary glands of cadavers and can contain a number of active viruses. Use in the US was banned after four patients developed Creutzfeldt-Jacob disease, a fatal virus that literally eats your brain.[6]

Then there is the bogus growth hormone. Some muscle magazines have run anecdotal stories that growth hormone has no effect. But when the Colgan Institute chased down some of the athletes involved, we found they had used bootleg growth hormone bought in Los Angles at $1100 per one month supply. Who knows what was in the stuff? Some bootleg vials have tested in the past turned out to be physiological saline.

Right now a German company in Mexico is offering shots of "growth hormone" at $150 each, with the claim that the stuff will work for three months after the shot. Can't be growth hormone or any steroid. All of them need to be injected every few days because the body neutralizes them to nothing very fast.

Does Growth Hormone Work?

If you give synthetic growth hormone to very short children they grow like weeds, towering over untreated control groups by six to nine inches within four years.[7] They also increase the number and size of their muscle cells. And they lose up to three-quarters of their body fat.[8] A new research report from Britain concluded that short children treated with growth hormone not only spring to normal height but also become "inappropriately muscular." The treated lads hotly disagree -- they love it!

The stuff also works with children who have no growth hormone deficiency.[9] And if you give adolescents higher doses than recommended by the manufacturer, they grow even faster.[10]

There is a lot of public scientific mumbling that these findings do not mean that children of normal height will end up any taller than their genes dictate. But that's mainly to dissuade parents from zapping their kids. It's a good bet from the evidence that a genetic 6-footer treated through childhood could grow to match eyeballs with Magic Johnson.

It also works with adults, though it doesn't make them taller. In old men aged 61-81 spectacular recent studies show that six months of synthetic growth hormone increased lean mass by 8.8%, decreased bodyfat by 14.4%, increased bone density, and rejuvenated their skin.[11] That's without any exercise program. And highly trained males and females aged 22-33 (the only study of growth hormone with athletes), showed a 4% increase in lean mass and a 12% reduction in bodyfat.[12]

Such evidence does not guarantee that synthetic growth hormone will work with athletes, or with anyone who does not fulfill a host of screening criteria used by physicians to select the patients who will benefit. To make a judgement call we need to dip into a bit of the science.

Growth hormone does not cause much growth directly because it is neutralized in the body by the liver in less than an hour after injection (You can't take growth hormone by mouth: digestion destroys it). It works by stimulating the liver to make a group of polypeptide chemicals called **somatomedins**. The most powerful of these is **somatomedin-C**, also called **insulin-like growth factor-1**. The somatomedins chug around the body for hours, causing all sorts of growth everywhere.[13]

But a lot of other organs also participate. You have to have a healthy liver to make the somatomedins in the first place. You have to have a healthy thyroid and pancreas to provide increased amounts of other hormones essential to growth. And you have to have a healthy liver and kidneys to handle all the waste products of the huge amounts of food you need to eat to provide the raw materials for growth.

Over 8,000 calories a day is the commonly quoted figure.

That disreputable but sometimes accurate publication, **The Underground Steroid Handbook,** recommends 10,000 calories per day, way beyond the average capacity to digest food or get rid of wastes. Together with the possible development of antibodies to the drug, explained above, this overeating is another reason why some bodybuilders, whose livers and kidneys are shot from steroids, don't like growth hormone and report it makes them sick.

A third reason for illness from the drug is excess use. In medical studies, levels of growth hormone and somatomedins are strictly monitored and the dose adjusted for each individual to keep somatomedins at the high end of the physiological range. With illegal use there is no such monitoring. Athletes whose growth hormone levels are usually at the high end of the range already, push them into the witchcraft range.

Some athletes, look around you can't mistake them, have already developed the gorilla-like overgrowth of facial bones, and the huge hands and feet of acromegaly. Acromegaly is the genetic disease of oversecretion of growth hormone (the Andre the Giant syndrome). A dead giveaway is development of gaps between the teeth as the jawbone grows wider. If any athlete you know suddenly gets bigger and starts whistling through his teeth, you know what he's doing.

In the healthy athlete who fulfills the above criteria, there is no doubt that synthetic growth hormone will produce more muscle growth than in his drug-free state, and probably more muscle growth than by use of any other drug. Anecdotal reports of gains of 30-40 lbs of lean mass in three months are commonplace.[14,15] But strength is another story.

Is It Good Muscle?

No one has tested the quality of human muscle gained by growth hormone use. It is definitely big, but is it proportionately strong? Doubtful. Cases of acromegaly do not produce people with muscles that are as strong as they look. Acromegalics have large muscles but show weakness for their size, are easily fatigued, and have low exercise tolerance.[16]

Animal studies also show that the strength and performance of muscles grown with exogenous growth hormone are not increased proportional to their size.[17] It is likely from the studies to date, that growth hormone causes a great increase in muscle connective tissue (**sarcoplasm**), and a much smaller increase in contractile elements (**myofibrils**) that give the muscle its strength. The upside of this effect is that growth hormone is also likely to strengthen tendons and ligaments. As we saw in Chapter 33, anabolic steroids build weak connective tissue, the biggest source of injury among steroid users. Growth hormone may reduce this problem.

Even though the strength increase is not ideal, if you get big enough, then sheer mass will dominate. Especially so, because growth hormone will also remove your fat and thicken your bones. Even if they don't get sick, long-term users can expect a bigger jaw, fatter nose and thickened shelf of ape-man bone above the eyes.

And hairy, very hairy. We have seen one case of an athlete taking prescribed growth hormone who grew copious body hair, especially on his butt and thighs. The hair is so thick he had to give up training at the gym, because after a few minutes of hard exercise he sweats so much it looks like he wet his pants. With the satyr Pan in mind, some mischevious soul couldn't help asking whether he had noticed any hoof-like changes in his feet. Really big, really lean, and downright primitive: I hope it doesn't become the new macho look.

The other popular sports advantage of synthetic growth hormone is that it cannot be detected by urine tests. But athletes don't get away totally clean. As well as the bone growth, one giveaway is that growth hormone brings on carpal tunnel syndrome, intense wrist nerve pain that pleads for operations to relieve it.[18] Look for wrist scars. In older athletes, diabetes is the key, because the drug also screws up insulin metabolism.[19] They kick the bucket early too. Folk with excess growth hormone running through their veins rarely last till 60.[20]

Don't use synthetic growth hormone. Far better to use the information in Chapters 30 and 32 to make your body increase it's own supply. It will be slower, thereby enabling the lean growth to get the exercise stimulation necessary to turn it into stronger growth. In the undersized children with low growth hormone levels, bringing them up to a mite above normal with injected growth hormone, spreads their growth over years. Unlike the athlete who uses excess growth hormone to produce size too quickly, these children develop strength that is proportional to the muscle size. That's the only kind of muscle that really works.

Chapter 36

Beta-Blockers: Beta-Boosters

We heard a lot about beta-blockers at the '88 Olympics. But since then they have faded from public sight. Shooters, archers, skiers, biathletes, skaters, and pentathletes use these drugs to "steady their nerves." Simply put, they block receptor sites on nerves, inhibiting the action of adrenalin and other stimulating hormones. In medicine they are used to treat migraine, anxiety, and stress-related hypertension.

In healthy athletes, beta-blockers can slow the heart to less than 30 beats a minute (one beat every two seconds!), and reduce the firing of nerves dramatically. For sports where motionless concentration is essential, such as shooting, hand tremor is eliminated. Former Chief Medical Officer of the US Olympic Committee, Dr Robert Voy, describes how shooters achieve unreal perfect scores as they squeeze a tremor-free trigger finger in the motionless space between each beat of their drug-slowed hearts.[1]

For extreme stress sports, such as ski-jumping, beta-blockers bring racing hearts and shaking legs under easy control. Figure skaters can complete their nerve-wracking discipline without a wobble. Any athlete suffering from nerves can gain relief. Beta-blockers are often prescribed to athletes of every stripe to calm them down in the few days before competition and enable them to get a decent sleep.

Propanolol hydrochloride (Inderal, made by Wyeth-Ayerst, Philadelphia), is the most common beta-blocker. The United States Olympic list of banned beta-blockers is given in Table 25. They are very difficult to detect in drug tests, so we don't hear a lot about them. Also, in preventing an athlete using them, the USOC may be interfering with his medical treatment for non-medical reasons, which could be very costly in a legal fight. But if they insist that an athlete can't compete while being medically treated with beta-blockers, then the Olympic Charter is in jeopardy. So it's Catch 22.

Table 25. Beta-blockers banned by the USOC.*

Chemical	Trade Name
Acebutolol	Sectral
Alprenolol	Aptine, Betacard
Atenolol	Tenormin
Labetalol	Normodyne, Trandate
Metoprolol	Lopressor
Nadolol	Corgard
Oxprenolol	Apsolox, Oxanol
Pindolol	Nisken
Propanolol	Inderal
Sotalol,	Sotalex, Beta-cardone
Timolol	Blocadren

*Source: USOC , Reference 2.

These drugs are officially banned from sports competition by the US Olympic Committee, because they confer a decided advantage on the user.[2] Nevertheless, they are frequently and legitimately prescribed to athletes. It's a borderline question whether preventing an athlete's migraine or anxiety attack, or allowing him a good sleep, is giving an unfair advantage. It's certainly *not* as unfair as the permitted and lauded practice of allowing selected athletes access to the superior training facilities of the Olympic Training Center at Colorado Springs, while denying access to others.

Side-effects of beta-blockers include inhibition of the central nervous system with all its problems, including depression, reduction of anaerobic power, and impotence. Any athlete in top condition, which always includes being super-calm and relaxed, is crazy to use these drugs. A great way to slow you down all round. And if your heart rate dips below 25 bpm under the influence of beta-blockers, it can go into fibrillation and precipitate a heart attack.[3]

Beta-Boosters

The research on beta-blockers hit a little serendipity in the early '80s. Researchers were using **beta-boosters**, that is, drugs that *increase* adrenergic stimulation of the nerves, to test the effectiveness of beta-blockers in preventing that stimulation. After a few weeks they noticed that the test animals were growing huskier, stronger, and more aggressive. The **beta-adrenergic agonists**, as these drugs are termed, were rapidly increasing muscle mass.

Since then, there has been a pile of studies in animals showing that beta-boosters are as effective as anabolic steroids at building muscle. In a recent study from the Rowett Research Unit, Aberdeen, Scotland, Dr P.J. Reeds and colleagues gave the beta-agonist **clenbuterol** to young rats and compared them with controls. They found that the clenbuterol increased growth in both skeletal and cardiac muscle. The animals also progressively lost bodyfat.[4]

In another recent study, Drs Peter MacLennan and Richard Edwards at the Muscle Research Center of the University of Liverpool, England, gave rats subcutaneous injections of clenbuterol (0.125 mg/kg bodyweight), or put it in their diet

(2 mg/kg of food). In both studies the rats rapidly gained muscle.[5] In an earlier study, rats given clenbuterol increased their muscle mass by 34% in just 19 days.[6]

Biochemical analyses of the animals in these studies showed that the muscle mass increase was caused by beta-adrenergic stimulation alone, via a completely different metabolic pathway to that used by anabolic steroids. Results also showed that clenbuterol had no effect on growth hormone or insulin, two of the major anabolic hormones in the body. The muscle built by clenbuterol was still there six weeks after the drug was stopped.

To date only three beta-agonists have shown marked muscle-building and fat-reducing properties, clenbuterol (the most studied), fenoterol, and cimeterol. But it isn't the muscle-building aspect that has excited researchers. Hordes of biochemists are busily at work in major pharmaceutical companies trying to be first with new fat-busting drugs for treatment of America's ever growing obesity. A new wave of diet drugs may soon hit the market, but it's unlikely that athletes will use them for that primary purpose.

Chapter 37

Cocaine: Manco Cepac's Revenge

After 50 years in short supply, following its ban by the Harrison Act in 1914, cocaine emerged again on the playing field in the late '60s, when illicit trafficking from South America became organized. By the mid '70s, its more powerful effects easily replaced amphetamines. Since then, cocaine has been the premium stimulant of professional athletes.

Popular athletes and role models like Eddie Johnson (NBA), Cliff Branch (NFL), Willie Aikens, Steve Howe (baseball), Mark Heaslip, Steve Durbano (hockey), Tyrell Biggs (boxing) were linked to cocaine in a media feeding frenzy. Basketball stars Terry Furlow, Len Bias, Hernell Jackson, football greats Don Rogers, Larry Gordon, Rico Marshall, are some of the best known of the host of top athletes who have died since 1980 for their love of cocaine.[1,2] What had long been a private vice well tolerated in top corporate and celebrity circles, became a public outrage.

The National Institute on Drug Abuse estimates that 30,000,000 Americans have used cocaine[3] and that over 600,000 use the drug *at least once a week!* For the first six months of 1991, hospital emergency rooms report 47,000 emergencies caused by cocaine.[4] The Incas of Peru revered coca in their rituals as the gift of Manco Cepac, the Sun God.[5] America is now seeing the wrath of Manco Cepac's revenge.

Worst Addiction

To understand why cocaine is so popular in sport today, we need to know a bit about its history and its chemistry. Unfortunately, few of our drug enforcement folk have had the wit to acquire this knowledge. With their tunnel vision for bigger and better drug busts, and their helicopter gun-ships shooting Peruvian farmers whose families have grown coca for a thousand years, they falsely believe they are fighting a winnable war of attrition against evil men. In fact, they are fighting an unquenchable public demand for the most addictive substance in existence.

It used to be thought that because cocaine has no clear physical withdrawal syndrome, it is non-addictive. The psychological addiction to cocaine, however, is stronger than addiction to heroin. If you give rats unlimited access to heroin, about one-third of them will neglect food and other activities until the heroin kills them. But if you give rats unlimited access to cocaine, 90% of them neglect everything else until the cocaine kills them.[6] Heroin is a marshmallow compared with cocaine.

Whole cultures have died for the love of cocaine. It has captured many of our greatest intellects. It has been lauded by pontiffs and kings. Unlike other narcotics, *controlled* use does not impair function and may even empower both mind and body. No surprise that Drug Czar William Bennett called cocaine America's "most dangerous and formidable foe."

Cocaine is extracted from the leaves of *Erythroxylon coca*, a shrub indigenous to the Peruvian Andes. The local people have chewed coca leaves since pre-Incan times to create euphoria and courage, and to mask pain and fatigue. The Incas restricted use of coca as a sacrament for the priesthood and nobility. Because of this restriction they easily rose to power midst all the other Indian tribes in the country, all of whom were ravaged by the drug.

The Incas maintained control for centuries and built an advanced civilization. Then there was an upsurge of illicit coca use among their own people that decimated the labor force. By the time of the so-called Spanish "conquest" of Peru, there was little left to conquer. The Incas were already a fast declining race. Cocaine was a major force in the demise of their great culture.

The Spaniards experimented with coca leaves for three centuries. But cocaine left in the leaf quickly degrades. Leaf transported to the Old World yielded only a mild buzz at best. Then in 1859, German chemist Friedrich Gaedche isolated the cocaine alkaloid, and a graduate student Albert Nieman determined the chemical formula as the work for his Ph.D. thesis.[4,7] They set the scene for devastation.

Cocaine began appearing everywhere. A fiendish Corsican chemist Angelo Mariani added the new alkaloid to wine, and "Vin Mariani", with 24 mg cocaine per 4 oz glass, became the overnight hit of Europe. Endorsed by Pope Leo XIII, the spiked wine addicted hundreds of thousands of people, including writers Jules Vern and Alexander Dumas.[8]

In America, John Pemberton in Atlanta added coca leaf to soda to form Coca-Cola, a cocaine spiked drink for all ages. With this addictive start, Coca-Cola became the most popular drink ever devised. Famous American surgeon Halstead recognized the excellent properties of cocaine as a topical anaesthetic and blood vessel constrictor. He used it extensively in operations and also became an addict. Soon cocaine was being used so widely in ear, nose, and throat surgery, that major American pharmaceutical companies petitioned the government for help in expediting shipments from Peru.[8]

By 1900, cocaine was used in thousands of lotions, medicines, and snake-oil potions worldwide. And its addicting effect and devastation of health had become painfully obvious. In 1906, cocaine was regulated under a new law, **The Pure Food and Drug Act**. After some protest, Coca-Cola removed the drug from its drink. In 1914, all but topical surgical use was banned by the

Harrison Act. Today, topical cocaine is *legally* used in America in about 200,000 ear, nose, and throat operations every year.[9]

Following the Harrison Act, it took until the 1960s for the *illegal* cocaine trade to build up and get organized. It also took some advances in chemistry, that have made cocaine easy to prepare and market and far more dangerous. Today it has no competition as the most dangerous and destructive drug in sports.

Most cocaine used in sport is in the form of **cocaine hydrochloride,** a dry white powder that is "snorted" into the nose for absorption through the nasal mucous membranes, or held under the tongue for absorption through the oral mucous membranes. The powder is convenient to use, simple to conceal, and very difficult to detect in drug tests. Either method of administration produces an effect which begins within a minute or two and lasts over an hour.[10]

Injection of the drug gets more of it into the brain faster (about 30 seconds) and produces a more intense, but shorter high. But it is an inconvenient and risky procedure compared with the simplicity of sniffing. So drug traffickers are always seeking alternatives that will give the most intense high that lasts for the shortest time. That way they can addict more people, and compel them to use cocaine more frequently.

The quickest route of absorption, even quicker than injection, is inhalation of cocaine smoke into the huge area of the vascular bed of the lungs. But cocaine hydrochloride cannot be smoked because it is degraded by heat. Hence the development of **"freebase"** and **"crack"**. The pure cocaine alkaloid is extracted from the hydrochloride with ammonia and ether (freebase) or ammonia and bicarbonate (crack). Both are smokeable and yield an intense effect that begins in 8-10 seconds and lasts 15-20 minutes.[11]

How Cocaine Works

Cocaine works directly on an area of the brain behind your nose called the **lateral hypothalamus,** a primitive part of the brain that mediates your feelings of confidence, pleasure, and sexual drive. When one type of nerve in this area fires, it releases a neurotransmitter called **dopamine**. This compound make the essential connection between the firing nerve and other nerves. The result is a sensation of euphoria. Most humans are euphoria addicts.

In normal life, the sensation occurs in bursts of only a few seconds. Orgasm is a prime example. After the short burst, the dopamine is reabsorbed into the nerve and sensation dies away. Cocaine works by holding the dopamine in place and prolonging intense sensations of pleasure and sexuality for minutes at a time. This unique action explains why it is the most addictive substance known, and why even one or two casual uses of the most intense form, crack, can addict a person for life.[12]

No one did any studies of cocaine with athletes before it was banned. So we have no systematic evidence that it improves athletic performance. The only reasonable studies were done by Sigmund Freud in the 1880s, using himself as a subject. In his famous paper **Uber Cocaine** he advocated its use as a cure for depression, as an intellectual stimulant, and as a means to increase courage, energy, and strength. His experiments showed that cocaine increased hand strength by 12-20%, quickened reactions by up to 40%, and increased energy by 8-10%.[13]

If these are true effects, they go a long way towards explaining why so many professional athletes believe cocaine improves their game.[1,14] Even without real increases in strength and speed, there is no doubt that increased confidence alone can improve performance. And the anaesthetic effect of cocaine certainly masks pain and fatigue. Despite the lack of direct evidence, you have to conclude that this drug is a prime candidate for an effective ergogenic aid.

The Dark Side of Cocaine

Tolerance to cocaine occurs so rapidly that the amount that got you high enough last week will not do it today.[12]

Professional athletes typically use ever increasing amounts, until a big proportion of their gargantuan salaries go to support the habit. With inevitable progression, it is not long before they cannot perform without cocaine, and become continuously moody and depressed when off the drug.

It gets worse. Many athletes who become addicted, increase or restore their high by combining alcohol with cocaine. This combination produces a substance inside the body called **cocaethylene**. Like cocaine, cocaethylene raises your heart rate while constricting its blood supply, a great combination for a heart attack. The action of cocaine is short and would probably destroy only an already weak heart. But the action of cocaethylene is prolonged over 24 hours or more, and is now thought to be responsible for many of the unexplained deaths by heart attack of healthy professional athletes.

It gets worse still. While controlled and measured use of cocaine, like that of Freud, appears to enhance performance, uncontrolled use by professional athletes quickly damages fine control mechanisms in the muscles and brain. Habitual cocaine heads become both slow and stupid.[15] Some examples: Lonnie Smith of the Kansas City Royals, "I think it slowed me down, not just running but my mental thinking." Tim Raines of the Montreal Expos, "It certainly hurt my performance. I struck out a lot more, my vision was lessened".[2] And the skill and smarts of Tyrell Biggs declined almost overnight after he won the Olympic gold medal in boxing, and took up cocaine.[1]

I knew a super-smart young athlete, dux of her school and a National class runner, who was turned onto cocaine by her footballer boyfriend. Within two years her whole life had become turning tricks on Sunset Boulevard in Los Angeles to support her habit. She died of it in 1989. If you believe cocaine couldn't do it to you, you're already thick as a brick.

Chapter 38

Speed Kills

In a group of club-level marathoners I was training in 1982, there was one weird standout. A quiet, middle-of-the-pack young guy with a best time for the 10K (6.2 miles) of 39 minutes 42 seconds, and a best time for the half-marathon (13.1 miles) of just under 90 minutes. But when we did our 20-mile or above training runs, sometimes he would jump into overdrive at about 10 miles and beat the pants off the rest of us.

At the end of the 18-week training program he ran the New York marathon, in his best time ever, a speedy 2 hours 49 minutes and change. As a long-time trainer, I knew that time was just not possible, given his best times at shorter distances. For any runner, you can plot a curve from his best times, that predicts the time he can expect for a marathon with an accuracy of 95%. There is no way a 39:42 10K, and an 89-minute half-marathon can yield a marathon time of 2 hours 49 minutes. His best marathon should have been about 3 hours 9 minutes, that is, 20 minutes slower.

So I asked him. He led me to a teapot on the mantle in his living room. "Try a few greenies Doc. I take 8 to 10 of them right before races. Have to restrict 'em to races or you get hooked." The pot was half-full of 10 mg Dexedrine (dextroamphetamine) tablets. He provided my first direct measurement of amphetamine's potent stimulant effects. It improved his marathon time by a huge 20 minutes, nearly a minute a mile.

In the years I followed this lad, he showed no adverse

effects. He knew enough about the dangers of habituation and addiction to restrict his use to occasional long training runs and competitions. Despite severe prescription regulations on amphetamines imposed by the Controlled Substances Act of 1970,[1] many athletes are able to obtain this drug today, and use it in the same way as our marathoner. He happened to have the biochemical individuality that got a really big ergogenic effect out of amphetamines, without the side-effects of irritability and anxiety. Most athletes who use this drug don't get as large a response. Nevertheless, it does provide a definite edge in sports competition.

Use of Speed

In his book **Drugs Sport and Politics**[2], Dr. Robert Voy, former Chief Medical Officer of the US Olympic Committee, writes, about amphetamines;

> ...scientific studies do not give us any definite con-
> clusions about how well stimulants can enhance
> performance... p. 37.

Like many writers who fudge the truth about drugs in well-meaning attempts to dissuade athletes from using them (that no one believes), he is 100% wrong. When amphetamines first became obvious in sports in the late '50s, the American Medical Association commissioned a detailed and very careful study at Harvard University. Subjects were elite runners, throwers, and swimmers. Dosages were low, only 10-15 mg. Even so, amphetamines significantly improved the performance of three-quarters of the athletes tested.[3]

Dr. Voy does acknowledge that he has seen football players on high-dose amphetamines, completely insensitive to pain and fatigue, who could maintain high energy and motivation to the last minute of a game, even after breaking fingers. And they didn't even notice the injury until trying to untie their shoelaces after the final whistle. That's a hell of an edge in any body contact sport. What Voy didn't mention is that these effects of amphetamines are all well documented in the scientific literature.[4,9]

Recent studies also report a performance edge with amphetamines in cycling and other aerobic exercise,[5] and in anaerobic exercise where strength is the dominant factor.[5] Animal experiments show clearly the physiological basis of these effects. Amphetamines stimulate both the peripheral and central nervous systems.

They increase hormone output from the pituitary gland, that pea of complex functions that hangs from the brain on a stalk, about an inch behind your nose. The pituitary output in turn, through what is called the **adrenal-pituitary axis,** stimulates the adrenal glands to increase output of the excitatory hormones, adrenalin and noradrenalin. This hormone output stimulates use of glycogen and glucose for anaerobic exercise, and use of bodyfat for fuel for endurance exercise.[7,8]

That's not all. Although high doses of amphetamines often cause notorious shaking and loss of balance, low doses (10-15 mg) *improve* steadiness and balance.[10] Low doses also improve alertness, attention, and eye-hand coordination, especially in subjects who are fatigued.[10,11] That's why long distance truck drivers often call amphetamines "co-pilots."

Downside of Speed

The inevitable price of stimulating the adrenal-pituitary axis with any drugs is a sharp reduction in its activity, once the drug has cleared from your body. Depending on dosage, you get mild to severe physiological (and psychological) depression. This depression can last 24-48 hours.

Therein lies the first problem of amphetamine use. Serious athletes need to train daily. Post-amphetamine depression makes training, or any other skilled activity, a real drag. So the athlete pops a little more amphetamine and in 30 minutes depression disappears and he is back in action. Pretty soon he is using the stuff every day.

Then the second problem kicks in. With daily or near daily use, within 2-3 weeks the body becomes more efficient at neutralizing the drug. So you have to up the dose to get any effect. After 2-3 months, it may take 10 times the initial dose to get the same effect. Soon you cannot operate without a daily fix of high-dose amphetamines. In the '60's and '70's hundreds of thousands of American women got into this severe drug addiction from amphetamines prescribed to them as a diet aid. That's why they were jerked from the market.

Athletes continued to use them. In a famous paper in 1981, Dr A.L. Mandell and colleagues reported that two-thirds of players in the National Football League admitted using amphetamines, up to 150 mg per game.[12] At that level you are risking it all. High doses combined with maximum performance are linked to numerous deaths of top athletes, such as French cyclist Yves Motten,[2] and British cyclist Tommy Simpson who collapsed and died after leading in the Tour de France.[13] Intra-cerebral hemorrhage (bursting of blood vessels in the brain) and stroke (obstruction of blood vessels in the brain), are both documented risks of amphetamine use.[14,15]

If they don't kill or disable you, high-doses of amphetamines are likely to cause permanent degeneration of the brain, because they damage what is called the dopaminergic system of neural transmission.[16] Simply put, the brain system responsible for much of your alertness and feelings of well-being is progressively and irreversibly damaged.

You become chronically fatigued, confused, and depressed. Even to get up in the morning becomes a major task. I have seen a few of these former speed freaks in mental hospitals. Not a pretty sight. Yet back in the '60s, Olympic coaches used to inject their athletes with amphetamines freely, in full view, right before competition.[17] I guess we live and learn.

Don't fall into the speed trap. Follow this book and you will do it right, do it clean, do it at least as well as by using drugs, and end up still in possession of your marbles.

Chapter 39

Erythropoietin: Blood Dope

$\mathbf{R}$ed blood cells are your oxygen carriers. If you have a deficient supply, then your capacity for exercise is severely limited, because insufficient oxygen gets to muscles and brain. Some folk think that this **hypoxia**, as it is called, affects only aerobic performance. Not so. Hypoxia is equally detrimental to anaerobic sports.

It's a common misconception that anaerobic exercise involves only muscle contractions beyond the oxygen delivery capacity of the body. The crucial word is *beyond*. Right up to that point, called the **anaerobic threshold**, the muscles are using all the oxygen they can get. So the level of your anaerobic threshold is a major determinant of your performance in every type of sport, because anaerobic power is additive on top of maximal aerobic power. And your red blood cell count is a major determinant of your anaerobic threshold. So athletes pursue anything that can boost their red cells.

In the '60s, researchers discovered that red cell production was controlled by a glycoprotein hormone produced in the kidneys called **erythropoietin.**[1] By 1977, erythropoietin had been isolated and purified,[2] permitting researchers to determine its amino acid structure.[3] Determining the chemical structure of anything is the first step in making a synthetic copy.

By the early '80s, scientists in the recombinant DNA industry succeeded in growing synthetic erythropoietin with the exact 165 amino acid sequence of human erythropoietin. This drug, called in America **Epoetin-alfa,** was approved by the Food and Drug Administration in 1989. It is now used worldwide for treatment of various kinds of anemia, including the anemia caused by the drug AZT in the treatment of AIDS.

The two commercial forms of Epoetin-alfa in America are Epogen, made by Amgen Inc. of Thousand Oaks, California, and Procrit made by Ortho Pharmaceuticals of Raritan, New Jersey. There is also a black market in European erythropoietin. The street name for this drug is EPO. It works extremely well.[4]

Biochemical effects of erythropoietin are measured by the hematocrit blood test. Hematocrit is the volume percentage of your blood that is made up of red cells. The normal range is 42-52% for males and 36-46% for females. At a dose of 150 units per kilogram bodyweight, erythropoietin raises hematocrit an average of 3.5 percentage points in two weeks.[5] That's a huge increase in capacity to deliver oxygen to muscles and brain.

Blood Doping

The only other way to raise hematocrit to the extent achieved by the erythropoietin is **blood doping.** About two months prior to competition, the athlete has two units of blood withdrawn (two bottles of a normal blood donation, about two pints). The red cells are separated from the plasma and preserved by glycerol freezing. About a week before competition, the red cells are thawed, mixed with physiological saline and reinfused into the athlete by a slow drip into a vein.

Blood doping works. That's why it's banned by the International Olympic Committee. The 1984 US Olympic cycling team, for example, performed way beyond expectations. Coaches knew it was more than the adrenalin of the Games. The team finally admitted they were blood doped.[6]

In controlled studies, Dr. Melvin Williams and colleagues at Old Dominion University, Norfolk, Virginia, have shown that blood doping improved performance on a five-mile treadmill run in the laboratory.[7] Taking this laboratory work into the real world of athletics, Dr. AJ Brien and TL Simon reinfused runners with 400 ml of their own red blood cells, drawn only nine days earlier. The runners' hematocrits rose by over 5 percentage points. More important, they improved their 10K race times by an average of 69 seconds.[8] That's big!

But, blood doping is not a popular ergogenic. Even though it is undetectable by drug tests, it takes a lot of careful work and requires clandestine access to medical facilities. Erythropoietin is equally undetectable in drug tests and involves just a simple injection. It didn't take athletes and coaches very long to embrace this new drug. And, with its widespread use in AIDS, and other diseases (Epogen sales in 1990-1991 totalled $304 million), black market supplies of erythropoietin, especially from Europe, are a snip.

Use and Abuse

Use of erythropoietin is not as simple as some athletes believe. It is no use stimulating the production of red cells if the body doesn't contain the necessary supplies of the hematopoietic (blood-building) nutrients required to make them. If even one of these nutrients is in short supply, then that becomes the rate-limiting step in red cell production.

Recent studies show that many athletes have depleted iron stores, for example.[9] **The Physicians Desk Reference** cautions that erythropoietin should not be used if serum ferritin (a measure of iron store) is below 100 ng/ml.[5] The normal range of serum ferritin is 30-160 ng/ml, but athletes, especially female athletes, frequently show serum ferritin levels below 20 ng/dl.[10]

In one study at the Colgan Institute, the average level of serum ferritin in apparently healthy male and female runners was 22.6 ng/dl.[9] They were also low in other hematopoietic nutrients, pyridoxine (B_6) cobalamin (B_{12}), folic acid, and vitamin C. Using erythropoietin with such athletes would be counter-productive. They don't have enough raw materials to build the extra red cells, without compromising the nutrition of other parts of the body that are equally important for performance.

There is only one study of erythropoietin with athletes, because most ethics committees would rightly turn down any proposal to use it on healthy people. This one squeaked through somehow. At the Karolinska Institute in Stockholm, Dr. Bjorn Ekblom, an expert in blood doping research, gave low doses of erythropoietin to 15 physical education students for seven weeks. He found that their red blood cell counts increased by the same amount as after a blood doping transfusion. And performance capacity increased by almost 10%.[11,12]

Risky business! The big problem with erythropoietin in healthy subjects is that it thickens your blood. Maximum increases in hematocrit with this drug exceed 10 percentage points. That means an athlete with a hematocrit of 48% could jump to 58%. In long athletic events, inevitable dehydration could raise hematocrit another 5 points to over 60%. That is blood as thick as syrup, a betting certainty for cardiovascular damage.

Case evidence indicates that erythropoietin has been responsible for at least 20 deaths of elite athletes in the last four years.[11,13] There is little absolute proof because the drug is not detectable by usual blood tests. In any case, it disappears from the body within 48 hours, though its effects may last 10 days. Most deaths have been in cyclists in Europe, where erythropoietin flooded the market for use in clinical trials in 1986.

In 1987, five Dutch cyclists died suddenly with no known cause. In 1988, two more Dutch and one Belgian cyclists died. In 1989, five more Dutch cyclists died. In 1990, two Dutch and three Belgian cyclists died. In one highly publicized case, Dutch cyclist Johannes Draaijer was known to be using the drug before he died of a heart blockage a few days after a race.[9] Erythropoietin is a real heart stopper.

Chapter 40

Grab Bag of Ergogenic Drugs

The 1990 Anabolic Steroids Control Act made steroid sale worth 5 years, and possession worth 1 year as a penitentiary guest of the government. That was the final impetus needed to ensure organized crime involvement in the illicit steroid trade. As always happens with such people, costs have soared and quality has vanished. A flood of fake steroids, stimulants, and hormones is pouring in from South America and Europe. Fakes now dominate the market.

Powerful lethal stimulants such as strychnine are being added to convince the buyer he is onto something good. These mixtures have pushed the risk of steroid use a lot higher than a slap-on-the-wrist sports suspension or even a term in jail. I was recently called on a case where one-time use of a street steroid/stimulant mix scrambled the athlete's brain - probably permanently.

So the smarter sports drug users are now thumbing the **Physician's Desk Reference**[1] in search of easy-to-get legal drugs that can pinch-hit some of the effects of steroids, growth hormone, cocaine, and amphetamines. For anyone with a little biochemistry, it's a veritable treasure trove.

Diuretics

Bodybuilders have known about diuretics for decades. But other athletes are newer at the game. Diuretics, such as **Lasix** and **Diuril**, work by increasing the rate of urine formation. So, provided you don't drink anything, you lose water weight fast. The potential advantages for muscular looks are obvious, as are the potential disadvantages of dehydration. Bodybuilding great Albert Beckles looked hard as iron in two recent contests. But each time, he was hospitalized afterwards for the side-effects of diuretics.

But looks are only the tip of it. Coaches learn in school these days that human bodies obey the laws of physics. The maximum speed you can move your body through space at maximum energy output is proportional to your body mass. Reduce body mass while maintaining strength, and speed increases. Diuretics reduce body mass. Less water, more speed.

Speed determines performance in most sports. How far you can cover a hundred meters, how high or far you can jump, the flash of Kim Zmeskal's double somersault from the floor, the acceleration of Carl Lewis, the dazzle of Evander Holyfield, all hinge on the relation between speed and body mass.

In endurance events, such as boxing, long distance running, and triathlons, diuretics are death to performance because of dehydration.[2] But in anaerobic events, from sprints through gymnastics, jumps, throws, wrestling, martial arts, weightlifting, reducing your water weight provides a definite edge. In some of these sports, diuretics provide a double edge. You get the greater speed by reducing body mass, and you also get to use it in a lower weight class by "making weight."

Diuretic Downside

The downside of diuretics is four-fold. First, users become more and more dependent on the drugs for a last-minute fix to compensate for deficiencies in their training and nutrition.

Second, with regular use the body adapts, demanding progressively higher doses of diuretics to get the same effect. Eventually, you can't pee without the drug. Third, effects are unpredictable. In one study, athletes lost an average of 4% of bodyweight in 24 hours. That big a weight loss thickened their blood, and wiped out the speed edge by biochemical turmoil.[3]

The last and most compelling reason not to use diuretics is they have no place in a healthy body. Long-term, they screw around with your hormone levels (that's how they work), leading to loss of control of body water distribution, edema, especially of the legs, and a marked decline in performance.

The trick of successful sports participation is to stay there for the long haul. That way you have the years required to learn the complex skills. Unlike some other drugs, diuretics will not kill you, but regular use will likely make your athletic career painful, brutish, and short.

Stimulants

Ever since amphetamines were withdrawn from the legitimate market because of their potential for addiction, pharmaceutical companies have been pushing stimulants that yield a less addicting buzz, but just enough to sell like goldbricks. The two main compounds are **phenylpropanolamine** (PPA) and **ephedrine**. They are in everything from cold remedies to over-the-counter weight-loss pills such as Dexatrim. By 1982, PPA became the fifth biggest selling drug in the U.S.[4]

PPA was often combined with caffeine and with the bronchodilator ephedrine, a potent addicting mix now banned by the Food and Drug Administration. But it doesn't take much thinking for athletes to continue to buy these three drugs separately and combine them. Ephedrine was partially banned for OTC sale in 1991, but Nevada opted out of the ban. Nevada registered companies now supply athletes everywhere from small, rapidly changing outlets scattered throughout the country.

Do these substitute stimulants work? At a very high dose

(150 mg) one study concluded that ephedrine does mimic amphetamine. The ephedrine produced equivalent responses of increased alertness and reports of euphoria, as one-fifth the same dose of amphetamine.[5] PPA appears to have much smaller effects.[6]

So we are back to the old amphetamine argument, does euphoria and alertness improve athletic performance? My gut feeling is yes, but the limited science available says no. The only good study to date measured effects of 24 mg of ephedrine on strength, endurance, VO2max, reaction time, speed of recovery, and a host of other athletic capacities, in a three-week double-blind trial. Result - zero.[7]

The 24 mg dose, however, was probably far too small. But athletes who use higher doses face all the risks of amphetamines outlined in Chapter 38. Use of both PPA and ephedrine cause irritability, anxiety, insomnia, headaches, hypertension, and addiction. High doses have produced paranoia, mania, hallucinations, heart attacks, and strokes.[8,9] Anyone who messes with this drug better be a careful messer.

Ephedrine may not be ergogenic but new studies indicate that even small doses may aid fat loss while preserving muscle.[10] In the latest study, Dr Arne Astrup and colleagues at the University of Copenhagen in Denmark gave overweight women a low-fat, low-calorie diet supplemented with 20 mg of ephedrine, three times daily for eight weeks. The ephedrine group lost 10.1 kg (22 lbs) compared with 8.4 kg (18.5 lbs) lost by a second group of women given the diet alone.

Doesn't seem like a whole lot of difference until you examine the loss of fat versus the loss of lean mass. The diet only group lost 3.9 kg (8.6 lbs) of lean mass and 4.5 kg (9.9 lbs) of fat. The ephedrine group lost only 1.1 kg (2.4 lbs) of lean mass and 9.0 kg (19.8 lbs) of fat.[11] In an already lean athlete, that ratio of fat to lean loss would cut you to the bone, while leaving most of your muscle intact.

This study also used 200 mg of caffeine along with each

dose of ephedrine. Caffeine is unsuccessful by itself as a weight-loss agent (except for water loss because it is diuretic). The main action of caffeine in this and similar studies, is to potentiate the effect of ephedrine, which it does very nicely if taken simultaneously with the ephedrine.[12,13]

The third compound that makes the mixture even more effective is regular aspirin. Like caffeine, aspirin is a methylzanthine. Methylzanthines potentiate the ephedrine activity by increasing release of the hormone nor-epinephrine.[13] This effect was first noticed when these mixtures were used to treat asthma and other respiratory complaints. The patients also lost fat.[13]

The herb Ma Huang contains ephedra the basis of ephedrine and is now available in standardized doses. Kola nut and guarana both contain caffeine. And white willow bark contains salycilic acid, the original base of aspirin. They should work equally as well as the more toxic synthetic drugs.

Bronchodilator Inhalers

We saw in Chapter 36 that injectable beta-adrenergic-agonist drugs, such as clenbuterol, probably build strength. Well there is another whole class of such drugs used as inhalants in treatment of asthma and similar diseases. The latest and highly logical venture by athletes is to examine whether sucking on asthma inhalers can benefit performance.

The first study of inhaled beta-adrenergic-agonists surfaced in the **Canadian Journal of Sports Medicine** in 1988.[14] The researchers used a single measured puff of **albuterol** (180 mcg), the commercial asthma medication Proventil. They found no effect on 1-hour endurance exercise, but a significant increase in anaerobic performance in the final sprint to the finish.

The latest study is by Dr. Joe Signorile and colleagues at the University of Miami in Florida. They gave two 90 mcg puffs of albuterol or a placebo to healthy male and female athletes, 10 minutes before they rode an ergometer bicycle. After a warm-up ride, the athletes were tested with a 15-second all out sprint. Results showed that the albuterol significantly increased peak power on the ride and significantly reduced fatigue. These data are a strong indication that beta-adrenergic-agonist inhalers, used to treat asthma, have a real ergogenic effect.

That's not the whole of it. It's a common misconception that bronchodilators affect performance by stimulating the lungs and increasing the amount of oxygen getting into the systems of athletes. Not so. The Signorile study showed that the increased power of the athletes was independent of the minor improvement in ventilation that occurred. Studies of isolated muscle tissue suggest that albuterol and similar drugs can directly increase the contractile force of muscle tissue itself.[15] If so, then it is no surprise that use is skyrocketing among anaerobic and power athletes.

The downside of these drugs include the usual stimulant problems of agitation, anxiety, elevated blood pressure, and heart irregularities. But the amount of albuterol used in the Signorile study (180 mcg), is a common prescribed dosage used several times daily by asthmatics with little risk. At least it's better than death drugs off the street.

Part VIII

Putting It All Together

The champions are not more gifted than you. They have simply analysed their strengths and practiced them to the exclusion of disrupting influences. Exclude the trivialities of everyday. Focus on all that you really have in life: Your body and your will.

Michael Colgan, Sports Medicine Lectures, 1992

Chapter 41

Your Personal Sports Nutrition Program

You are using this book because you want to excel. Excellence is never an accident. It develops only by careful design, by constant, meticulous attention to detail. Excellence in sport relies equally on an optimal nutrition program and an optimal training program. This book gives you the detail to design one half of the picture - your nutrition.

How Nutrients Create the Structure

Part I gave you the principles of **synergy, completeness, biochemical individuality, lifestyle dynamics, precision,** and **physiological dynamics** to guide your design. We stressed the importance of your biochemical and lifestyle uniqueness, and how they demand an individual nutrient program, designed to fit your body, your sport, your environment, and your lifestyle.

Part I also showed you how your body is precisely made and re-made constantly, out of all the chemicals, both nutrient and toxic, that get into your body by eating drinking and breathing. To the exact extent that your water, food and air is defective or polluted with toxic substances, so your body structure will be defective and polluted also. I gave you strategies to avoid the bad and obtain the good. To the extent that you follow these strategies your body will progress towards excellence.

Gas and Parts

Part II showed you how your body uses fuel, and what types and mix of fuels to put in it. I detailed strategies to limit fat intake and to use the best carbohydrates to optimize energy for training and competition. Don't put junk fuel in your Masserati.

I also gave you the rules to minimize bodyfat (dead weight) while maximizing muscle (dynamic weight). Initially the rules are tough to follow, but eminently worth it. Each time you sit down to eat, remember your body in motion obeys the laws of physics. More waist, less speed.

Part III emphasized how proteins provide the parts, the building blocks of muscle, and how optimal development of strength is dependent on a daily mix of top quality parts, such as whey protein and egg white protein. Chapter 12 showed how much you need for your personal sports nutrition program.

Part III also covered the vitamins and minerals and how much athletes need of each to offset the increased nutrient demands of exercise. We saw that many athletes are deficient in a variety of nutrients. I stressed how vitamins are the nuts and bolts that hold your body together, and minerals are the framework that holds it up.

We saw that numerous supplements offered to athletes are like fake car parts, with the wrong ingredients, and the wrong forms of nutrient, or just plain fraud with no ingredients at all. I stressed how obtaining the right supplements requires constant vigilance and attention to detail.

We saw also, that in any sensible amounts, vitamins and minerals are not dangerous substances like drugs, despite raucous media reports, and uninformed pronouncements by the FDA.

They are nutrients that the human body evolved on. Vitamins and minerals are about as toxic as lemonade.

Optimal Performance

Part IV showed you how vitamins and minerals are related to performance purely by providing an optimal base of nutrients for growth, maintenance and repair. Studies purporting to find ergogenic effects of this or that vitamin or mineral, have almost always been simply correcting a deficiency caused by the trauma of training and the poor nutrition of the athlete. These nutrients are not effective ergogenic substances. They are building and maintenance department, and the body uses them accordingly.

Part IV also showed you how a synergic mix of antioxidants can combat athletic injury, and how another synergic mix can help you optimize your red blood system, and thus your capacity to carry and use oxygen. We covered a third group of nutrients also, mainly antioxidants together with specific animo acids, that help you achieve the strong immunity that prevents illness and injury, and so maintains the regular training progress essential to excellence.

Ergogenics/Anabolics

Part V covered some specific substances that, unlike drugs, are minimally toxic to your body, and that do provide an ergogenic edge. I stressed how these substances are ergogenic rather than nutrient in function, and should be used sparingly. The real business of optimal sports nutrition is not to boost a competiton day, but to build a better body.

Part VI covered the important new resarch on the **anabolic drive**, how neuroendocrine influences of nutrition release growth hormone, stimulate production of insulin-like growth factor, stimulate the **insulin drive** and stimulate manufacture of testosterone. We discussed in detail nutrient anabolics such as arginine, ornithine alpha-ketoglutarate, ketoisocaproate, and chromium picolinate, that can strengthen your anabolic drive and increase muscle growth.

Part VI also exposed the plethora of snake oil "anabolic alternatives" now foisted on athletes by the latest generation of carpetbaggers. Everything from yohimbe bark to dubious hormones from cockroach hindquarters litter the sports marketplace. Chapter 31 saves you from wasting your money on this morass of hogwash and flapdoodle.

Drugs Work But . . . . . .

For the first time in a documented book, Part VII told you the truth about drugs in sport, and gave you the evidence and the scientific references to back it up. There is no doubt that a wide variety of drugs improve sports performance. Anyone who tells you different is either a liar or a fool. But they also pose serious dangers for both physical and mental health. And anyone who tells you different is also a liar or a fool.

But the worst consequence of drug use is that it destroys your pride, your integrity, your concept of self. Drugs inhibit the pursuit of excellence, because you never know whether you could have done it without them. You can never escape the knowledge that you rely on a drug crutch of deception for your status in the world.

You do not have to use drugs to achieve your potential. In Chapter 32 I gave you a nutrition program that will equal or surpass effects of drugs, and leave your body sound, your mind sane, and your integrity intact. In Chapter 42 I expand that program to incorporate strength training that needs no steroids to support it. Follow it patiently and you will achieve a degree of excellence in sport that is the true expression of the power of your will.

Shape Your Will

Beyond the trivial trappings of our culture, you have only **your body and your will**. Treat both with respect. Put nothing in your mouth unless it strengthens your structure. A difficult habit, but worth the cultivation. Nothing tastes as good as lean and mean feels.

Put nothing in your mind unless it strengthens your will. Be careful what you watch and what you read, for that becomes what you know. Continually watch the daily soaps and you will become a soap opera character with the willpower and integrity of a wet noodle. But watch real strength and courage such as Fred Lebow fighting brain cancer to complete the 1992 New York Marathon, and your will grows stronger automatically.

It is always so, because the information that makes you what you are remains long after the source is forgotten. Even the most private beliefs that drive your life, even belief in God, you learned from other people. Were you born into a different culture you would believe with all your will in different Gods.

It is crucial, therefore, to your pursuit of excellence that you acquire the best information. The basis of information presented here is science from peer-reviewed medical and scientific journals, plus eighteen years of hands-on work with athletes. Contrast that with the daily media reports of unexamined speculation that shape much of public belief. Rely on television for your knowledge and you will eat burgers for nutrition.

Much of popular writing and programming is entertainment, designed to stimulate emotional reactions and capture market share, not to inform your mind. It is aimed at an obtuse middle-class who have surrendered their intellect to entrepreneurs and their will to politicians. Don't become one of them. March to your own drummer.

Already much of your potential may lie buried beneath false doubts and fears, sown by poor instruction during childhood. If you desire to excel you must wipe the slate clean and start anew. Practice resisting external influences every day. Practice internal calm, silence, stillness in the midst of the daily static, the noise that passes for fact. Practice being driven only from within.

Those who excel are not more gifted than you. They have simply cleared their minds of former fears, analysed their strengths, and practiced them to the exclusion of disrupting inflluences. You must do the same.

Three easy-to-read books that will help you with this task are, **The Way of the Peaceful Warrior** by Dan Millman, **Zen in the Martial Arts** by Joe Hyams, and Mark Allen's **Total Triathlete.** [1,2,3] As I write Mark Allen has just won the Hawaii Ironman Triathlon, the premier contest of that sport, - *again*! From these elite athletes who are masters of the mental side of training you can learn the degree of focus and concentration essential to be a champion.

Seek A Teacher

You have within you the seeds of excellence. How far those seeds will grow depends on the instruction you receive. Do not try to go it alone. It will not come from mere effort and diligence. Practice does not make perfect. Practice makes permanent. Each time you repeat something incorrect in your nutrition or your training, you are making the mistake more ingrained in your mind. So it is crucial to have the right programs before you start.

If you try to do it alone each step becomes a tortuous and exhausting labor, because the teacher is also the student. Take this book and the Colgan Institute hotline for nutrition, and take only the best of coaches for training. Then trust them completely to lead your athletic life. Let no outside influences interfere.

But before you do, examine your teachers minutely. I invite you to examine everything about me and what I say. If anyone giving you advice is not a living example of what they say, reject them utterly.

Only those who know excellence can let you glimpse it also. Without such guides you are lost in a morass of conflicting advice. You cannot separate the truth from the hokum of hidden agendas that will pull you for profit into aquiescent mediocrity.

Form Specific Goals

Make your athletic goals specific, detailed. Write them down. Make them measurable so that you know at regular intervals how far you are progressing. Make them time-limited, so that you strive to reach particular stages by particular dates. Divide you goals into subgoals, so that you have one to strive for each four weeks. Make them public so that there is shame if you fail and pride if you succeed.

But share your goals only with those who will help you reach them. Avoid anyone who belittles your program. Only failures belittle others, to compensate their own mediocrity. If you associate with the mediocre you will become mediocre also.

You Will Succeed

Do not fear failure. Fear does not exist in objects or situations that confront you. It is an obstacle to action created by your mind, created solely by false ideas of weakness that have been taught to you by others. Whenever you are afraid, you have frightened yourself. Once you understand that you create your own fear, then you can learn to eliminate it.

The will to excel is of far greater strength than any inborn talent. But you cannot do it halfway. Excellence is never achieved by moderation. While you have the youth, make your athletic goals the focus of your life. Do not reach old age only to accuse yourself in the mirror, "You never even let me try".

Go for the gusto while Nature will allow it. I can promise you it is the finest feeling you will know, as fine as the faith in the hug of your child, as fine as the gentle gaze of your lover. A thing of ecstasy.

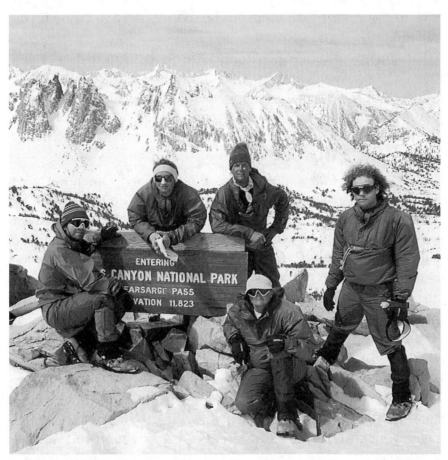

Left to right: Michael Colgan with champion endurance athletes Andre Boesel, Rex Keep, Jaqueline Shaw and Emile van der Moevre on a week-long ski mountaineering project across the Sierra Mountains in winter to test multi-vitamin/mineral/amino acid tablets for possible use by the U.S. Armed Forces. During the seven days of 12-14 hours climbing and cross-country skiing daily, they lived without solid food, existing entirely on nutrient pills and water. Photo shows day 7 on the way out.

Chapter 42

Strength Program To Beat Steroids

To beat steroids your nutrition has to fit your training, like a pair of custom running shoes fit your feet. This book is focussed on the nutrition half of the formula, but I want to leave you with one more goodie: the most effective strength program ever.

Why strength? Because all athletes should include strength training in their programs. For the primary strength sports like weightlifting, shot putting, jumps, sprints, it's obvious. But some coaches still question its relevance for speed or endurance, and warn their athletes away from the weights. Big mistake! Thirty years ago, expert in human physiology Dr Lawrence Morehouse, was the first to show how strength of a working muscle is the limiting factor on development of endurance in that muscle.[1] His findings have since been confirmed many times.[2,3] Strength is the primary requirement for achieving your full endurance potential.

It's simple physics. And your body, like rocks and rivers and every speck of dust on Earth, obeys the laws of physics. Consider two runners, both equally endurance trained and both with a best time of 30 minutes in the 10K. One now adopts the Colgan Institute strength program for runners, and his legs grow 25% stronger in six months, without increasing his bodyweight.

That's a snip to do. Now the maximum load his legs can carry is 25% more than before the program. At his old maximum endurance speed, the muscles are now being stressed about 25% less than they were previously. So, given the right endurance training, he makes a big improvement and leaves his former companion in the dust.

We have done this job with athletes many, many times at the Colgan Institute. It's so simple and so effective, that we have developed strength programs for all major sports. They work every time.

What about speed? Some coaches of boxers, wrestlers, martial artists, still quote the old musclebound myth that weight training slows you down. The *wrong* training, which stresses hypertrophy (growth) of the **red, slow-twitch fibers** of muscles, *does* slow you down. But the *right* weight training for speed, which stresses the **white, fast-twitch fibers** of muscles, can make you a whole lot faster.

Again, it's simple physics. If you make the speed fibers of a muscle stronger, then they can apply more sudden force to a limb. It has to move faster. Evander Holyfield was always good, even when he was wrongly disqualified in the Olympics and took it like the noble man he is. But since he went to Lee Haney's gym and took some serious weight training, he has become totally awesome.

The Program

The first step is **complete nutrition**. Work out your individual requirements for fats, carbohydrates and proteins, using Chapters 8, 9 and 12. Then work out your individual requirments for each vitamin and mineral using Chapters 14 and 15. I would have liked to include in the book our more accurate analysis of individual needs for vitamins and minerals, but we have to use a massive computer program just to contain it. To write it out would take another book at least this size. If you have trouble assessing your needs, call our hotline at (619) 632-7722.

Ask for the **Optimal Sports Nutrition Analysis**.

The second step is to get your food right. All your food has to be top quality as detailed throughout this book. Work out your meals precisely, so that you never miss, or have to eat the wrong food, or eat at the wrong time. This task takes a bit of planning. Draw up a chart of cooked meals, protein/carb drinks and other food on a precise schedule.

You don't have to become a monk. Food is one of life's great pleasures. Over the years the Colgan Institute, has worked out great-tasting diet plans, and recipes, and foods to support your program while on the road. All is revealed in our book **Sports Gourmet**.

The third step is to adopt the **Anabolic Drive Program** in Chapter 32. Shape your life around it. It will not let you down. But remember, it is an experimental program. The long-term safety of using amino acids has not been determined. So you should read the scientific references and decide for yourself. I am giving you the latest science. What you do with the information is at your own choice and risk.

We have had no problems with athletes using various versions of this program in the last 10 years. Quite the opposite. High levels of growth hormone, insulin-like growth factor and testosterone are dynamite for performance. Why do you think that most stallions today are gelded before they are a year old. Their hormones are chopped because otherwise no one could catch them or control their strength. The Anabolic Drive Program creates stallions.

The Exercise

The last step is the weight training itself. You have to be very specific and you have to be an experienced weight trainer to get the most benefit. This stuff is not for beginners.

1. Use your two workouts per day to cover the widest range of exercises possible. That way you hit the most white fibers. The

Colgan Institute program contains up to 180 different exercises. For every possible variation on weight exercises see Bill Pearl's book, **Keys to the Inner Universe.**[4]

2. Exercise only one muscle system per day. I say system rather than the old idea of bodypart, because you need to train your whole body to work in synchrony, not as isolated bits. Unless you train the connections and reciprocal movements of muscles with each other, you are asking for inefficiency and injury. Systems for a 4-day per week program are:

        a. Shoulders, chest and upper back.
        b. Arms and shoulders.
        c. Chest, back and abs.
        d. Lower back and legs.

3. Do exercises in pairs. This strategy permits you to use supersets of opposing muscle groups, and takes advantage of the temporary exhaustion of reciprocal inhibition to lift more weight. For example, a set of shoulder barbell presses from the neck is immediately followed by a set of lat pulldowns to the neck. Then back to shoulder presses, and so on until the set quota for both exercises is complete.

4. Do a four set routine for each exercise. First set is a warm up of the maximum weight you can use for 12-15 reps. Second set is the maxiumum weight you can use for 6-8 reps. Third set is the maximum weight you can use for 4-6 reps. Fourth set flushes the system with the maximum weight you can use for 20 reps.

5. Crucial strategy for maximum strength and speed. *Accelerate* the concentric movement of each rep. Do it at maximum speed consistent with good form. That's how your speed develops. *Slow* the eccentric movement of each rep to a 2-second count. The lengthening of muscles under load is how maximum strength develops.

6. Do each exercise only *once* per week. Muscle remodelling for speed and strength goes this way. For 24-48 hours after exercise, traumatized muscle tissue breaks down and is excreted. For the next 48-72 hours, muscle cells rebuild. Maximum strength **in that**

movement is achieved 5-9 days after the exercise. If you recover faster than that, you are not working hard enough.

7. Don't overtrain. Keep each training session to 11/2 hours maximum. And that's the program. I can't cover the hundreds of exercise studies we have reviewed to come to these rules. That's all in the **Colgan Institute Power Program**. Suffice to say here it works - big!

"Yeah," you say. "But does it beat steroids?" Try it! We know that ours and similar programs work better than drugs. Other coaches in the know also use similar work to produce drug-free athletes that beat the world. Bobby Kersee is a great example. Think of his students, Florence Griffith Joyner, Gail Devers, and Jackie Joyner Kersee. They are not only the best in the world, they are the best that have ever existed in human history. They are what sport is really about: the pursuit of excellence by hard work, by patient perfection of your body, by triumph of the human spirit.

References

Chapter 1. Nutrition Basics

1. Levander OA, Cheng L, eds. **Micronutrient Interactions: Vitamins, Minerals, and Hazardous Elements.** New York: New York Academy of Sciences, 1980.
2. Hickson J, Wolinsky I. **Nutrition in Exercise and Sport.** Boca Raton, Florida: CRC Press, 1989.
3. Mertz W. **Trace Elements in Human and Animal Nutrition. Fifth Edition.** New York: Academic Press, 1987.
4. **Recommended Dietary Allowances. 10th Ed.** Washington, D.C.: National Academy Press, 1989.
5. Lindenbaum JE, et al. Neuropsychiatric disorders caused by cobalamin deficiency in the absence of anemia or macrocytosis. **N Engl J Med** 1988;318:1720-1728.
6. Norman AW, ed. **Vitamin D: Basic Research And Its Clinical Applications.** Berlin: Walter de Gruyter, 1979.
7. Sauberlich HE. Interaction of thiamin, riboflavin, and other B-vitamins. In: Levander OA, Cheng L, eds. **Micronutrient Interactions.** New York: New York Academy of Sciences, 1980:80.
8. Machlin J, Gabriel E. Interaction of vitamin E with vitamin C, vitamin B_{12} and zinc. In: Levander OA, Cheng L, eds. **Micronutrient Interactions.** New York: New York Academy of Sciences, 1980:98.
9. Shils M. Mangesium, calcium, and parathyroid hormone interactions. In: Levander OA, Cheng L, eds. **Micronutrient Interactions.** New York: New York Adademy of Sciences, 1980:165.
10. Smith CJ. The vitamin A-zinc connection: A review. In: Levander OA, Cheng L, eds. **Micronutrient Interactions.** New York: New York Academy of Sciences, 1980:62.
11. Goode HF, et al. The effect of dietary vitamin E deficiency on Plasma Zinc and Copper Concentrations. **Clin Nutr** 1991;10:233-235.
12. Philips M, Baetz A, eds. **Diet and Resistance To Disease: Advances In Experimental Medicine and Biology. Vol 35.** New York: Plenum, 1981.
13. Colgan M. **Your Personal Vitamin Profile.** New York: Morrow, 1982.
14. Williams RJ. **Biochemical Individuality.** New York: Wiley, 1956.
15. Williams RJ, Deason G. **Proc Nat Acad Sci USA** 1967;57:1638.
16. Albanese AA, ed. **Protein and Amino Acid Nutrition.** New York: Academic Press, 1959.

17. Williams RJ. **Physicians Handbook of Nutritional Science.** Springfield, IL:Thomas, 1975.
18. Burns JJ, et al., eds. **Third Conference on Vitamin C.** Ann NY Acad Sci. 498. New York: New York Academy of Sciences, 1987.
19. **Recommended Dietary Allowances.** Food & Nutrition Board, Washington D.C.: National Academy of Sciences, 1980:1.
20. Harper AE. Official dietary allowances: those pesky RDAs. **Nutrition Today** 1974;9:15-25.
21. Dressendorfer RH, Wade CE, Amersterdam EA. Development of pseudoanemia in marathon runners during a 20-day road race. **JAMA** 1981;246:1215.
22. Colgan M, Fiedler S, Colgan L. Micronutrient status of endurance athletes affects hematology and performance. **J Appl Nutr** 1991; 43: 16-30.
23. Hathcock JN, ed. **Nutritional Toxicology.** New York: Academic Press, 1982.
24. Colgan M.Effects of multinutrient supplementation on athletic performance. In: Katch FI, ed. **Sport, Health, and Nutrition.** Champaign IL:Human Kinetics, 1986, Chapter 3.
25. Maloney T. Pie in the face. **Cycling** 1992;September/October:9.
26. Barcelona! **Track and Field News** 1992;October:6-86.

Chapter 2. A Hairy Bag of Water

1. Oser BL, ed. **Hawke's Physiological Chemistry.** New York: McGraw-Hill, 1965.
2. Colgan M. Effects of multi-nutrient supplementation on athletic performance. In: Katch FI, ed. **Sport Health and Nutrition, Vol 2, I**llinois: Human Kinetics. 1986:21-50.
3. Sargent F, Weinman K. Physiological variability in young men. In: Consolazio CF, et al, eds. **Physiological Measurements of Metabolic Functions in Man.** New York: McGraw-Hill 1963, 453-480.
4. Sawka MN, et al. Influence of hydration level and body bluids on exercise performance in the heat. **Journal of the American Medical Association** 1984; 252:1165-1169.
5. Armstrong, LE, Costill DL, Fink WJ. Influence on diuretic-induced dehydration on competitive running performance. **Medicine and Science in Sports and Exercise.** 1985;17:456-461.
6. Fink WJ. In Haskell W, et al, eds. **Nutrition and Athletic Performance.** Palo Alto, CA: Bull Publishing, 1981, 52-63.

7. Norman C. Wastes seep round the law. **Science** 1983;220:34.
8. Raloff J. **Science News** 1990;137:169.
9. **Technologies and Management Strategies for Hazardous Waste Control** Washington DC: Government Printing Office, 1983.
10. Fine JC. A crisis of contamination. **The Sciences** 1984;24:2, 22.
11. Lawrence CE, et al. Trihalomethanes in drinking water and human colorectal cancer. **J Nat Cancer Institute** 1984;72:563-568.
    See also: Raloff J. Chlorination residues cloud water safety. **Science News** 1989;135:65.
12. Studlick JR, Bain RC. Bottled water: expensive ground water. **Well water Journal** 1980;7:15-79.
13. Weissman JD. **Choose to Live**, New York: Penguin Books, 1988.
14. Underwood EJ. **Trace Elements in Human and Animal Nutrition, Fourth Edition**. New York: Academic Press, 1977, 466.

Chapter 3. Play It Cool

1. Leithead CS, Lind AR. **Heat Stress and Heat Disorders**. Philadelphia: Davis, 1964.
2. Costill DL. **A Scientific Approach to Distance Running.** Track and Field News Publishing, 1979.
3. Nadel ER. Circulatory and thermal regulation during exercise. **Fed Proc** 1980;39:1491.
4. American College of Sports Medicine. Position statement of prevention of heat injuries during distance running. **Med Sci Sports** 1975;7:7-9.
5. Greenleaf JE, Castle BL. Exercise temperature regulation in man during hypohydration and hyperhydration. **J Appl Physiol** 1971;30:847-853.
6. Fink W, Costill DL, Van Handel, PJ. Leg muscle metabolism during exercise in the heat and cold. **European J Appl Physiol** 1975;24:183-190.
7. Costill DL, Miller JM. Nutrition for endurance sport: Carbohydrate and fluid balance. **Int J Sports Med** 1980;1:2-14.
8. Locksley R. Fuel utilization in marathons: Implications for performance. **West J Med** 1980;133:493-502.
9. Greenleaf JE, Olsson K, Saltin B. Muscle glycogen content and its significance for the water content of the body. **Acta Physiol Scand** 1969: 330.
10. Moroff SV, Bass DE. Effects of overhydration on man's physiological responses to work in the heat. **J Appl Physiol** 1965; 20:267-270.
11. Fortney SM, et al. Effect of acute alterations of blood volume on circulatory performance in humans. **J Appl Physiol** 1981;50:292-298.

12. Fink W. Fluid intake for maximizing athletic performance. In:Haskell W, et al., eds. **Nutrition and Athletic Performance**. Palo Alto: Bull Publishing, 1982.

13. Pitts GC, Johnson RE, Consolazio FC. Work in the heat as affected by intake of water, salt and glucose. **Am J Physiol** 1984;142:253-259.

14. Pugh LG, Corbett JI, Johnson RH. Rectal temperature, weight losses and sweat rates in marathon running. **J Appl Physiol** 1967;23:347-352.

15. Coyle EF, Costill DL, Fink WJ. Gastric emptying rates for selected athletic drinks. **Res Quart** 1978;49:119-124.

16. Evans Wj, Hughes VA. Dietary carbohydrate and endurance exercise. **Am J Clin Nutr** 1985;41:1146-1154.

17. Murray R. The effects of consuming carbohydrate/electrolyte beverages on gastric emptying and fluid absorption during a flollowing exercise. **Sports Med** 1987;4:322-351.

18. Seiple RS, et al. Gastric emptying characteristics of two glucose polymer-electrolyte solutions. **Med Sci in Sports and Exercise** 1983;15:366-369.

19. Davis JM, et al. Fluid availability of sports drinks differing in carbohydrate type and concentration. **Am J Clin Nutr** 1990;51: 1054-1057.

20. Koivisto V, Karonen S, Nikkila E. Carbohydrate ingestion before exercise: comparison of glucose, fructose, and sweet placebo. **J Appl Physiol** 1981;51:783-787.

21. Levine L, et al. Fructose and glucose ingestion and muscle glycogen use during submaximal exercise.**J Appl Physiol** 1983;55:1767-71.

22. Davenport HW. **Physiology of the Digestive Tract: 5th Ed.** Chicago: Yearbook Medical Publishers, 1982.

23. Costill DL, et al. Water and electrolyte replacement during repeated days of work in the heat. **Aviat, Space, Environ Med** 1975;45:795-800.

Chapter 4. Real Food

1. Colgan M. We have poisoned the land. **Nutrition & fitness** 1990;9: 170-171.

2. **Recommended Dietary Allowances 10th Edition.** Washington DC: National Academy Press, 1989.

3. Harris R, Karmas E, eds. **Nutritional Evaluation of Food Processing.** Westport CT: Avi Publishing, 1975.

4. Hulme AC, ed. **The Biochemistry of Fruits and Their Products Vol 1.** NY: Academic Press, 1970.

5. Hartman AM, Dryden LP. **Vitamins in Milk.** Champaign IL: Am Dairy Sci Assoc, 1965.
6. Schroeder HA. **Amer J Clin Nutr** 1971;24:562.
7. Geselwitz G. **Health Foods Business**. February 1990: 46.
8. **Composition of Foods. Beef Products.** USDA Handbook No 8-13, Washington DC: USDA Information Service, 1986.
9. **Composition of Foods. Pork Products.** USDA Handbook No 8-10, Washington DC: USDA Information Service, 1983.
10. **Wellness Letter** 1991, December, 4.
11. **FSIS Monitoring and Controlling Pesticide Residues in Domestic Meat and Poultry Products.** Washington DC: USDA Information Service, 1988.
12. Is our fish fit to eat? **Consumers Reports.** February, 1992:103-120.
13. Food and Drug Administration Office of Seafood. Personal Communication, May, 1992.
14. See, for example, Foran JA. **Amer J Public Health** 1989, March.
15. Protein quality evaluation. Report of a joint FAO/WHO expert consultation. **Food and Nutrition Paper No 51**. Rome: FAO/WHO, 1990.
16.. Young VR, Pellet PL. Protein evaluation, amino acid and scoring and the Food and Drug Administration's proposed food labelling regulations. **J Nutr** 1991;121:145-150.
17. Young VR. Soy protein in relation to human protein and amino acid nutrition. **J Am Dietet Assoc** 1991;91:828-835.
18. Henley EC. Food and Drug Administration's proposed labelling rules for protein. **J Am Dietet Assoc** 1992;92:293-296.
19. Colgan M. **Your Personal Vitamin Profile.** New York: Morrow, 1982.
20. Spiller GA, Kay RP, eds. **Medical Aspects of Dietary Fiber.** New York: Plenum, 1980.
21. Camarini-Davalos RA, Hanover R, eds. **Treatment of Early Diabetes. Advances in Experimental Medicine and Biology, Vol 119.** New York Plenum, 1979.
22. Colgan M. **Prevent Cancer Now. Second Edition.** San Diego: CI Publications, 1992.
23. Marshall E. A scramble for data on Artic radioactive dumping. **Science** 1992;257:608-609.

Chapter 5. Give Me Air

1. Ostro B. Paper presented to the Annual Convention of the Society for

Occupational and Environmental Health at Arlington VA, March, 1991.

2. Raloff J. Air pollution: A respiratory hue and cry. **Science News** 1991;139:203.

3. Stone R. Immunology: Pollutants a growing threat. **Science** 1992;256:28.

4. **Biologic Markers in Immunotoxicology.** Washington DC: National Research Council, 1992.

5. Hall JV. Valuing the health benefits of clean air. **Science** 1992;255:812-816.

6. Vander AJ. **Nutrition Stress and Toxic Chemicals.** Ann Arbor: University of Michigan Press, 1981.

7. McDonnell WF, et al. Pulmonary effects of ozone exposure during exercise; dose-response characteristics. **J Appl Physiol** 1983;54: 1345-1352.

8. Folinsbee LJ, Bedi JF, Horvath SM. Respiratory responses in humans repeatedly exposed to low concentrations of ozone. **Ann Rev Respir Dis** 1980;121:431-439.

9. Folinsbe LJ, Silverman F, Shepard RI. Decrease of maximum work performance following ozone exposure. **J Appl Physiol** 1977;42:5 31-536.

10. Adams WC, Schelegle ES. Ozone and high ventilation effects of pulmonary function and endurance performance. **J Appl Physiol** 1983; 55:805-812.

11. Folinsbee LJ, Silverman F, Shephard RJ. Decrease of maximum work performance following ozone exposure. **J Appl Physiol** 1977;42:531-536.

12. Horvath SM, Gliner JA, Matsen-Twisdale JA. Pulmonary function and maximum exercise responses following acute ozone exposure. **Aviat Space Environ Med** 1979;40:901-905.

13. Calabrese E, et al. Influence of dietary vitamin E on susceptibility to ozone exposure. **Bull Environ Contam Toxicol** 1985;34:417-422.

14. Chow EK, et al. **Environmental Res** 1981;24:315.

15. Colgan M. Junk food Olympics. **Penthouse,** August, 1984.

16. Murphy P. Coaches hazy about training for smog. **Physician and Sportsmed** 1984;12:182-183.

17. Ekblom B, et al. Effect of changes in arterial oxygen content on circulation and physical performance. **J Appl Physiol** 1975;39:71-75.

18. Vogel JA, et al. Carbon monoxide and physical work capacity. **Arch Environ Health** 1972;24:198-203.

19. Raven PR, et al. Effect of carbon monoxide and peroxyacetyl nitrate on man's maximal aerobic capacity. **J Appl Physiol** 1974;36:288-293.

20. Horvath SM, et al. Maximal aerobic capacity at different levels of carboxyhemoglobin. **J Appl Physiol** 1975;38:300-303.

21. Nicholson JP, Case DB. Carboxyhemoglobin levels in New York City

runners. **Physician and Sportsmed** 1983;11:135-138.

22. Stanitski C. Air pollution affects exercise performance. **Clinics in Sports Medicine.** 1986;4:725-726.

23. Mohammed Z, et al. **FASEB Proc** 1986, No. 4344.

Chapter 6. Body Pollutants

1. **J Occup Med** 1985;27:19.
2. **Health Letter Supplement** 1985, Public Citizen, 2000 P Street NW, Washington DC 20036. (202) 872-0320.
3. Sunderman FW. **Biol and Trace Element Res** 1979;1:63.
4. Colgan M. **Prevent Cancer Now.** San Diego: CI Publications, 1990.
5. Norel S, et al. **Lancet** 1983;1:462.
6. The Surgeon General **Healthy People** DHEW Publications Nos. 79-55071,79-55071A.
7. Fishbein L. **Sci Total Environ** 1974;2:341.
8. Costa L, et al.. **Nature** 1975;254:238.
9. Mitchell DG, Aldous KM. **Environ Health Perspect** 1974;7:59.
10. **Consumer Reports** 1981;July:376.
11. Needleman H, et al. **N Engl J Med** 1979;300:689.
12. Waldron H, Stofen D. **Subclinical Lead Poisoning.** New York Academic Press, 1974.
13. Levander OA, Cheng L. **Micronutrient Interactions**. New York: New York Academy of Sciences, 1982.
14. Byrce-Smith D, Stephens R. **Lead or Health**. London: The Conservation Society, 1981.
15. Crapper DR, Krishman SS, Dalton AJ. Brain aluminum distribution and experimental neuro-fibrillary degeneration. **Science** 1973;180:May.
16. Spencer H, et al. In: Levander OA, Cheng L., eds. **Micronutrient Interactions**. New York: New York Academy of Sciences 1980;181-194.
17. Parkinson IS, et al. Fracturing dialysis osteodystrophy and dialysis encephalopathy: an epidemiological survey. **Lancet** 1979;1:406-409.
18. Salusky IB, Foley J, Nelson P, Goodman WG. Aluminum accumulation during treatment with aluminum hydroxide and dialysis in children and young adults with chronic renal disease. **N Engl J Med** 1991;324:527-531.
19. Altmann P, et al. Disturbance of cerebral function by aluminum in haemodialysis patients without overt aluminum toxicity. **Lancet** 1989;2:7-12.
20. **Physicians Desk Reference 46th Edition**. Montvale, NJ: Medical Economics Co., 1992.

21. Latham PM. Quoted in Wadler GI, Hainline B. **Drugs and the Athlete.** Philadelphia: FA Davis, 1989:ix.

Chapter 7. Rest And Sleep

1. Hickson JF, Wolinsky I, eds. **Nutrition in Exercise and Sport.** Boca Raton, FL: CRC Press, 1989.
2. Costill DL. **A Scientific Approach to Distance Running.** Los Altos, CA:Track & Field News, 1979.
3. Bompa TO. **Theory and Methodology of Training.** Dubuque, Iowa: Kendall/Hunt Publishing, 1983.
4. Fry RW, Morton AR, Keast D. Overtraining in athletes. **Sports Medicine** 1991;12:32-65.
5. Karpovitch PV. **Physiology of Muscular Activity.** Philadelphia: WB Saunders, 1965.
6. Viru A. **Hormones in Muscular Activity.** Boca Raton, FL: CRC Press, 1985.
7. Noakes TD. **Love of Running.** London: Oxford University Press, 1989.
8. Jokl E. The immunological status of athletes. **J Sports Med** 1984;14: 165-167.
9. Galloway J. **Galloway's Book on Running.** Bolinas, CA: Shelter Publications, 1984.
10. Fitzgerald L. Exercise and the immune system. **Immunology Today** 1988;9:337-339.
11. Liu Y, Wang S. The enhancing effect of exercise on the production of antibody to salmonella typhi in mice. **Immunological Letters** 1987;14: 117-120.
12. Sheehan G. **Medical Advice for Runners.** Mountain View, CA: World Publications, 1978.

Chapter 8: Smart Fats

1. US National Research Council. **Report of the Committee on Diet and Health, Food and Nutrition Board.** Washington, DC: National Academy Press, 1989.
2. Brisson GJ. **Lipids in Human Nutrition.** Inglewood, NY: Burgess, 1981.
3. Mattson RH, Grundy SM. **J Lipid Res** 1985;26:194.
4. Mensink RP, Katan MB. **N Engl J Med** 1989;321:436.

5. Erasmus U. **Fats and Oils.** Vancouver: Alive Books, 1986.

6. **Lancet.** 1980, 8 March, 534.

7. Grain Research Laboratory, **Crop Bull No. 181,** Winnipeg, Canada: Canadian Grain Commission, 1989.

8. Slover HT, et al. **J Am Oil Chem Soc** 1985;62:775.

9. Enig MG, et al. **J Am Chem Soc** 1983;60:1788.

10. **N Engl J Med** 1991;325:No.24.

11. Sacks FM, et al. Plasma lipids and lipoproteins in vegetarians and controls. **N Engl J Med** 1975;292:1148.12.

12. **Food Additive Petition No. 743997.** Cincinnati, OH: Proctor & Gamble, 1987.

13. **J Am Coll Toxicol** 1991;10:357.

14. Roy CC, et al. **J of Pediatrics** 1975;86:446.

15. Bach AC, Babayan VK. **Am J Clin Nutr** 1982;36:950.

16. Foster DW. **Diabetes** 1984;33:1188.

17. Wilson DE, et al. **J Clin Endocrinology Metab** 1983;57:517.

18. Bergen SS. **Diabetes** 1966;15:723.

19. Dias VC, et al. Effects of Medium-Chain Triglyceride Feeding on Energy Balance in Adult Humans. **Metabolism** 1990;39:887-891.

Chapter 9. Carbohydrates: Premium Fuel

1. Astrand PO. Diet and athletic performance. **Fed Proc** 1967;26:1772-1777.

2. Hultman E, Sjoholm H. Biochemical causes of fatigue. In: Jones H, et al, eds. **Human Muscle Power.** Champaign, IL: Human Kinetics, 1986: 215-238.

3. Ivy JL, Costill DL, Maxwell BD. Skeletal muscle determinants of maximum aerobic power in man. **Eur J Appl Physiol** 1980;44:1-8.

4. Ahlborg B, et al. Muscle glycogen and electrolytes during prolonged physical exercise. **Acta Physiol Scand** 1967;70:129-142.

5. Newsholme EA. Application of knowledge of metabolic integration to the problem of metabolic limitations in middle distance and marathon running. **Acta Physiol Scan** 1986;556:93-97.

6. Bergstrom J, Hultman E. A study of the glycogen metabolism during exercise in man. **Scand J Clin Lab Invest** 1967;19:218-226.

7. Valeriani A. The need for carbohydrates during endurance exercise. **Sports Medicine** 1991;12:349-358.

8. Siliprandi N. Il fegato nell 'esercizio fisico. **Rassenga Internat Med Sport** 1986;4:1-7.

9. Hultman E. Studies on muscle metabolism of glycogen and active phosphate in man with special reference to exercise and diet. **Scand J Clin Lab Invest** 1967;19:1-63(Suppl).

10. Ivy JL, et al. Muscle glycogen synthesis after exercise affect of time of carbohydrate ingestion. **J Appl Physiol** 1988;64:1480-1485.

11. Ivy JL, et al. Muscle glycogen storage after different amounts of carbohydrate ingestion. **J Appl Physiol** 1988;65:2018-2023.

12. Bergstrom J, Hultman E, Roch-Norlund AE. Muscle glycogen synthase in normal subjects. **Scand J Clin Lab Invest** 1972;29:231-236.

13. Bonen A, et al. Glucose ingestion before and during intense exercise. **J Appl Physiol** 1980;50:766.

14. Murray R. The effect of consuming carbohydrate/electrolyte beverages on gastric emptying and fluid absorption during and following exercise. **Sports Med** 1987;4:322-351.

15. Costill DL, et al. The role of dietary carbohydrate in muscle glycogen resynthesis after strenuous running. **Am J Clin Nutr** 1981;34:1831-1836.

16. Browns F, et al. Eating, drinking, and cycling: a controlled Tour de France simulation study. Part I and Part II. **Int J Sports Med** 1989;10:S32-S48 (Suppl).

17. Mitchell JB, et al. Influence of carbohydrate dosage on exercise performance and glycogen metabolism. **J Appl Physiol** 1989;67: 1843-1849.

18. Costill DL, Miller JM. Nutrition for endurance sport: carbohydrates and fluid balance. **Int J Sports Med** 1980;1:2.

19. Welle S, et al. Stimulation of protein turnover by overfeeding in men. **Am J Physiol** 1989;257:E413-E417.

20. Juy JL. Muscle glycogen synthesis before and after exercise. **Sports Medicine** 1991;11:6-19.

21. Young AA, et al. Insulin response of components of whole-body and muscle carbohydrate metabolism in humans. **Am J Physiol** 1988;254: 231-E236.

22. Jenkins DJA. Lente carbohydrate: a newer approach to the management of diabetes. **Diabetes Care** 1982;5:634-639.

23. Costill, DL. Carbohydrate nutrition before, during, and after exercise. **Fed Proc** 1985;44:364-368.

24. Costill DL. Carbohydrates for exercise; dietary demands for optimal performance. **Int J Sports Med** 1988;9:1-18.

25. Blom PCS, et al. Effect of different post-exercise sugar diets on the rate of muscle glycogen synthesis. **Med Sci Sports Ex** 1987;19:491-496.

26. Kritchevsky D, et al. Influence of type of carbohydrate on atherosclerosis in baboons fed semi-purified diet plus 0.1% cholesterol. **Am J Clin Nutr** 1980;33:1869.

27. Emmerson BT. Effect of oral fructose on urate production. **Ann Rheumatic Dis** 1974;33:276.

28. Maehlum S, Felig P, Wahren J. Splanchnic glucose and muscle glycogen metabolism after glucose feeding post exercise recovery. **Am J Physiol** 1978;235:E255-E260.

29. Nilsson LH, Hultman E. Liver and muscle glycogen after glucose and fructose infusion. **Scad J Clin Lab Invest** 1974;33:5-10.

30. Saris W, Van Erp-Baart M, Brouns F, et al. Study on food intake and energy expenditure during extreme sustained exercise: The Tour de France. **Int J Sports Med** 1989;10:S26-S31.

31. Brouns F, Saris W, Beckers E, et al. Metabolic changes induced by sustained exhaustive cycling and diet manipulation. **Int J Sports Med** 1989;10:S49-S62.

32. Deuster PA, et al. Nutritional survey of highly trained women runners. **Am J Clin Nutr** 1986;45:954-962.

33. Brotherhood JR. Nutrition and sports performance. **Sports Med** 1984; 1:350.

34. Nieman DC, et al. Nutrient intake of marathon runners. **J Am Dietet Assoc** 1989;89:1273-1278.

35. Pallikarakis N, et al. Remarkable metabolic availability of oral glucose during long duration exercise in humans. **J Appl Physiol** 1986;60:1035-1042.

36. Veufer PD, et al. Improvement in exercise performance: effects of carbohydrate feedings and diet. **J Appl Physiol** 1987;62:983-988.

37. Coggan AR, Coyle EF. Metabolism and performance following carbohydrate ingestioin late in exercise. **Med Sci Sports Ex** 1989; 21:59-65.

38. Costill DL. Carbohydrates for exercise. Dietary demand for optimal performance. **Int J Sports** 1988;9:1-18.

39. Koivisto V, Harkonen J, Karone, et al. Glycogen depletion during prolonged exercise: Influence of glucose, fructose or placebo. **J Appl Physiol** 1985;58:731-737.

40. Coggan AR, Coyle EF. Metabolism and performance following carbohydrate ingestion late in exercise. **Med Sci Sports Ex** 1989; 21:59-65.

41. David J. Fluid availability of sports drinks differing in carbohydrate type and concentration. **Am J Clin Nutr** 1990;51:1054-1057.

Chapter 10. Carbo Loading

1. Bergstrom J, et al. Diet, muscle glycogen, and physical performance. **Acta Physiol Scand** 1967;71:140-150.
2. Hermansen L, Hultman E, Saltin B. Muscle glycogen during prolonged severe exercise. **Acta Physiol Scand** 1967;71:334-346.
3. Karlsson J, Saltin B. Diet, muscle glycogen, and endurance. **J Appl Physiol** 1971;31:203.
4. Sherman WM, et al. Effect of exercise - diet manipulation on muscle glycogen and its subsequent utilization during performance. **Int J Sports Med** 1981;2:114-118.
5. Sherman W, Costill D. The marathon: dietary manipulation to optimize performance. **Am J Sports Med** 1984;12:44.
6. Zachwieja JJ, Costill DL, et al. Influence of muscle glycogen depletion on the rate of resynthesis. **Med Sci Sports Ex** 1991;23:44-48.
7. Williams MH. The role of carbohydrates on physical activity. In: Williams, MH, ed. **Nutritional Aspects of Human Physical and Athletic Performance**. Springfield, IL: CC Thomas, 1985:58.
8. Soderling TR, Park CR. Recent advances in glycogen metabolism. In: Greengard P, Robinson GA, eds. **Advances in Nucleotide Research Vol 4**. New York: Raven 1974:283-333.
9. Bergstrom J, Hultman E. Muscle glycogen synthesis after exercise; an enhancing factor localized to the muscle cells in man. **Nature** 1967;210:309-310.
10. Richter EA, et al. Enhanced muscle glycogen metabolism after exercise: modulation by local factors. **Amer J Physiol** 1984;246:E476-E482.
11. Locksley B. Fuel utilization in marathons: implications for performance. **Western J Med** 1980;133:493-502.
12. Danforth, WH. Glycogen synthase activity in skeletal muscle: interconversion of two forms and control of glycogen synthesis. **J Biol Chem** 1965;240:588-593.
13. Ivy JL. Muscle glycogen synthesis before and after exercise. **Sports Med** 1991;11:6-19.
14. Kochan RG, et al. Glycogen synthase activation in human skeletal muscle: effects of diet and exercise. **Am J Physiol** 1979;236:E660-E666.

Chapter 11. Battling The Bulge

1. Wilmore JH. Body composition in sport and exercise: directions for future research. **Med Sci Sports Exer** 1983;15:21-31.
2. Tipton CM. **Physician & Sports Med** 1987;15:160.
3. Tipton CM, Olinger RA. **Iowa Medicine** 1984;74:381.
4. Zambraski E, et al. **Med Sci Sports** 1976;8:105.
5. Steen SN, McKinney S. **Physician & Sports Med** 1986:14:100.
6. Evers CL. **J Amer Dietetic Assoc** 1987;87:66.
7. Moffat RJ. **J Amer Dietetic Assoc** 1984;84:136.
8. Deuster PA, et al. Nutritional intakes and status of highly trained amenorrheic and enmenorrheic women runners. **Fertil Steril** 1986; 46:636.
9. Colgan M, Fielder S, Colgan LA. Micronutrient status of endurance athletes affects hematology and performance. **J Appl Nutr** Vol 43, No. 1 1991:17-36.
10. Faber M, Spinnler Benade AJ. Mineral and Vitamin Intake in Field Athletes (Discus-,Hammer-, Javelin-Throwers and Shotputters). **Int J Sports Med** Vol 12, No. 3 1991:324-327.
11. Short SH. Dietary surveys and nutrition knowledge. In: Hickson JF, Wolinsky I, eds. **Nutrition in Exercise and Sport**. Boca Raton, FL: CRC Press, 1989:309-343.
12. **US News and World Report**, 3 February 1992, 55-60.
13. Fisher MC, La Chance PA. Nutrition evaluation of published weight reducing diets. **J Amer Dietet Assoc** 1985;85:450-454.
14. Report of National Institute of Health Expert Panel on Weight-loss. Meeting at Bethesda, MD, 31 March - 2 April 1992.
15. **Amer J Publ Health**, 1988, Sept/Oct. ANN - GET AT LIB.
16. Oskai LB. The role of exercise in weight control. In: Wilmore JH, ed. **Exercise and Sport Science Reviews** Vol 1. New York: Academic Press, 1975:105-123.
17. Enzi G, et al., eds. **Obesity: Pathogenesis and Treatment.** New York: Academic Press, 1981.
18. Lohman TG. Skinfolds and body density and their relation to body fatness: A review. **Human Biol** 1991;53:181-225.
19. Kern PA, et al. The effect of weight loss on the activity and expression of adipose tissue lipoprotein lipase in very obese humans. **N Engl J Med** 1990;322:1053.
20. Elliot DL, et al. **Am J Clin Nutr** 1989;49:93.
21. Herberg L, et al. **J Lipid Res** 1974;15:580.

22. Jen KL, et al. **Physiol Behav** 1981;72:161.

23. Wade GN. **Physiol Behav** 1983;29:710.

24. Miller WC, et al. **Growth**. 1984;48:415.

25. Schultz Y, Flatt JP, Jequier E. Failure of dietary fat intake to promote fat oxidation: a factor favoring the development of obesity. **Am J Clin Nutr** 1989;50:307-314.

26. Acheson KJ, et al. Glycogen storage capacity and de novo lipogenesis during massive carbohydrate overfeeding in man. **Am J Clin Nutr** 1988; 48:240-247.

27. Jones PJ, Scholler DA. Polyunsaturated: saturated ratio of diet fat influences energy substrate utilization in the human. **Metabolism**, 1988;37:145-151.

28. Pi-Sunyer FX. Effect of the composition of the diet on energy intake. **Nutr Rev** 1990;48:94-105.

29. Colgan M. **Your Personal Vitamin Profile.** New York: Morrow, 1982.

30. Greenway FL, Bray GA. Regional fat loss from the thigh in obese women after adrenergic modulation. **Clin Ther** 1987;9:663-669.

31. Horowitz JD, et al. **Lancet** 1980;1:60.

32. Beunett W, Gurn J. **The Dieter's Dilemma**. New York: Basic Books, 1982.

33. Winick M, ed. **Childhood Obesity.** New York: Wiley, 1975.

34. Gordon T, Kannel WB. **Geriatrics** 1973;28:80.

35. Cahill GF Jr. Physiology of insulin in man. **Diabetes** 1971;20:785-799.

36. Schultz Y, Flatt JP, Jequier E. Failure of dietary fat to promote fat oxidation: a factor favoring the development of obesity. **Am J Clin Nutr** 1989;50:307-314.

37. Lennon D, et al. Effects of acute moderate intensity exercise on carnitine metabolism in men and women. **J Appl Physiol** 1983;55: 489-495.

38. McCarty MF. Orthomolecular aids for dieting. **Medical Hypotheses** 1982;8:269.

39. Gorostiaga E, Maurer C, Eclache J. Decrease in respiratory quotient during exercise following L-carnitine supplementation. **Int J Sports Med** 1989;10:169-174.

40. Mertz W, Shapcott D, Hubert J, eds. **Chromium in Nutrition and Metabolism.** Amsterdam: Elseviar N. Holland 1979:11.

41. **Recommended Dietary Allowances. 10th Ed.** Washington DC, National Academy Press, 1989.

42. Tipton Stewart PL. In: Hamphill DD, ed. **Trace Substances in Environmental Health.** Vol 3. Columbia, MO: University of Missouri, 1970.

43. Campbell WW, Anderson RA. Effects of aerobic exercise on the trace minerals chromium, zinc, and copper. **Sports Med** 1987;4:9-18

44. Levine R, Luft R, eds. **Advances in Metabolic Disorders**. Vol 9. New York: Academic Press, 1978.

45. Wallace G, Bell L, eds. **Fiber in Human and Animal Nutrition.** Wellington: The Royal Society of New Zealand, 1983.

46. Albrink MJ. Dietary fiber, plasma insulin, and obesity. **Am J Clin Nutr** 1978;31:S277-S279.

47. Katts GR, et al. The short-term efficacy of treating obesity with a plan of improved nutrition and moderate caloric restriction. **Curr Ther Res** 1992;51:261-274.

48. Storlien LH. **Science** 1987;237:885.

49. Lennon D, et al. Diet and exercise training effects on resting metabolic rate. **Int J Obesity** 1985;9:39-47.

50. Lawson S, et al. Effect of a 10-week aerobic exercise program on metabolic rate, body composition, and fitness in lean sedentary females. **Brit J Clin Prac** 1987;41:684-688.

Chapter 12. Protein For Growth

1. **Recommended Dietary Allowances, 10th Edition.** Washington, D.C.: National Academy Press, 1989.

2. Davis BD. Frontiers of the biological sciences. **Science** 1980;209:88.

3. Lemon PWR, Mullin JP. Effect of initial muscle glycogen levels on protein catabolism during exercise. **J Appl Physiol** 1980;48:624-629.

4. Colgan M, Fielder MS, Colgan LA. Micronutrient status of endurance athletes affects hematology and performance. **J Applied Nutr** 1991;43: 17-36.

5. Lemon PWR. Protein and exercise update, 1987. **Med Sci Sports Exer** 1987;19(Suppl):S179-S190.

6. Gontzea I, Sutzescu P, Dumitrache S. The influence of muscular activity on nitrogen balance and on the need of man for proteins. **Nutr Rep Int** 1974;10:35.

7. Gontzea I, Sutzescu R, Dumitrache S. The influence of adaptation to physical effort on nitrogen balance in man. **Nutr Rep Int** 1975;11:231.

8. **Tufts University Diet & Nutrition Letter.** How much protein do athletes reall need? 1987;5:1.

9. Meredith CN, Zackin MJ, Frontera WR, Evans WJ. Dietary protein requirements and body protein metabolism in endurance-trained men. **J Appl Physio 1989;66:2850-2856.**

10. Friedman JE, Lemon PWR. Effet of chronic endurance exercise on retention of dietary protein. **Int J Sports Med** 1989;10:1180123.

11. Brouns F, et al. Eating drinking, and cycling: a controlled Tour de France simulation study, part 1. **Int J Sports Med** 1989;10(Suppl. 1): S32-S40.

12. Brouns F, et al. Eating, drinking, and cycling: a controlled Tour de France simulation study, part II. Effect of diet manipulation. **Int J Sports Med** 1989;10(Suppl. 1):S41-S48.

13. Brouns F, et al. Metabolic changes induced by sustained exhausstive cycling anddiet manipulation. **Inter J Sports Med** 1989;10:(suppl 1): S49-S62.

14. Oddoye EB, Margen S. Nitrogen balance studies in humans: long-term effect of high nitrogen intake on nitrogen accretion. J Nutr 1979;109: 363-377.

15. Consolazio GF , et al. Protein metabolism during intensive physical training in the young adult. **Am J Clin Nutr** 1975;28:29-35.

16. Dragan GI, Vasiliu A, Georgescu E. Effects of increased supply of protein on elite weightlifters. In: Galesloot TE, Tinbergen BJ, eds. **Milk Proteins**. Pudoc, Wageningen, The Netherlands 1985:99-103

17. Albanese AA, ed. **Protein and Amino Acid Metabolism.** New York: Academic Press, 1959.

18. Pearl B. **Keys to the Inner Universe.** Phoenix, OR: Physical Fitness Architects, 1982.

19. Passwater R. **Supernutrition**. New York: Dial Press, 1975.

20. Holland B, et al., eds. **McCance & Widdowson's Composition of Foods Fifth Edition**. Cambridge: The Royal Society of Chemistry, 1991.

21. Young VR, Pellet PL. Protein intake and requirements with reference to diet and health. **Am J Clin Nutr** 1987;45:1323-1343.

22. Vegetarian diets. Position paper of the American Dietetic Association. **J Am Dietet Assoc** 1988;88:351-355.

Chapter 13. Protein Supplements

1. Crampton RF, et al. Rates of absorption by rat intestine of pancreatic hydrolysates of proteins and their corresponding amino acid mixtures. **Clin Sci** 1971;41:409-417.

2. Grimble GK, et al. Effect of peptide chain length on absorption of egg protein hydrolysates in the normal human jejunum. **Gastroenterology** 1987;92:136-42.

3. Zaloga GP. Physiologic effects of peptide-based enteral formulas. **Nutr Clin Pract** 1990;5:231-237.

4. Meredith JW, Ditesheim JA, Zaloga GP. Visceral protein levels in trauma

patients are greater with peptide diet than intact protein diet. **J Trauma** 1990;30:825-9.

5. Smith JL, Arteaga C, Heymsfield SB. Increased ureagenesis and imparied nitrogen use during infusion of a synthetic amino acid formula. **N Engl J Med** 1982;306:1013-8.

6. Beer WH, Fan A, Halsted CH. Clinical and nutritional implications of radiation enteritis. **Am J Clin Nutr** 1985;41:85-91.

7. Poullain MG, et al. Effect of whey proteins, their oligopeptide hydrolysates and free amino acid mixtures on growth and nitrogen retention in fed and starved rats. **J Parenteral and Enteral Nutr** 1989;13:382-386.

8. Holaday JW, Malcolm DS. Endogenous opioids and other peptides: evidence for their clinical relevance in shock and CNS injury. In: Chernow B, et al., eds. **The Pharmacological Approach To The Critically Ill Patient. 2nd Ed**. Baltimore: Williams and Wilkins 1988;718-732.

9. Parker NT, Goodrum KJ. A comparison of casein, lactalbumin, and soy protein effect on the immune response to a T-dependent antigen. **Nutrition Research** 1990;10:781-792.

10. Felig P, Wahren J. Amino acid metabolism in exercising man. **J Clin Invest** 1971;50:2703.

11. Roth E, et al. Glutamine: An anabolic effector? **J Parent Ent Nutr** 1990;14:1305-1365.

12. Felig P. The glucose-alanine cycle. **Metabolism** 1973;22:179.

13. Lemon PWR, Nagle FJ, Mullin JP, Benevenga NJ. In vivo leucine oxidation at rest and during two intensities of exercise. **J Appl Physiol** 1982;53:947-954.

14. Henderson SA, Black AL, Brooks GA. Leucine turnover and oxidation in trained rats during exercise. **Am J Physiol** 1985;249:E137-E144.

15. Babij P, Matthews SM, Rennie MF. Changes in blood ammonia, lactate and amino acids in relation to workload during bicycle ergometer exercise in man. **European J of Appl Physiol** 1983;50:405-411.

16. Evans WJ, Fisher EC, Hoerr RA, Young VR. Protein metabolism during exercise. **Physician and Sports Med** 1983;11:63.

17. **Recommended Dietary Allowances 10th Edition**. Washington DC: National Academy Press, 1989.

18. Kasperek GJ, Snider RD. Effect of exercise intensity and starvation on activation of branched-chain keto acid dehydrogenase by exercise. **Am J Physiol** 1987;252:E33-E37.

19. Matthews DE, Motil KJ, Rohrbaugh DK, et al. Measurement of leucine metabolism in man from a primed, continuous infusion of L-(1-C)leucine. **Am J Physiol** 1980;238:E473.

20. Meguid MM, et al. Leucine kinetics at graded leucine intakes in young

men. **Am J Clin Nutr** 1986;43:770.

21. Meguid MM, Matthews DE, Bier DM, Meredith CN, Young VR. Valine kinetics at graded valine intakes in young men. **Am J Clin Nutr** 1986;43: 781.

22. Carli G, et al. Changes in the exercise-induced hormone response to branched chain amino acid administration. **Eur J Appl Physiol** 1992; 64:272-277.

23. Kraemer WJ. Endocrine response to resistance exercise. **Med Sci Sports Exer** 1988;(Suppl)20:S152-S157.

24. Wagenmakers AJM, et al. Exercise-induced activation of branched-chain 2-oxo acid dehydrogenase in human muscle. **Eur J Appl Physiol** 1989;59:159-167.

Chapter 14. Vitamins Are Nuts And Bolts

1. Goodman DS. Vitamin A and retinoids in health and disease. **N Engl J Med** 1984;310:1023-1031.

2. **Recommended Dietary Allowances 10th Edition**. Washington DC: National Academy Press, 1989.

3. Steen SN, McKinney S. **Physician and Sports Med** 1986;14:100.

4. Ten State Nutritional Survey. USDHEW Publications Nos. 72-8130 to 72-8133. Rockville MD: DHEW, 1972.

5. Hathcock JN, ed. **Nutritional Toxicology**. New York: Academic Press, 1982.

6. Sauberlich HE, Skala JH, Dowdy RP. **Laboratory Tests for the Assessment of Nutritional Status**. Cleveland, OH: CRC Press, 1976.

7. Colgan M. Effects of multi-nutrient supplementation on athletic performance. **IFBB Special Report**. Montreal, Canada, IFBB, 1987.

8. Harris RS, Karmas E, eds. **Nutritional Evaluation of Food Processing**. Westport CT: AVI Publishing, 1975.

9. US Department of Agriculture Survey. **Food Technology** 1981;35:9.

10. Belko AZ, et al. Effects of exercise on riboflavin requirements of young women. **Am J Clin Nutr** 1983;37:509-517.

11. Haralambie G. Vitamin B_{12} status in athletes and the influence of riboflavin administration on neuromuscular irritability. **Nutr Metab** 1976;20:1.

12. McCormick DB. Riboflavin. In: Shils ME, Young VR. **Modern Nutrition in Health & Disease**. Philadelphia: Lea and Febiger 1988:362-369.

13. Kaijser L, et al. The relation between carbohydrate extraction by the forearm and arterial free fatty acid concentration in man. **Scand J Clin Lab Invest** 1978;38:41.

14. Nationwide Food Consumption Survey 1977-78. Preliminary Report No. 2. Washington CD: USDA, 1980.

15. Colgan M, Fielder MS, Colgan LA. Micronutrient status of endurance athletes affects hematology and performance. **J Appl Nutr** 1991;43:16-30.

16. Kishi H, Folkers K. Improved and effective assays of glutamic oxaloacetic transaminase by the coenzyme - apoenzyme principle. **J Nutr Sci Vitamin** 1976;22:225-234.

17. Dalton K, Dalton MJT. Characteristics of pyridoxine overdose neuropathy syndrome. **Acta Neurol Scand** 1987;76:8-11.

18. De Vos A, Leklem J, Campbell D. Carbohydrate loading, vitamin B6 supplementation and fuel metabolism during exercise in man. **Med Sci Sports Ex** 1982;14:37.

19. Tarr JB, Tamura T, Stokstad ELR. Availability of vitamin B6 and pantothenate in an average American diet in man. **Am J Clin Nutr** 1981;34:1328-1337.

20. Ralli EP, Dumm ME. Relation of pantothenic acid to adrenal cortical function. **Vitam Horm** 1953;11:133-158.

21. Litoff D, Scherzer H, Harrison J. Effects of pantothenic acid on human exercise. **Med Sci Sports Ex** 1985;17:287.

22. Colgan M. **Your Personal Vitamin Profile**. New York: Morrow, 1982.

23. Milne DB, Johnson LK, Mahalko MS, Sanstead HH. Folate status of adult males living in a metabolic unit: possible relationships with iron nutriture. **Am J Clin Nutr** 1983;37:768-773.

24. Scott JM, et al. Trouble-free neurobiological serum and red cell folate assays. **Am J Med Tech** 1974;40:125-134.

25. Hoffbrand AV, et al. Method of assay of red cell folate activity and the value of the assay as a test for folate deficiency. **J Clin Path** 1966;19:17-22.

26. Butterworth CE, et al. Zinc concentration in plasma and erythrocytes of subjects receiving folic acid supplementation. **Am J Clin Nutr** 1988;47: 484-486.

27. Skeggs HR. *Lactobacillus leichmanni* assay for vitamin B12. In: Kavanagh E, ed. **Analytical Microbiology**. New York: Academic Press, 1963;551-572.

28. Keith RE. In: Hickson JF, Wolinsky I, eds. **Nutrition in Exercise and Sport**. Boca Raton, FL: CRC Press, 1989:234-249.

29. Bonjour JP. Biotin in human nutrition. **Ann New York Acad Sci** 1985;447:97-104.

30. Baugh CM, Malone JW, Butterworth CE. Human biotin deficiency. **Am J Clin Nutr** 1968;21:173-182.

31. Marshall MW, Judd JT, Baker H. Effects of low and high fat diets varying in ratio of polyunsaturated to saturated fats on biotin intakes and biotin in serum, red cells, and urine of adult men. **Nutrition Res** 1985;5:801-814.

32. Krishnamurti D, Bhagavan HN. **Biotin.** New York: New York Academy of Sciences, 1985.

33. Roe JH. Appraisal of methods of the determination of L-ascorbate. **Ann New York Acad Sci** 1961;92:277-283.

34. Omaye S, et al. Measurement of vitamin C in blood by HPLC. **Ann New York Acad Sci** 1987;498:389-401.

35. Williams MH. Vitamin, iron, and calcium supplementation: effect on human physical performance. In: Haskell W, et al., eds. **Nutrition and Athletic Performance.** Palo Alto, CA: Bull Publishing 1981:106-153.

36. Berven H. The physical working capacity of healthy children seasonal variation and effect of ultra-violet radiation and vitamin D supply. **Acta Paediatrica** 1963;148:1-22(Suppl).

37. Farrell PM, et al. Plasma tocopherol levels and tocopherol lipid relationships in a normal population of children, as compared to healthy adults. **Am J Clin Nutr** 1978;31:1720-1726.

38. Farrell PM, et al. Evaluation of vitamin E deficiency in children with lung disease. **Ann New York Acad Sci** 1982;393:96-108.

39. Bendich A, Machlin LJ. Safety of oral intake of vitamin E. **Am J Clin Nutr** 1988;48:612-619.

40. Ansell JE, et al. The spectrum of vitamin K deficiency. **J Am Med Assoc** 1977;238:40-42.

41. Olson RE. Vitamin K. In: Shils, ME, Young VR. **Modern Nutrition in Health and Disease 7th Edition.** Philadelphia: Lea and Febiger 1988: 328-339.

42. Almquist HJ. Vitamin K: Discovery, identification, syntheses, functions. **Fed Proc** 1979;38:2687-2689.

43. Owen CA. Pharmacology and toxicology of the vitamin K group. In: Sebrell WH, Harris RS, eds. **The vitamins, Vol III.** New York: Academic Press 1971;492-509.

44. Colgan M. **Improve Your Memory.** San Diego; CI Publications, 1989.

45. Wurtman RJ. Sources of choline and lecithin in the diet. In: Barbeau A, et al., eds. **Nutrition and the Brain Vol 5. Choline and Lecithin in Brain Disorders.** New York: Raven Press 1979;73-81.

46. American Academy of Pediatrics. **Pediatric Nutrition Handbook.** Elk Gove, IL: AAP, 1985.

47. Conaly LA. Decreased plasma choline concentrations in marathon runners. **N Engl J Med** 1986;315:892.

48. Prentki M, Matshcinsky FM. Ca, cAMP, and phospholipid derived messengers in coupling mechanisms of insulin secretion. **Physiol Rev** 1987;67:1186-1235.

49. Agranoff BW. Inositol triphosphate and related metabolism. **Fed Proc** 1986;45:2627-2652.

50. Draper HH, ed. **Advances in Nutritional Research Vol 4.** New York: Plenum 1982;107-141.

51. Pfeiffer CC. **Mental and Elemental Nutrients.** New Canaan CT: Keats, 1975.

52. Folkers K, Wolaniuk A. **Drugs Under Exper Clin Res** 1985;11:539-546.

53. Liebovitz B. Coenzyme Q. **Nutrition & fitness** 1991;10:47-48.

54. Folkers K, Yamamura Y, eds. **Biomedical and Clinical Aspects of Coenzyme Q Vol IV.** New York: Elsevier 1984:201-208:291-300.

55. Kamei M, et al. The distribution and content of ubiquinone in foods. **Int J Vit Nutr Res** 1986;56:57-63.

56. Folkers K, Yamamura Y, eds. **Biochemical and Clinical Aspects of Coenzyme Q. Vol V.** New York; Elsevier. 1986:291-302.

57. Folkers K, et al., eds. **Biomedical and Clinical Aspects of coenzyme Q.** London: Elsevier Science Publishers 1991:513-520.

58. **University of California Wellness Letter** 1991;7:2.

59. Pearson WN. Flavonoids in human nutrition and medicine. **J Amer Med Assoc** 1957;164:301.

60. Gabor M. Pharmacologic effect of flavonoids on blood vessels. **Angiologica** 1972;9:355-374.

61. Kilgore J, et al. **Science** 1989;245:850.

Chapter 15. Minerals Are The Framework

1. Colgan M. **Your Personal Vitamin Profile** New York: Morrow, 1982.

2. Sheehan G. Eat to live; eat to win. **Runners World.** 1991 June 22.

3. **Recommended Dietary Allowances 10th Edition.** Washington DC: National Academy Press, 1989.

4. Sibtain M. Gastrointestinal absorption of calcium from milk and calcium salts. **N Engl J Med** 1987;317:532.

5. Woo SL, et al. The effect of prolonged physical training on the properties of long bone. A study of Wolf's Law. **J Bone Joint Surg** 1981;63:780.

6. Avioli LV. Calcium and osteoporosis. **Am Rev Nutr** 1984;4:471.

7. Wallach S. Effects of magnesium on skeletal metabolism. **Magnesium Trace Elem** 1990;9:1-14.

8. Carlisle EM. Silicon. In: Mertz W, ed. **Trace Elements in Human and Animal Nutrition 5th Edition Vol 2.** New York: Academic Press 1986; 373-390.

9. Krisnamachari KA. Fluorine. In: Mertz W, ed. **Trace elements in Human and Animal Nutrition 5th Edition Vol 1.** New York Academic Press

1987;365-415.

10. Hambidge KM. Zinc. In: Mertz W, ed. **Trace Elements in Human and Animal Nutrition.5th Edition. Vol 2.** New York: Academic Press, 1986: 1-137.

11. Davis GK, Mertz W. Copper. In: Mertz W, ed. **Trace Elements in Human and Animal Nutrition 5th Edition. Vol 1.** New York: Academic Press, 1987:301-364.

12. Neilsen FH. Effect of dietary boron on mineral, estrogen, and testosterone in postmenopausal women. **FASEB J** 1987;1:394-397.

13. Hurley JS, Keen CL. Manganese. In: Mertz W, ed. **Trace Elements in Human and Animal Nutrition. 5th Edition. Vol 1.** New York: Academic Press, 1987:185-223.

14. Parfitt AM, et al. Vitamin D and bone health in the elderly. **Am J Clin Nutr** 1982;36:1014-1031.

15. Bobb A, Pringle D, Ryan AJ. A brief study of this diet of athletes. **J Sports Med** 1969;9:255.

16. Moffat RJ. **J Amer Dietet Assoc** 1984;84:136.

17. Rucinski A. Relationship of body image and dietary intake of competition ice skaters. **J Am Dietet Assoc** 1989;89:58-63.

18. Lane NE, et al. Long distance running bone density and osteoporosis. **J Amer Med Assoc** 1986;255:1147.

19. Linnel SL, et al. Bone mineral content and menstrual regularity in female runners. **Med Sci Sports Mex** 1984;16:343.

20. Hegsted M, et al. Urinary calcium and calcium balance in young men as affected by level of protein and phosphorus intake. **J Nutr** 1981;111:553.

21. Gregor JL. Effect of variation in dietary protein phosphorus electrolytes and vitamin D on calcium and zinc metabolism. In: Bodwell CE, Erdman JW, eds. **Nutrient Interactions.** New York: Marcel Dekker 1988;205-227.

22. Nishiyama T. Effects of calcium on muscular training. **J Nutr Sci Vitaminol** 1985;31:545.

23. Richardon JH, Palmenton T, Chenan H. The effect of calcium on muscle fatigue. **J Sports Med** 1980;20:149.

24. Aikawa JK. **Magnesium: Its biological significance.** Boca Raton, FL: CRC Press, 1981.

25. Marier JR. Magnesium content of the food supply in the modern-day world. **Magnesium** 1986;5:1-8.

26. Wohl MG, Goodheart RS. **Modern Nutrition in Health and Disease 3rd Edition.** Philadelphia.

27. Lui L, et al. Hypomagnesemia in a tennis player. **Phys Sportsmed** 1983;11:79.

28. Steen SN, McKinney S. Nutrition assessment of college wrestlers. **Physician and Sports Med** 1986;14:100.

29. Bazzarre TL, et al. Incidence of poor nutritional status among triathletes endurance athletes and controls. **Med Sci Sports Ex** 1986;18:S90.

30. Benson J, et al. Inadequate nutrition and chronic caloric restriction in adolescent ballerinas. **Phys Sportsmed** 1985;13:79.

31. Recheigl M, ed. **Nutritional Disorders Vol 1.** Boca Raton, FL: CRC Press, 1978.

32. Lotz ME, et al. Evidence for a phosphorus-depletion syndrome in man. **N Engl J Med** 1968;278:409-415.

33. Kirby CR, Convertino VA. Plasma aldosterone and sweat sodium concentration after exercise and heat acclimatization. **J Appl Physiol** 1986;61:967.

34. Williams MH, ed. **Nutritional Aspects of Human Physical and Athletic Performance.** Springfield, IL: CC Thomas, 1985.

35. **Sodium/Potassium Ratios in Common Foods.** San Diego: The Colgan Institute, 1989.

36. Khaw KT, Barrett-Connor E. Dietary potassium and stroke associated mortality. A 12-year prospective population study. **N Engl J Med** 1987;316:235-240.

37. Knochel JP. Potassium deficiency during training in the heat. In: Milvey P, ed. **The Marathon.** New York: New York Academy of Sciences 1977:175.

38. Short SH, Short WR. Four year study of university athletes' dietary intake. **J Amer Dietet Assoc** 1983;82:632.

39. Dallman PR, Yip R, Johnson C. Prevalence and causes of anemia in the United States 1976-1980. **Am J Clin Nutr** 1984;39:437-445.

40. Gillooly M, et al. The effects of organic acids phytates and polyphenols on the absorption of iron from vegetables. **Brit J Nutr** 1983;49:331-342.

41. Murphy SP, Calloway DH. Nutrient intakes of women in NHANES II emphasizing trace minerals fiber and phytase. **J Am Dietet Assoc** 1986;86:1366-1372.

42. **Recommended Dietary Allowances 9th Edition.** Washington, DC: National Academy of Sciences, 1980.

43. Hambidge KM, et al. Zinc. In: Mertz W, ed. **Trace Elements in Human and Annual Nutrition 5th Edition Vol 2.** New York: Academic Press, 1986:1-137.

44. Holden JM, Wolf WR, Mertz W. Zinc and copper in self-selected diets. **J Am Dietet Assoc** 1979;75:23-28.

45. Netter A, et al. Effect of zinc administration on plasma testosterone, dehydrotestosterone and sperm count. **Arch Androl** 1981;7:69.

46. Couzy F, Lafargue P, Guezennec CY. Zinc metabolism in the athlete: Influence of training, nutrition and other factors. **Int J Sports Med** 1990;11:263-266.

47. Deuster PA, et al. Nutritional survey of highly trained women runners.

Am J Clin Nutr 1986;44:954.

48. Grace SJ, Jeffrey DM. Iron zinc and copper intakes of women track team members. **Fed Proc** 1983;42:803.

49. Shils ME, Young VR. **Modern Nutrition in Health and Disease 7th Edition**. Philadelphia: Lea and Febiger 1988.

50. Prasad AS, et al. Hypocupremia induced by zinc therapy in adults. **J Am Med Assoc** 1978;240:2166-2168.

51. Ohno H, et al. Changes in dopamine-beta-hydroxylase, and copper, and catecholamine concentrations in human plasma with physical exercise. **J Sports Med** 1984;24:315.

52. Pennington JAT, et al. Nutritional elements in US diets: Results from the Total Diet Study 1982-1986. **J Am Dietet Assoc** 1989;89:659-664.

53. Dowdy RP, Burt J. Effect of intensive long-term training on copper and iron nutriture in man. **Fed Proc** 1980;39:786.

54. Mason KE. A conspectus of research on copper metabolism and requirements of man. **J Nutr** 1979;109:1979-2066.

55. Uauy RC, et al. Red cell superoxide dismutase activity as an index of human copper nutrition. **J Nutr** 1985;115:1650-1655.

56. **Recommended Dietary Allowances 7th Edition.** Washington DC: National Academy of Sciences 1968:61.

57. Anderson RA. Chromium. In: Mertz W, ed. **Trace Elements in Human and Annual Nutrition Fifth Edition Vol 1.** New York: Academic Press, 1987:225-244.

58. Hoekstra WG. Biochemical function of selenium and its relation to vitamin E. **Fed Proc** 1975;34:2083-2089.

59. Colgan M. Trace Elements. **Science** 1981;214:744.

60. Whanger PD, et al. Blood selenium and glutathione peroxidase activity of population in New Zealand, Oregon, and South Dakota. **FASEB** 1988;2:2996-3002.

61. Matovinovic J. Endemic goiter and cretinism at the dawn of the third millennium. **Ann Rev Nutr** 1983;3:341-412.

62. Consolazio CF, et al. Comparison of nitrogen, calcium, and iodine excretion in arm and total body sweat. **Am J Clin Nutr** 1966;18:443.

63. Hunt CD, Nielsen FH. Interaction between boron and cholecalciferol in the chick. In: McHowell, J, Hawthorne JM, White CL, eds. **Trace Element Metabolism in Man and Animals Vol 4**, 1981. Canberra: Australian Academy of Science 1981:597-600.

64. Neilsen FH. Possible future implication so ultra trace elements in health and disease. In: Prasad AS, ed. **Essential and Toxic Trace Elements in Human Health & Disease. Vol 18.** New York: Alan R. Liss 1988:277-292.

65. Nielsen FH, et al. Effect of dietary boron on mineral, estrogen, and testosterone metabolism in postmenopausal women. **J Fed Am Soc**

Ex Biol 1987;1:394-397.

66. Colgan M. Boron. **Nutrition & Fitness** 1988;7:33,46.

67. Varo P, et al. **Acta Agric Scand** 1980;22: 27-171(Suppl).

68. Neilsen F. Other elements. In: Mertz W, ed. **Trace Elements in Human and Animal Nutrition 5th Ed Vol 2**. New York: Academic Press, 1986: 415-463.

69. Pinto J, et al. **J Lab Clin Med** 1978;92:126-134.

70. Rajagopalan KV. Molybdenum: an essential trace element in human nutrition. **Ann Rev Nutr** 1988;8:401-427.

71. Mills, CF, Davis GK. Molybdenum. In: Mertz W, ed. **Trace Elements in Human and Animal Nutrition 5th Edition Vol 1**. New York: Academic Press 1988;429-463.

Chapter 16. The Right Supplements

1. Bell LS, Fairchild M. **J Amer Dietet Assoc** 1987;87;341.

2. Horwitt MK, et al. Serum concentrations of alpha-tocopherol after ingestion of various forms of vitamin E preparation. **Amer J Clin Nutr** 1984;40:240.

3. Ogihara T, et al. Comparative changes in plasma and RBC alpha-tocopherol after administration of D,L-alpha-tocopherol and D-alpha-tocopherol. **J Nutr Sci Vitaminol** 1985;31:169.

4. **Recommended Dietary Allowance 10th Edition**. Washington DC: National Academy Press, 1989.

5. Lonsdale D. Thiamin and its fat-soluble derivatives as therapeutic agents. **Int Clin Nutr Rev** 1988;7:187.

6. **Food Chemicals Codex. 3rd Edition**. Washington DC: National Academy Press, 1981.

7. Holland B, et al., eds. **McCance and Widdowson's. The Composition of Foods**. Letchworth, Herts England: The Royal Society of Chemistry, 1991.

8. Bush MJ, Verlangiari AJ. An acute study of the relative gastrointestinal absorption of a novel form of calcium ascorbate. **Res Comm Chem Path Pharm** 1987;57:1.

9. Verlangiari AJ, Fay MJ, Bannon AW. Comparison of the antiscorbutic activity of L-ascorbic acid and Ester C in the non-ascorbate synthesizing osteogenic disorder Shionogi (ODS) rat. **Life Sciences** 1991;48:2275-2281.

10. Report by Irvine Analytical Laboratory, Irvine, CA to Elliot Balbert of Natrol Inc., Chatsworth, CA. 24 January 1991.

11. **Food and Drug Administration Bulletin**. 23 September 1991.

12. Interview with Dr Linus Pauling. **Muscular Development** 1991;28:62-64.
13. Sibtain M. Gastrointestinal absorption of calcium from milk and calcium salts. **N Engl J Med** 1987;317:532.
14. Liebowitz B, ed. **J Optimal Nutr** 1992;1:1-3.

Chapter 17. What Nutrient Toxicity?

1. Hathcock JH. Vitamin safety: A current appraisal. **Vitamin Issues**. 1984;5:1-6.
2. Hayes KC, Hegsted MD. Toxicity of the vitamins. **Toxicants Occurring Naturally in Foods**. Washington DC: National Academy of Sciences, 1973.
3. Costas K, et al. Use of supplements containing high-dose vitamin A. **J Amer Med Assoc** 1987;257:1292-1297.
4. Herbert V, Jacob E, et al. **Am J Clin Nutr** 1978;31:253-258.
5. Hines JD. **J Amer Med Assoc** 1975;234:24.
6. Newmark HL, Scheiner J, et al. **Am J Clin Nutr** 1976;29:645-649.
7. Hagenkamp HP. **Amer J Clin Nutr** 1980;33:1.
8. Colgan M. Consequences of ingestion of large quantities of vitamins and trace elements - nine years of studies. Paper presented at the Cancer and the Environment symposium of the International Study Center for Environmental Health Sciences, Washington, DC, December, 1982.
9. Schmidt KH, et al. Urinary oxalate excretion after large intakes of ascorbic acid in man. **Am J Clin Nutr** 1981;34:305-311.
10. Hanck A, Rizel G. **Re-evaluation of Vitamin C**. Stuttgart: Verlag Hans Huber, 1977.
11. Honig DH, Moser U. The safety of high vitamin C intakes in man. In: Counsell JN, Honig DH, eds. **Vitamin C**. New York: Applied Sciences Publishers, 1981.
12. Anderson TW. **Acta Vitamin Enzymologica** 1977;31:43.
13. Haskell BE. Toxicity of vitamin B6. In: **Effects of Nutrient Excesses and Toxicities in Animals and Man**. Boca Raton, FL: CRC Press, 1978.
14. Shaumberg H, et al. Sensory neuropathy from pyridoxine abuse: a new mega-vitamin syndrome. **N Engl J Med** 1983;309:8.
15. Dalton K, Dalton MJT. Characteristics of pyridoxine overdose syndrome. **Acta Neurol Scand** 1987;76:8-11.
16. Hathcock JN, et al. Evaluation of vitamin A toxicity. **Am J Clin Nutr** 1990;52:183-202.
17. American Association of Poison Control Centers, **Annual Reports** 1985-1990.

Chapter 18. Vitamins And Performance

1. Colgan M, Fiedler S, Colgan LA. Micronutrient status of endurance athletes affects hematology and performance. **J Appl Nutr** 1991;43:16-30.
2. Dossey L. **Space, Time, and Medicine**. Boulder, CO: Shambala Publications, 1982.
3. Herbert V. **Nutrition Cultism**. Philadelphia: George F Stickley, 1980.
4. Kallman B. Micronutrient intakes in laboratory animals and humans. **J Appled Nutr** 1989;41:23-25.
5. Colgan M. **Your Personal Vitamin Profile**. New York: Morrow, 1982.
6. Rosenberg H. **The Book of Vitamin Therapy**. New York: Putnam and Sons, 1974.

Chapter 19. Minerals and Performance

1. Bobb A, Pringle D, Ryan AJ. A brief study of this diet of athletes. **J Sports Med** 1969;9:255.
2. Moffat RJ. **J Amer Dietet Assoc** 1984;84:136.
3. Rucinski A. Relationship of body image and dietary intake of competition ice skaters. **J Am Dietet Assoc** 1989;89:58-63.
4. Steen SN, McKinney S. Nutrition assessment of college wrestlers. **Physician and Sports Med** 1986;14:100.
5. Bazzarre TL, et al. Incidence of poor nutritional status among triathletes endurance athletes and controls. **Med Sci Sports Ex** 1986;18:S90.
6. Benson J, et al. Inadequate nutrition and chronic caloric restriction in adolescent ballerinas. **Phys Sportsmed** 1985;13:79.
7. Short SH, Short WR. Four year study of university athletes' dietary intake. **J Amer Dietet Assoc** 1983;82:632.
8. Colgan M, Fiedler S, Colgan LA. Micronutrient status of athletes affects hematology and performance. **J Appl Nutr** 1991;43:16-30.
9. Couzy F, Lafargue P, Guezennec CY. Zinc metabolism in the athlete: Influence of training, nutrition and other factors. **Int J Sports Med** 1990;11:263-266.
10. Grace SJ, Jeffrey DM. Iron zinc and copper intakes of women track team members. **Fed Proc** 1983;42:803.
11. Anderson RA. Chromium. In: Mertz W, ed. **Trace Elements in Human and Annual Nutrition. Fifth Edition. Vol 1.** New York: Academic Press, 1987;255-244.

12. Colgan M. Boron. **Nutrition & Fitness** 1988;7:33,46.
13. Richardson JH, Palmenton T, Chenan H. The effect of calcium on muscle fatigue. **J Sports Med** 1980;20:149.
14. **J Amer Coll Nutr** 1992; July: 326-329.
15. Keen C, et al. Dietary magnesium intake influences exercise capacity and hematologic parameters in rats. **Metabolism** 1987;36:788-793.
16. Anderson RA, et al. Effect of exercise (running) on serum glucose, insulin, glycogen, and chromium excretion. **Diabetes** 1982;31:212-216.

Chapter 20. Antioxidants Combat Injury

1. Ernster L. Oxygen as an environmental poison. **Chemical Scripta** 1986;26:525-534.
2. Gerutti A, et al., eds. **Oxy-radicals in Molecular Biology and Pathology** New York: AR Liss, 1988.
3. Brooks GA, Fahey TD. **Exercise Physiology**. New York: John Wiley and Sons, 1984.
4. Quintanilha A. In: Miguel J, et al., eds. **Handbook of Free Radicals and Antioxidants**. Boca Raton, FL:CRC Press, 1989:133.
5. Gullnick PD, et al. **European Journal of Physiology** 1990;415:407-413.
6. Loschen E, et al. Superoxide radicals as precursors of mitochondrial hydrogen peroxide. **FEBS Letters** 1974;42:68-72.
7. Karlsson J. Heart and skeletal muscle ubiquinone or CoQ10 as a protective agent against radical formation in man. In: Benzi R, Libby B., eds. **Advances in Myochemistry**, Eurotext Ltd, 1987:305-318.
8. Gohill K, et al. Effect of exercise training on tissue vitamin E and ubiquinone content. **J Applied Physiol** 1987;63:1638-1641.
9. Folkers K, ed. **Biomedical and Clinical Aspects of Coenzyme Q Vol 3**. Amsterdam: Elsevier, 1981.
10. Beyer RE, et al. Elevation of coenzyme Q and cytochrome C concentrations by endurance exercise in the rat. **Arch Biochem Biophys** 1984;234:323-329.
11. Maughan RJ, et al. Delayed onset muscle damage and lipid peroxidation in man after a downhill run. **Muscle and Nerve** 1989;12:332-336.
12. Homan-Muller JW, et al. **J Lab Clin Med** 1975;85:198.
13. Kauter MM, et al. Serum enzyme levels and lipid peroxidation in ultramarathon runners. **Annals of Sports Med** 1986;3:39-41.
14. Apple FS, Rhodes MJ. **J Applied Physiol** 1988;65:2598.
15. Hoper C. Free radicals: research on biochemical bad boys comes of age. **J Nat Inst Health Res** 1989;1:101.

16. Zidenberg-Cherr S, et al. Dietary superoxide dismutase does not affect tissue levels. **Am J Clin Nutr** 1983;37:5.

17. Pyke S, Lew H, Quintanilha A. Severe depletion in liver glutathione during physical exercise. **Biochem Biophys Res Comm** 1986; 139:926-931.

18. Meister A. Selective modification of glutathione metabolism. **Science** 1983; 220:472-477.

19. Tsan MF. Modulation of endothelial GSH concentration: effect of exogenous GSH and GSH monoethyl ester. **J Applied Physiol** 1989; 66: 1029-1034.

20. Schneider D, et al. Blood glutathione: a biochemical index of aging women. **Fed Proc Am Soc Exp Biol** 1982;41:3570.

21. Varyshkin S, et al. Blood glutathione: a biochemical index of human aging. **Fed Proc Am Soc Exp Biol** 1981;40:3179.

22. Tappel AL. Will antioxidant nutrients slow the aging process. **Geriatrics** 1968; 23:97-105.

23. Ganther HE. In: Zinagaro RA, Cooper WS, eds. **Selenium.** New York: Van Nostrand, 1974:546-614.

24. **Recommended Dietary Allowances 10th Edition**. Washington DC: National Academy Press, 1989.

25. Diplock A. Dietary supplementation with antioxidants. Is there a case for exceeding the Recommended Dietary Allowances. **Free Radicals in Biol & Med** 1987;3:199-201.

26. Bendich A, Macklin LJ. Safety of oral intake of vitamin E. **Am J Clin Nutr** 1988;48:612-619.

27. Colgan M. Trace elements. **Science** 1981;214:744.

28. Yang G, et al. Endemic selenium intoxication of humans in China. **Am J Clin Nutr** 1983; 37:872-881.

29. Marsten R, Raper N. Nutrient content of the US food supply. **National Food Rev** 1987; NFR36:18-23.

Chapter 21. Good Red Blood

1. Martin RP, Haskell WL, Wood PD. Blood chemistry and lipid profiles of elite distance runners. **Ann NY Acad Sci** 1977;301:346-351.

2. Brotherhood J, Brozovic B, Pugh LG. Hematological status of middle and long distance runners. **Clin Sci Mole Med** 1975;48:139-147.

3. Expert Scientific Working Group. Summary of a report on assessment of the iron nutritional status of the United States population. **Am J Clin Nutr** 1985;42:1318-1330.

4. Colgan M, Fielder S Colgan LA. Micronutrient status of endurance

athletes affects hematology and performance. **J Appl Nutr** 1991;43:17-30.

5. Hunding A, Jordal R, Paulev PE. Runners anemia and iron deficiency. **Acta Med Scand** 1981;209:315-320.

6. Plowman SA, McSwegin PC. The effects of iron supplementation on female cross-country runners. **J of Sports Med** 1981;21:407-416.

7. Solvell L. Oral iron therapy. In: Hallbery L, et al., eds. **Iron Deficiency - Pathogenesis Clinical Aspects Therapy**. New York: Academic Press, 1970.

8. Emory T. **Iron and Your Health: Facts and Fallacies**. Boca Raton, FL: CRC Press, 1991.

9. Weinberg ED. Iron and susceptibility to infectious disease. **Science** 1975;188:1038.

10. Bullen JJ, Griffiths E., eds. **Iron and Infection**. New York: John Wiley & Sons, 1987.

11. Celsing F, et al. Effects of anemia and stepwise-induced polyeythemia on maximal aerobic power in individuals with high and low hemoglobin concentration. **Acta Physiol Scan** 1987;129:47-54.

12. Ekblom B, Goldberg AN, Gullbring B. Response to exercise after blood loss and reinfusion. **J Applied Physiol** 1972;33:75-180.

13. Berglund B, Hemingson P. Effect of reinfusion of autologous blood on exercise performance in cross-country skiers. **Int J Sports Med** 1987;8: 231-233.

14. **Recommended Dietary Allowances Tenth Edition.** Washington, DC: National Academy Press, 1989.

15. Vellar OD. Studies on sweat loss of nutrients. **Scad J Clin Lab Invest** 1968;21:157-167.

16. Ehn L, Carlmark B, Hoglund S. Iron status in athletes involved in intense physical activity. **Med Sci Sports Exer** 1980;12:61-70.

17. Williamson MR. Anemia in runners and other athletes. **Physician Sports Med** 1981;9:73-78.

18. Davidson RJ. March or exertional hemoglobinura. **Sem Hematol** 1969;6:150.

19. Refsum HE, Jordfald G, Stromme SB. Hematological changes following prolonged heavy exercise. In: Jokl E, Anand RL, Stoboy H, eds. **Advances in exercise physiology**. Vol 9. Basel: Karger, 1976:91-99.

20. Colgan M, Fielder S, Colgan LA. Effects of multi nutrient supplementation on athletic performance. In: Katch F., ed. **Sport, Health and Nutrition**. Champaign IL: Human Kinetics 1986:59-80.

21. Selby GB, Eichner ER. Endurance swimming, intravascular hemolysis anemia and iron depletion. **Amer J Medicine** 1986;81:791-794.

22. Eichner ER, Strauss RH, Sherman WM, Dernbach A, Lamb DR. Intravascular hemolysis in elite college rowers. Abstract no. 466. **Med Sci Sports Exer** 1989;S8:21(Suppl).

23. Fisher RL, et al. Gastrointestinal bleeding in competitive runners. **Digest Dis Sci** 1986;31:1226.

24. Puhl JL, Runyan WS. Hematological variations during aerobic training of college women. **Res Quar Exer Sport** 1980;51:533-541.

25. Jenkins RR. Free radical chemistry: relationship to exercise. **Sports Med** 1988;5:156-170.

26. Clement DB, Asmundson RC. Nutritional intake and hematological parameters in endurance runners. **Physician and Sports Med** 1982;10: 37-43.

27. Russer WL, et al. Iron deficiency in female athletes. **Med Sci Sports Exer** 1988;20:116-121.

28. Levander OA, Cheng L, eds. **Micronutrient interactions.** New York: New York Academy of Sciences, 1980.

29. Bates CJ, Black AE, Phillips DR, Wright AJ, Southgate DA. The discrepancy between normal folate intakes and the folate RDA. **Human Nutr Appl Nutr** 1982;63:422-429.

30. Rodriguez MS. A conspectus of research on folacin requirements of man. **J Nutr** 1981;108:1983-2130.

31. Milne DB, Johnson LK, Mahalko MS, Sanstead HH. Folate status of adult males living in a metabolic unit: possible relationships with iron nutriture. **Am J Clin Nutr** 1983;37:768-773.

32. Herschko C, Grossowicz N, Racmilewitz M, Kester S, Izak G. Serum and erythrocyte folates in combined iron and folate deficiency. **Am J Clin Nutr** 1975;28:1217-1222.

33. Pennington JAT, Wilson DB, Newell RF, Harland BF, Johnson RD, Vanderveen JE. Selected minerals in foods, surveys, 1974 to 1981/82. **J Am Dietet Assoc** 1984;84:771-780.

34. Holden JM, Wolf WR, Mertz W. Zinc and copper in self-selected diets. **J Am Dietet Assoc** 1979;75:23-28.

35. Patterson KY, Holbrook JT, Bodner JE, Kelsay JC, Smith JC Jr, Veillon C. Zinc, copper, and manganese intake and balance for adults consuming self-selected diets. **Am J Clin Nutr** 1984;40:1397-1403.

36. Baer MT, King JC. Tissue zinc levels and zinc excretion during experimental zinc depletion in young men. **Am J Clin Nutr** 1984;39:556-570.

37. Worme JD. Dietary patterns, gastrointestinal complaints and nutrition knowledge of recreational triathletes. **Am J Clin Nutr** 1990;51:690-697.

38. Couzy F, Lafargue P, Guezennec CY. Zinc metabolism in the athlete: Influence of training, nutrition, and other factors. **Int J Sports Med** 1990; 263-266.

39. Stokstad EL, Chan MM, Watson JE, Brody T. Nutritional interactions of vitamin B_{12}, folic acid. and thyroxine. In: Levander OA, Cheng L, eds. **Micronutrient interactions.** New york: New York Academy of Sciences

1980:119-129.

40. Nationwide food consumption survey of 1977-78. Preliminary report No. 2. Washington DC: USDA, 1980.

41. Folkers K, Watanabe T, Ellis J. Studies on the basal specific activity of glutamic oxaloacetic transaminase of erythrocytes in relationship to a deficiency of vitamin B5. **Res Comm Chem Path Pharm** 1977;17:187-189.

42. Woodring MJ. Storvick CA. Effect of pyridoxine supplementation on glutamic-pyruvic transaminase and in vitro stimulation in erythrocytes of normal women. **Am J Clin Nutr** 1970;23:1385-1391.

43. Baker EM, Canham JE, Numes WT, Sauberlich HE, McDowell ME. Vitamin B5 requirement for adult men. **Am J Clin Nutr** 1964 ;15:59-66.

44. Leklem JE, Schultz TD. Increased plasma pyridoxal-5'-phosphate and vitamin B6 in male adolescents after a 4,500 meter run. **Am J Clin Nutr** 1983;38:541-548.

45. Cox EV, Meynell BE, Northam BE, Cooks WT. The anemia of scurvy. **Am J Med** 1966;42:220-227.

46. Golberg A. The anemia of scurvy. **Q Med J** 1963;32:51-64.

47. Stokes PL, Melikan V, Leeming RL, Portman-Graham H, Blair JA, Cooke WT. Folate metabolism in scurvy. **Am J Clin Nutr** 1975;28:126-129.

48. Irwin MI, Hutchins BK. A conspectus of research on vitamin C requirements of man. **J Nutr** 1976;106:823-879.

49. Visagie ME, DuPlessies JP, Laubscher NF. Effects of vitamin C supplementation on black mineworkers. **S Afr Med** 1975;49:889-892.

50. Bowles DK, et al. Effects of acute submaximal exercise on skeletal muscle vitamin E. **Free Rad Res Comm** 1991;14:139-143.

51. Leonard PJ, Losowsky MS. Relationship between plasma vitamin E level and peroxide hemolysis test in human subjects. **Am J Clin Nutr** 1967;20:795-802.

52. Oski FA, Barnes LA. Hemolytic anemia in vitamin E deficiency. **Am J Clin Nutr** 1968;20:45-53.

53. Machlin LJ, Gabriel E. Interactions of vitamin E with vitamin C, vitamin B12 and zinc. In: Levander OA, Cheng L, eds. **Micronutrient Interactions.** New York: New York Academy of Sciences 1980;98-108.

54. Sumida S, et al. Exercise induced lipid peroxidation and leakage of enzymes before and after vitamin E supplementation. **Int J Biochem** 1989;21:835-838.

55. Cook JD, Finch CA. Assessing iron status of a population. **Am J Clin Nutr** 1979;32:2115-2121.

56. Clement DB, Asmundson RC. Nutritional intake and hematological parameters in endurance runners. **Physician Sports Med** 1982;10:37-43.

57. Colgan M, Fiedler SA, Colgan LA. Micronutrient status of endurance athletes: effects on blood status and performance. **Sports Medicine in**

Track and Field Athletes. Partridge Green, West Sussex: International Amateur Athletics Federation, 1988:59-80.

Chapter 22. Strong Immunity

1. Heiss F. **Unfallverhutung Beim Sport.** Schorndorf: Karl Hoffman, 1971: 17-19.
2. Fitzgerald L. Exercise and the immune system. **Immunology Today** 1988;9:337-339.
3. Herberman RB, Ortaldo JR. Natural killer cells: their role in defenses against disease. **Science** 1981;214:24-30.
4. Golub ES, Green DR. **Immunology: A Synthesis. 2nd Edition.** Sunderland, Mass: Sinauer, 1991.
5. Sharmanov AT, et al. Effect of vitamin E on oxidative metabolism of macrophages. **Bull Exper Biol Med** 1986;101:810.
6. Peterson BK. Influence of physical activity on the cellular immune system. **Int J Sports Med** 1991;12:S23-S29.
7. Nieman DC, et al. Effects of long endurance running on immune system parameters and lymphocyte function in experienced marathoners. **Int J Sports Med** 1989;5:317-323.
8. Tvede N, et al. Effect of physical exercise on blood mononuclear cell subpopulations and in vitro proliferative responses. **Scand J Immunol** 1989;29:383-389.
9. Pederson BK, et al. Indomethacin in vitro and in vivo abolished post exercise suppression of natural killer cell activity in peripheral blood. **Int J Sports Med** 1990;11:127-131.
10. Pederson BK, et al. Modulations of natural killer cell activity in peripheral blood by physical exercise. **Scand J Immunol** 1988;26:673-678.
11. Surkina ID. Stress and immunity among athletes. **Soviet Sports Rev** 1982;17:198-202.
12. Pederson BK, et al. Natural killer cells in peripheral blood of highly trained and untrained persons. **Int J Sports Med** 1989;10:129-131.
13. Lui Y, Wang S. The enhancing effect of exercise on the production of antibody to salmonella typhi in mice. **Immunol Lett** 1987;14:117-120.
14. Watson RR, et al. Modifications of cellular immune functions in humans by endurance exercise training during beta adrenergic blockade with antenolol or propanolol. **Med Sci Sports Ex** 1986;18:95.
15. Asgiersson G, Bellanti JA. Exercises immunity and infection. **Sem Adolescent Med** 1987;3:199-204.
16. Fitzgerald L. Overtraining increases the susceptibility to infections.

Int J Sports Med 1991;12:S5-S8.

17. Salo DC. Does swimming make you sick? **Swimming World** 1989; October:59.
18. Peters EM, Bateman ED. Ultra-marathon running and upper respiratory tract infections - an epidemiological survey. **South African Medical Journal** 1983;64:582-584.
19. Heath GW, et al. Exercise and the incidence of upper respiratory tract infections. **Med Sci Sports Ex** 1991;23:152-157.
20. Reilly T, Rothwell J. Correlates of illness and injury in female distance runners. Paper presented at The British Association of Sport and Medicine Congress. University of Liverpool, 1987.
21. Johanssen C. Individually programmed training and prevention of injuries in elite orienteers. **Abstracts of the 23rd FIMS World Congress** 1986:49.
22. Green RL, et al. Immune function in marathon runners. **Ann Allergy** 1981;47:73-75.
23. Tomasi TB, et al. Immune parameters in athletes before and after strenuous exercise. **J Clin Immunol** 1982;2:173-178.
24. Fry RW, Morton AR, Keast D. Overtraining in athletes. **Sports Medicine** 1991;12:32-65.
25. Chirico G, et al. Deficiency of neutrophil phagocytosis in premature infants: effect of vitamin E supplementation. **Acta Paediatr Scand** 1983;72:521.
26. Lehmann LJ, McGill M. **J Lipid Res** 1982;23:299.
27. Hoffeld JT. Agents which block membrane lipid peroxidation enhance mouse spleen cell immune activities in vitro. **Eur J Immunol** 1981;11:371.
28. Hoffeld JT. Inhibition of lymphocyte proliferation and antibody production by silica, talc, bentonite, or corynebacterium parvum. **Eur J Immunol** 1983;13:365.
29. Bendich A, et al., eds. **Antioxidant Nutrients and Immune Functions.** New York: Plenum, 1989.
30. Tengerdy RP. In: Philips M, Baetz A, eds. **Diet and Resistance to Disease. Advances in Experimental Medicine and Biology. Vol 135**. New York: Plenum Press, 1981:27.
31. Hill HR, et al. Defective monocyte chemotactic responses in diabetes mellitus. **J Clin Immunol** 1983;3:70.
32. Chavance M, et al. Immunological and nutrient status among the elderly. In: De Weck AL, ed. **Lymphoid Cell Functions In Aging**. Rijswijk: Eurage, 1984.
33. Meydani SN, et al. Antioxidants and the aging immune system. In: Bendich A, et al., eds. **Antioxidant Nutrients and Immune Functions.** New York: Plenum Press, 1989.

34. Bendich A, Machlin LJ. Safety of oral intake of vitamin E. **Am J Clin Nutr** 1988;48:612-619.
35. Moser U, Weber F. Uptake of ascorbic acid by human granulocytes. **Int J Vit Nutr Res** 1983;54:47.
36. Goldschmidt MC. The effect of ascorbic acid deficiency on leucocyte phagocytosis and killing actinomyces viscosus. **Int J Vit Nutr Res** 1988;58: 326.
37. Anderson R, Lukey PT. A biological role for ascorbate in the selective neutralization of extracellular phagocyte-derived oxidant. **Ann NY Acad Sci** 1987;498;229.
38. Beisel WR. Single nutrients and immunity. **Am J Clin Nutr** 1982;35:417.
39. Panush RS, et al. Modulation of certain immunologic responses by vitamin C: Potentiation of in vitro and in vivo lymphocyte responses. **Int J Vit Nutr Res** 1982;23:35.
40. Ursini F, et al. A newly discovered enzyme links selenium more closely to vitamin E. Paper presented at the Fourth International Symposium on Selenium in Biology and Medicine. Tubingen, Germany. July, 1988.
41. Shamberger RJ. **Biochemistry of Selenium**. New York Plenum Press, 1983:239-243.
42. Spallholtz JE, et al. **Proc Soc Exp Biol Med** 1973;143:685.
43. Bendich A. Antioxidant vitamins and immune responses. In: Chandra RK ed. **Nutrition and Immunology**. New York: Alan R. Liss, 1988:125-147.
44. Eskew ML, et al. Effects of vitamin E and selenium deficiencies on rat immune function. **Immunol** 1985;54:173.
45. Fernandes C, et al. Impairment of cell-mediated immunity functions by dietary zinc deficiency in mice. **Proc Nat Acad Sci** 1979;76:457-461.
46. Fraker PJ, et al. Regeneration of T-cell helperfunction in zinc deficient adult mice. **Proc Nat Acad Sci** 1978;75:5600-5604.
47. Gaworski CL, Sharma RP. The effects of heavy metals on H thymidine uptake in lymphocytes. **Toxicol Appl Pharmacol** 1978;46:305-313.
48. Dachateau J, Delespesse G, Verecke P. Influence of oral zinc supplementation on the lymphocyte response to mitogens of normal subjects. **Am J Clin Nutr** 1981;34:88-93.
49. Colgan M. **Prevent Cancer Now. 2nd Edition**. San Diego, CA: CI Publications, 1992.
50. DeVet HC. The puzzling role of vitamin A in cancer prevention. **Anticancer Res** 1989;9:145-151.
51. Tomita Y, et al. Augmentation of tumor immunity against syngenic tumors is by beta-carotene. **J Nat Cancer Inst** 1987;78:679-681.
52. Schwartz J, Suda D, Light G. Beta-carotene is associated with regression of hamster buccal pouch carcinoma and the induction of tumor necrosis factor in macrophages. **Biochem Biophys Res Comm** 1986;136:1130-1135.

53. Schwartz JL, Shklar G. Prevention and regression of hamster oral squamous cell carcinoma following administration of carotenoids. In: Bendich A, et al., eds. **Antioxidant Nutrients and Immune Function.** New York: Plenum Press, 1989.

54. Leslie CA, Dubey DP. Carotene and natural killer cell activity. **Fed Proc** 1982;41:331.

55. Bendich A, Shapiro SS. Effect of beta-carotene and canthaxanthin on the immune responses of a rat. **J Nutr** 1986;116:2254.

56. Alexander M, et al. Oral beta-carotene increases the number of OKT4 cells in human blood. **Immunol Lett** 1985;9:221.

57. Watson RR, et al. Effects of beta-carotene on lymphocyte sub-populations in elderly humans. **Am J Clin Nutr** 1991;53:90-94.

58. Folkers K, et al., eds. **Biomedical and Clinical Aspects of Coenzyme Q. Vol 6.** New York: Elsevier Science Publishers, 1991.

59. Leibowitz BE. Coenzyme Q. **Nutrition Update** 1988:3:1:1-9.

60. Bliznakov E, et al. Stimulants of phagocytic activity in rats and immune response in mice. **Experientia** 1970;26:953-954.

61. Block L, et al. Non-specific resistance to bacterial infections: enhancement by ubiquinone-B. **J Exper Med** 1978;148:1228-1240.

62. Bliznakov E. Immunological senescence in mice and its reversal by coenzyme Q10. **Med Age Deut** 1978;7:189-197.

63. Folkers K, Yamamura Y, eds. **Biomedical and Clinical Aspects of Coenzyme Q. Vol 3.** New York: Elsevier Science Publishers, 1981;399-412.

64. Bliznakov E. Effect of stimulation of the hot defense system on dibenzpyrene-induced tumors and infection with Friend leukemia virus in mice. **Proc Nat Acad Sci** 1973;70:390-392.

65. Kishimoto C, et al. The protection of coenzyme Q10 against experimental viral myocarditis in mice. **Japanese Circ J** 1984;48: 1358-1361.

66. Borman A, et al. The role of arginine in growth with some observations on the effect of arginoic acid. **J Biol Chem** 1946;166:585-594.

67. Seifter E, et al. Arginine: An essential amino acid for injured rats. **Surgery** 1978;84:224-230.

68. Barbul A. Arginine and immune function. **Nutrition** 1990;6:S53-S58

69. Kirk SJ, et al. Role of arginine in trauma, sepsis and immunity. **J Parent Ent Nutr** 1990;14:226S-229S.

70. Barbul A, et al. Wound healing and thymotrophic effects of arginine: A pituitary mechanism of action. **Am J Clin Nutr** 1983;37:786-794.

71. Moncada S, et al. Biosynthesis of nitric oxide fromL-arginine. A pathway for the regulation of cell function and communication. **Biochem Pharmacol** 1989;11:1709-1715.

72. Ardawi MS, Newsholme EA. Metabolism in lymphocytes and its

importance in the immune response. **Essays in Biochemistry** 1985;21:
1-43.

73. Newsholme EA. Psychoimmunology and cellular nutrition: an
alternative hypothesis. **Biol Psychiat** 1990;27:1-3.

74. Griffiths M, Keast D. The effect of glutamine on murine splenic
leucocyte responses to T- and B-cell mitogens. **Cell Biology** 1990;68:
405-408.

75. Roth E, et al. Glutamine: An anabolic effector. **J Parent Ent Nutr** 1990;
14:1305-1365.

76. Parry-Billings M, et al. A communicational link between skeletal muscle,
brain, and cells of the immune system. **Int J Sports Med** 1990;11:Suppl,
1-7.

77. Lacey J, Wilmore D. Is glutamine a conditionally essential amino acid?
Nutrition Reviews 1990;48:297-309.

78. Wernerman J, et al. Alpha-ketoglutarate and postoperative muscle
catabolism. **Lancet** 1990;335:701-703.

79. Milward DJ, Rivers PW. The need for indispensable amino acids: The
concept of the anabolic drive. **Diabetes Metab Rev** 1989;5:191-211.

80. Thenen SW. **J Nutr** 1978;108:836.

81. Axelrod AE. Pruzansky J. **Ann New York Acad Sci** 1955;63:202.

82. Schroeder HA. Chromium deficiency in rats: a syndrome simulating
diabetes mellitus with retarded growth. **J Nutr** 1966;88:439-445.

83. Barone J, et al. Dietary fat and natural killer cell activity. **Am J Clin Nutr**
1989;50:861-867.

84. Bounous G, Amer MA. The immunoenhancing effect of dietary whey
protein concentrate. **Clin Invest Med** 1988;11:271-278.

Chapter 23. Beating The Burn

1. Hermansen L, Osnes JB. Blood and muscle pH after maximal exercise
in man. **J Appl Physiol** 1972;32:304-308.

2. Porter R, Whelan J, eds. **Human Muscle Fatigue Physiological
Mechanisms.** London: Pitman Medical, 1981.

3. Danforth WH. Activation of the glycolytic pathway in muscle. In: Chance
B, Estabrook RW, eds. **Control of Energy Metabolism.** New York:
Academic Press, 1965:287-298.

4. Miller R, et al. 31p nuclear magnetic resonance studies of high energy
phosphate and pH in human muscle fatigue. **J Clin Invest** 1988;81:1190-
1196.

5. Brodan V, et al. Effects of sodium glutamate infusion on ammonia

formation during intense exercise in man. **Nutr Rep Int** 1974;9:223-232.

6. Kvamme E. Ammonia metabolism in the CNS. **Prog Neurobiol** 1983; 20:109-132.

7. Wilkerson JE, Batterson DL, Horvath SM. Exercise induced changes in blood ammonia levels in humans. **Eur J Appl Physiol** 1977;37:255-263.

8. Kreider RB, et al. Effects of phosphate loading on oxygen uptake, ventilatory anaerobic threshold and in performance. **Med Sci Sports Exer** 1990;22:250-255.

9. Dale G, et al. Fitness, unfitness, and phosphate. **Brit Med J** 1987;294:939.

10. McCully K, et al. Detection of muscle injury in humans with 31p magnetic resonance spectroscopy. **Muscle and Nerve** 1988;11:212-216.

11. Chasiotis D. Role of cyclic AMP and inorganic phosphate in the regulation of glycogenolysis during exercise. **Med Sci Sports Exer** 1988;20:545-550.

12. Farber M, et al. Effect of decreased O_2 affinity of hemoglobin on work performance during exercise in healthy humans. **J Lab Clin Med** 1984;104:166-175.

13. Kaijser L. Limiting factors for aerobic muscle performance. The influence of varying oxygen pressure and temperature. **Acta Physiol Scand**1970;(Suppl)346:1-96.

14. Jain SC, et al. Effect of phosphate supplementation on oxygen delivery at high altitude. **Intern J Biometeorol** 1987;31:249.

15. Brien AJ, Simon TL. The effects of red blood cell infusion on 10 km race time. **J Amer Med Assoc** 1987;257:2761.

16. Bremer J. Carnitine metabolism and function. **Physiol Rev** 1983;63: 1420-1480.

17. Lennon DLF, et al. Effects of acute moderate intensity exercise on carnitine metabolism in men and women. **J Appl Physiol** 1983;55: 489-495.

18. Warhol MJ, et al. Skeletal muscle injury and repair in marathon runners after competition. **Am J Pathol** 1985;118:331-339.

Chapter 24. Bicarbonate Buffers Acid

1. Davey C. **Biochem Biophys** 1960;89:303.

2. Lavender G, Bird SR. Effects of sodium bicarbonate ingestion upon repeated sprints. **Brit J Sports Med** 1989;23:41-45.

3. Shils ME, Young VR, eds. **Modern Nutrition in Health & Disease** Philadelphia: Lea & Febiger, 1988.

4. Johnson WR, Black DH. Comparison of effects of certain blood

alkalinizer and glucose upon competitive endurance. **J Appl Physiol** 1953;5:577-578.

5.   Hood VL, Schubert C, Keller U, Muller S. Effect of systemic pH on pHi and lactic acid generation in exhaustive forearm exercise. **Am J Physiol** 1988;255(24):F479-F485.

6.   Mainwood GW, Cechetto D. The effect of bicarbonate concentration on fatigue and recovery in isolated rat diaphragm muscle. **Canadian Journal of Pharmacology** 1980;58:624-632.

7.   Sutton JR, Jones NL, Toews CJ. Effect of pH on muscle glycolysis during exercise. **Clin Sci** 1981;61:331-338.

8.   Wilkes D, Gledhill N, Smyth R. Effect of induced metabolic alkalosis on 800-m racing time. **Medicine and Science in Sports and Exercise** 1983;15(4):277-280.

9.   Costill DL, et al. Acid base balance during repeated bouts of exercise. Influence of HC03. **Int J Sports Med** 1984;5:225-231.

10.   Sutton JR, Jones NL, Toews CJ. Effect of pH on muscle glycolysis during exercise. **Clin Sci** 1981;61:331-338.

11.   Rupp JC, Bartels RL, Zuelzer W, Fox EL, Clark RN. Effect of sodium bicarbonate ingestion on blood and muscle pH and exercise performance. **Medicine and Science in Sports and Exercise** 1983;15:115.

12.   McKenzie DC, et al. Maximal work production following two levels of induced metabolic alkalosis. **J Sports Sciences** 1986;4:35-38.

13.   Inbar O, et al. The effects of alkaline treatment on short-term maximal exercise. **J Sports Sciences** 1983;1:95-104.

14.   Horswill CA, et al. Influence of sodium bicarbonate on sprint performance:relationship to dosage. **Medicine and Science in Sports and Exercise** 1988;20(6):556-569.

15.   George KP, MacLaren DPM. The effect of induced alkalosis and acidosis on endurance running at an intensity corresponding to 4mM blood lactate. **Ergonomics** 1988;31(11):1639-1645.

16.   McNaughton LR, Cedaro R. The effect of sodium bicarbonate on rowing ergometer performance in elite rowers. **The Australian Journal of Science and Medicine in Sport** 1991;23(3):66-69.

17.   **Recommended Dietary Allowances 10th Edition**. Washington DC: National Academy Press, 1989.

Chapter 25. Phosphate Loading

1.   Kreider RB, et al. Effects of phosphate loading on oxygen uptake, ventilatory anaerobic threshold and in performance. **Med Sci Sports**

Exer 1990;22:250-255.

2. Dale G, et al. Fitness, unfitness, and phosphate. **Brit Med J** 1987;294: 939.

3. McCully K, et al. Detection of muscle injury in humans with 31p magnetic resonance spectroscopy. **Muscle and Nerve** 1988;11:212-216.)

4. Ljinghall S, et al. Plasma, potassium, and phosphate concentration - influence by adrenalin infusion, beta blockade, and physical exercise. **Acta Medica Scand** 1987;221:83-93.

5. **Recommended Dietary Allowances 10th Edition.** Washington DC: National Academy Press, 1989.

6. Miller GW, et al. Effects of phosphate loading on anaerobic threshold. **Med Sci Sports Exer** 1991;23:S35.

7. Chasiotis D. Role of cyclic AMP and inorganic phosphate in the regulation of glycogenolysis during exercise. **Med Sci Sports Exer** 1988;20:545-550.

8. Farber M, et al. Effect of decreased O_2 affinity of hemoglobin on work performance during exercise in healthy humans. **J Lab Clin Med** 1984;104:166-175.

9. Cade R, et al. Effects of phosphate loading on 2,3-diphosphoglycerate and maximal oxygen uptake. **Med Sci Sports Exer** 1984;16:263-268.

10. Stewart I, McNaughton L. Phosphate loading and effects on VO_2max in trained cyclists. **Res Quart** 1990;61:80-84.

11. Kreider RB, et al. Effects of phosphate loading on metabolic and myocardial responses to maximal and endurance exercise. **Int J Sports Nutr** 1992;2:20-47.

12. Bredel D, et al. Phosphate supplementation, cardiovascular function, and exercise performance in humans. **J Appl Physio** 1988;65:1821-1826.

13. Mannix E, et al. Oxygen delivery and cardiac output during exercise following oral phosphate-glucose. **Med Sci Sports Exer** 1990;22:341-347.

14. Lloyd G, et al. Effects of a commercial supplement containing sodium phosphate and bicarbonate on hematological responses to swim performance. Paper presented to the American College of Sports Medicine Meeting in Dallas, Texas. May 27-30, 1992.

Chapter 26. Carnitine Moves More Than Fat

1. Coyle EF. Carbohydrate supplementation during exercise. **J Nutr** 1992;122:788-801.

2. Strack E, Rotzsch W, Lorenz I. Biological action of carnitine in animal bodies. In: Peters H, ed. **Protides of the Biological Fluids.** New York:

Elsevier, 1964: 234.

3. Bremer J. Carnitine metabolism and function. **Physiol Rev** 1983;63: 1420-1480.

4. Stumpf DA. Carnitine deficiency organic acidemias and Reye's syndrome. **Neurology** 1985;35:1041-1045.

5. Brevetti G, et al. Increases in walking distance in patients with peripheral vascular disease treated with L-carnitine: a double-blind crossover study. **Circulation** 1988;77:767-773.

6. Lennon DLF, et al. Effects of acute moderate-intensity exercise on carnitine metabolism in men and women. **J Appl Physiol** 1983;55:489.

7. Siliprandi N, et al. Metabolic changes induced by maximal exercise in human subjects following L-carnitine administration. **Biochem Biophys Acta** 1990;1034:17-21.

8. Engle AG, Angelini C. Carnitine deficiency of human muscle with associated lipid storage myopathy: A new syndrome. **Science** 1973;179: 899-902.

9. Chalmers RA, et al. Urinary excretion of L-carnitine and acylcarnitines by patients with disorders or organic acid metabolism: evidence for secondary insufficiency of L-carnitine. **Pediat Res** 1984;18:1325-1328.

10. Lennon DLF, et al. Dietary carnitine intake related to skeletal muscle and plasma carnitine concentrations in adult men and women. **Amer J Clin Nutr** 1986;43:234-238.

11. **Physicians Desk References. 46th Edition**. Montvale, NJ: Medical Economics, 1992.

12. Cherci A, et al. Effects of L-carnitine on exercise tolerance in chronic stable angina: a multicenter, double-blind, randomized, placebo controlled crossover study. **Int J Clin Pharmacol Ther Tox** 1985;23:569-572.

13. Kosolcharoen P, et al. Improved exercise tolerance after administration of L-carnitine. **Curr Ther Res** 1981;30:753.

14. Canale C, et al. Bicycle ergometer and echocardiographic study in healthy subjects and patients with angina pectoris after administration of L-carnitine: semiautomatic computerized analysis of M-mode tracing. **Int J Clin Pharmacol Terh Toxicol** 1988;26:221.

15. Dal Negro R, et al.-Carnitine and rehabilitative physiokinesitherapy: metabolic and ventilatory response in chronic respiratory insufficiency. **Int J Clin Pharmacol Ther Toxicol** 1986;24:453.

16. Dal Negro R, et al. Effects of L-carnitine on physical performance in chronic respiratory insufficiency. **Int J Clin Pharmacol Ther Toxicol** 1988;26:269.

17. Arenas J, et al. Carnitine in muscle, serum, and urine of non-professional athletes: effects of physical exercise training and L-carnitine administration. **Muscle & Nerve** 1991;14:598-604.

18. Liebovitz B. **Carnitine: The Vitamin B$_T$ Phenomenon.** New York: Dell Publishing, 1984

19. Marconi C, et al. Effects of L-carnitine loading on the aerobic and anaerobic performance of endurance athletes. **Eur J Appl Physiol** 1985;54:131-135.

20. Angeline C, et al. Clinical study of efficacy of L-carnitine and metabolic observations in exercise physiology. **Clinical Aspects of Human Carnitine Deficiency.** Pergamon Press, NY: 1986:38.

21. Borum PR. Carnitine in human nutrition. **Nutrition and the MD** 1982;9:1.

22. Bazzato G, et al. Myasthenia-like (muscle weakness) Syndrome After Dl - but not L-carnitine **Lancet** 1981;1:1209.

23. DeGrandis D, et al. Myasthenia (muscle weakness) Due to Dl-carnitine treatment. **J Neurol Sci** 1980;46:365-371.

24. Health Effects of Dietary Carnitine. Prepared for Bureau of Foods, Food and Drug Administration. Department of Health and Human Services. Washington, DC. November, 1983.

25. Keith R. Carnitine in a runner. **J Amer Med Assoc** 1986;255:1137.

Chapter 27. Caffeine: The Right Way

1. Bucci LR. Nutritional Ergogenic Aids. In: Hickson JF, Wolinsky I. **Nutrition In Exercise and Sport.** Boca Raton, FL: CRC Press, 107-185.

2. Colton T, Gosswlin RE, Smith RP. The tolerance of coffee drinkers to caffeine. **Clin Pharmacol Ther** 1968;9:31.

3. Robertson D, Wade D, Workman R, et al. Tolerance to the humoral and hemodynamic effects of caffeine in man. **J Clin Invest** 1981;67:1111.

4. Fisher SM, McMurray RG, Berry M, et al. Influence of caffeine on exercise performance in habitual caffeine users. **Int J Sports Med** 1986; 7:276-280.

5. Voy R. **Drugs, Sport, and Politics.** Champaign, IL: Leisure Press, 1991.

6. Stillner V, Popkin MK, Pierce DM. Caffeine induced delirium during prolonged competitive stress. **Am J Psychiatr** 1978;135:855.

7. Cadarette BS, Levine L, Berube CL, et al. Effects of varied dosages of caffeine on endurance exercise to fatigue. In: Knuttgen HG, Voge JA, Poortmans J, eds. **Biochemistry of Exercise.** Champaign IL: Human Kinetics Publishers, 1983: 871.

8. Essig D, Costill DL, Van Handel PJ. Effects of caffeine ingestion on utilization of muscle glycogen and lipid during leg ergometer cycling. In **J Sports Med** 1980; 1:70-74.

9. Van Handel P. Caffeine. In: Williams MH, ed. **Ergogenic Aids in Sports.**

Champaign IL: Human Kinetics Publishers, 1983:128.

10. Williams MH. Drug foods - alcohol and caffeine. In: **Nutritional Aspects of Human Physical and Athletic Performance 2nd Ed**. Springfield IL: Charles C Thams, 1985: 272.

11. Wager-Srdar SA, Oken MM, Morley JE, Levin AS. Thermoregulatory effects of purines and caffeine. **Life Sci** 1983;33:2431-2438.

12. Curaldo PW, Robertson D. The health consequences of caffeine. **Ann Intern Med** 1983;98:641.

13. Falk, B, Burstein R, Rosenblum J, et al. Effects of caffeine ingestion on body fluid balance and thermoregulation during exercise. **Can J Physiol Pharmacol** 1990;68:889-892.

14. Costill DL, Dalsky GP, Fink WJ. Effects of caffeine ingestion on metabolism and exercise performance. **Med Sci Sports Exer** 1978;10: 155-158.

15. Ivy JL, Costill DL, Fink WJ, Lower RW. Influence of caffeine and carbohydrate feedings on endurance performance. **Med Sci Sports Exer** 1979;11:6.

16. Weir J, Noakes TD, Myburgh K, Adams B. A high carbohydrate diet negates the metabolic effects of caffeine during exercise. **Med Sci Sports** Exer 1987;19:100-105.

17. Belect S, et al. Responses of free fatty acids to coffee and caffeine. **Metabolism** 1968;17:702-707.

18. Flinn S, Gregory J, McNaughton LR, Tristram S, Davies P. Caffeine ingestion prior to incremental cycling to exhaustion in recreational cyclists. **Int J Sports Med** 1990; 11:188-193.

Chapter 28. Real Ginseng Works

1. Kim SK, et al. **Planta Medica** 1981;42:181.

2. Schulten HR, Soldati F. Identification of ginsenosides from panax Ginseng in fractions obtained by HPLC by FD-MS, MIR-JR and TLC. **J of Chromatography** 1981; 212:37-49.

3. Tyler VE. **The New Honest Herbal**. Philadelphia, George F Stickley, 1987.

4. Teves MA. Effects of ginseng on repeated bouts of exhaustive exercise. **Med Sci Sports Exer** 1983; 15:162.

5. Knapik JJ, et al. The influence of Panax ginseng on indices of substrate utilization during repeated exhaustive exercise in man. **Fed Proc** 1983;42: 336.

6. Hickson J, Wolinsky I, eds. **Nutrition in Exercise and Sport**. Boca Raton, FL: CRC Press, 1989: 146-147.

7. Samura MM, et al. Effect of standardized ginseng extract G115 on the metabolism and electrical activity of the rabbit's brain. **J Int Med Res** 1985;13:342-348.

8. Kaku T, et al. Chemicopharmacological studies on saponins of P ginseng CA Meyer. **Arzniem Forsch** 1975;25:539-547.

9. D'Angelo L, et al. A double-blind, placebo controlled clinical study on the effect of standardized ginseng extract on psychomotor performance in healthy volunteers. **J Ethnopharmacol** 1986;16:15-22.

10. Avakian EV, Sugimoto BR. Effect of panax ginseng on energy substares during exercise. **Fed Proc** 1980;39:287.

11. Avakian EV, et al. Effect of Panax ginseng extract on energy metabolism during exercise in rats. **Planta Medica** 1984;50:151.

12. Singh VK, et al. **Planta Medica** 1984;50:462.

13. Dorling E, et al. Do ginsenosides influence performance. Results of a double-blind study. **Notabene Medici** 1980;10:241-246.

14. Forgo I, Shimert G. The duration of effect of the standardized ginseng extract G115 in healthy competitive athletes. **Notabene Medici** 1985;15:636-640.

15. Sahlin K. In: Knuttgen HG, Vogel H, eds. **Biochemistry of Exercise**. Champaign, IL: Human Kinetics, 1983: 151-160.

16. Forgo I, Kirchdorfer AM. On the question of influencing the performance of top sportsmen by means of biologically active substances. **Arztliche Praxis** 1981;33:1784-1786.

17. McNaughton L, Egan G, Caelii G. A comparison of Chinese and Russian ginseng as ergogenic aids to improve various facets of physical fitness. **Int Clin Nutr Rev** 1989;9:32-37.

Chapter 29. Chromium Boosts Insulin Efficiency

1. **Recommended Dietary Allowances 7th Ed.** Washington DC: National Academy of Sciences, 1968: 61.

2. Mertz W, Shapcott D, Hubert J, eds. **Chromium in Nutrition and Metabolism**. Amsterdam: Elsevier N Holland, 1979.

3. Drazmin B, et al., eds. **Insulin Action**. New York: Alan R Liss, 1989.

4. Rudman D. Growth hormone, body composition and aging. **J Am Geriat Soc** 1985;33:800-807.

5. Camarini-Davalos RA, Hanover R, eds. Treatment of Early Diabetes. **Advances In Experimental Medicine and Biology Vol 119**. New York: Plenum Press, 1979.

6. **Recommended Dietary Allowances 10th Edition.** Washington DC:

National Academy Press, 1989: 241.

7. Tipton IH, Stewart PL, Analytical methods for the determination of trace elements -- standard man studies. In: Hemphill DD, ed. **Trace Substances in Environmental Health**. Columbia MO: University of Missouri, 1970: 305-330.

8. Kumpulainen JT, Wolf WR, Veillon C, Mertz W. Determination of chromium in selected United States diets. **J Agric Food Chem** 1979;27: 490-494.

9. Anderson RA, Kozlovsky AS. Chromium intake absorption and excretion of subjects consuming self selected diets. **Am J Clin Nutr** 1985;41:1177-1183.

10. Anderson RA, Polansky MM, Bryden NA, et al. Chromium supplementation of human subjects: effects on glucose, insulin, and lipid variables. **Metabolism** 1983; 32:894-899.

11. Riales P, Albrink R. Effect of chromium chloride supplementation on glucose tolerance and serum lipids including high density lipoprotein of adult men.. **Amer J Clin Nutr** 1981;34:2670-2678.

12. Anderson RA, Polansky MM, et al. Effect of exercise (running) on serum glucose, insulin, glycogen and chromium excretion. **Diabetes** 1982;31: 212-216.

13. Campbell WW, Anderson RA. Effects of aerobic exercise and training on the trace minerals chromium, zinc, and copper. **Sports Medicine** 1987;4:9-18.

14. Anderson RA, Bryden NA, Polansky MM, Deuster PA. Exercise effects on chromium excretion of trained and untrained men consuming a constant diet. **J Appl Physiol** 1988;64:249.

15. Mertz W. Chromium occurrence and function in biological systems. **Physiol Rev** 1969;49:163-239.

16. **Toxicity of the Essential Minerals**. Food & Drug Administration, Washington DC, 1975;125: 3.

17. Lefavi R, et al. Lipid lowering effect of a dietary nicotinic acid chromium complex in male athletes. **FASEB J** 1991;5:A1645.

18. Anderson RA. Chromium metabolism and its role in disease processes in man. **Clin Physiol Biochem** 1986;4:31.

19. Press RI, Geller J, Evans GW. The effect of chromium picolinate on serum cholesterol and apolipoprotein fractions in human subjects. **Western J Med** 1990;152:41-45.

20. Hasten DL, et al. Effects of Chromium Picolinate on Beginning Weight Training Students. **Int J Sports Nutr** 1992 (in press).

21. Page TG, Ward TL, Southern LL. Effect of chromium picolinate on growth and carcass characteristic of growing-finishing pigs. **J Animal Science** 1991;69:403.

22. Page TG, et al. Effect of chromium picolinate on growth hormone, cholesterol, insulin, and other components in serum of growing-finishing pigs. **J Animal Science** 1991;69:404.
23. Evans GW, Bowman T. A comparison of biological effects of chromium picolinate, chromium nicotinate, and chromic chloride on skeletal muscle cells. **J Inorganic Biochemistry** 1992;45 (in press).
24. Hambidge KM. Chromium nutrition in man. **Am J Clin Nutr** 1974;27: 505-514.

Chapter 30. Real Anabolics

1. Gambetta V, ed. **TAC Track & Field Coaching Manual**. West Point, NY: Leisure Press, 1981.
2. Duchaine D. Ask the guru. **Muscle Media 2000** 1992;Summer 63-67.
3. Daughaday WH, ed. **Endocrine Control of Growth**. New York: Elsevier, North Holland Press, 1981.
4. Rudman D, et al. Effects of human growth hormone in men over 60 years old. **N Engl J Med** 1990;323:1.
5. Crist DM, et al. Body composition response to exogenous GH during training in highly conditioned athletes. **J Appl Physiol** 1988;65:579.
6. Colgan M. Human growth hormone. **Muscle & Fitness** 1988;January:241.
7. Macintyre JG. Growth Hormone. **Sports Medicine** 1987;4:129.
8. Guillemin R, et al. Somatocrinin, the growth hormone releasing factor. In: Greep. **Recent Progress in Hormone Research** Proceedings of the 1983 Laurentian Hormone Conference, Academic Press Inc, New York, 1983;40:233-299.
9. Wurtman RJ, Hefti F, Melamed E. Precursor control of neurotransmitter synthesis. **Pharmacol Rev** 1980;32:315-335.
10. Reichlin S. Neuroendocrinology. Wilson & Foster, eds. **Williams Textbook of Endocrinology** 1985;7:514-531.
11. Woolf PD, Lee L. Effect of the serotonin precursor, tryptophan on pituitary hormone secretion. **J Clin Endocrinol Metab** 1977;45:123.
12. Fraser WM, et al. Effect of l-tryptophan on growth hormone and prolactin release in normal volunteers and patients with secretory pituitary tumors. **Horm Metab Res** 1979;11:149.
13. Sandy R, Consroe PF, Iacono RP. L-tryptophan in drug-induced movement disorders with insomnia. **N Engl J Med** 1986;314:1257.
14. Belongia EA, et al. An investigation of the cause of the eosinophilia-myalgia syndrome associated with tryptophan use. **N Engl J Med** 1990;323:357-365.

15. Sakimoto K. The cause of the eosinophilia-myalgia syndrome associated with tryptophan use. **N Engl J Med** 1990;323:992-993.

16. Chaikelis AS. The effect of glycocoll (glycine) ingestion upon the growth, strength and creatinine-creatine excretion in man. **Am J Physiol** 1941;132:578.

17. Coyle JT. Neurotoxic amino acids in human degenerative disorders. **Trends Neurosci** 1982;5:287-288.

18. Thomson AM. Glycine modulation of the NMDA receptor channel complex. **Trends Neurosci** 1989;12:349-353.

19. Kasai K, et al. Glycine stimulates growth hormone in man. **Acta En docrinol** 1980;93:283.

20. Kasai K, Kobayashi M, Shimoda S. Stimulatory effect of glycine on human growth hormone secretion. **Metabolism** 1978;27:201.

21. Braverman ER, Pfeiffer CC. Glycine. In: **The Healing Nutrients Within. Facts, Findings and New Research on Amino Acids**. Keats Publishing, New Canaan, 1986: 237.

22. Lane RJM, et al. An abnormality of glycine metabolism in ALS patients. **J Neurol Neurosurg Psychiat** 1990;52:180.

23. Giordano G, Marugo M, Minuto F. It test dell'arginina nella semeiologia funzionale dell'increzione dell'ormone somatotropo. **Folia Endocrinol** 1971;24:247.

24. Jackson D, Grant DH, Clayton BE. A simple oral test of growth-hormone secretion in children. **Lancet** 1968;2:373.

25. Pololsky S, Sivaprasad R. Assessment of growth hormone reserve: comparison of intravenous arginine and subcutaneous glucagon stimulation tests. **J Clin Endocrinol Metab** 1972;35:4.

26. Penny R, Blizzard RM, Davis WJ. Sequential study of arginine monochloride and normal saline as stimuli to growth hormone release metabolism. **Metabolism** 1970;19:165.

27. Dussault J, et al. Effect of somatostatin on thyrotropin, prolactin, growth hormone and insulin responses to thyrotropin releasing hormone and arginine in healthy, hypothyroid and acromegalic subjects. **Can Med Assoc J** 1977;117:478.

28. Raptis S, et al. Somatostatin and pentoxifylline modulation of insulin, glucagon and growth hormone following stimulation by arginine. **Acta Endocrinol (Copenh)** 1977;84:51.

29. Santander R, Garcia E. Comparative effects of glucagon and arginine upon growth hormone secretion in children and adolescents. **Acta Cient Fenez** 1977;28:290.

30. Masuda A, et al. Insulin-induced hypoglycemia, L-dopa and arginine stimulate GH secretion through different mechanisms in man. **Regulatory Peptides** 1990;31:53.

31. Ghigo E, et al. Combined administration of arginine and GHRH elicits similar GH responses in children, adults and elderly subjects. **J Endorcinol Invest** 1990;13:19.

32. Sneid DS, et al. Radioreceptor-inactive growth hormone associated with stimulated secretion in normal subjects. **J Clin Endocrinol Metab** 1975;41:471.

33. Isidori A, Lo Monaco A, Cappa, M. A study of growth hormone release in man after oral administration of amino acids. **Current Medical Research and Opinion** 1981;7:475-481.

34. Elam RP. Morphological changes in adult males from resistance exercise and amino acid supplementation. **J Sports Med Phys Fit** 1988;28:35.

35. Evian-Brion D, et al. Simultaneous study of corticotrophic pituitary secretions during ornithine infusion test. **Clin Endocrinol** 1982;17:119.

36. Braverman ER, Pfeiffer CC, eds. **The Healing Nutrients Within Facts, Findings, and New Research on Amino Acids.** New Canaan: Keats, 1986:186.

37. Cynober L, et al. Action of ornithine alpha-ketoglutarate on protein metabolism in burn patients. **Nutrition** 1987;3:187-191.

38. Wernerman J, et al. Ornithine alpha-ketoglutarate improves skeletal muscle protein synthesis as assessed by ribosome analysis and nitrogen balance postoperatively. **Ann Surgery** 1987;206:674-678.

39. Cynobar L, et al. Action of ornithine alpha-ketoglutarate, ornithine hydrochloride, and calcium alpha-ketoglutarate on plasma amino acid and hormonal patterns in healthy subjects. **J Amer Coll Nutr** 1990;9:2-12.

40. Vaubourdolle M, et al. Action of enterally administered ornithine alpha-ketoglutarate on protein breakdown in skeletal muscle and liver of the burned rat. **J Parent Ent Nutr** 1991;15:517-520.

41. Bucci L, et al. Ornithine ingestion and growth hormone release in bodybuilders. **Nutr Res** 1990;10:239-245.

42. Griffith RS, et al. A multi-centered study of lysine therapy in herpes simplex infection. **Dermatologica** 1978;156:257-267.

Chapter 31. Anabolics/Ergogenics & Snake Oil

1. Voy R. **Drugs, Sport and Politics.** Champaign IL: Leisure Press, 1991.

2. **Physicians Desk Reference.** 46th Ed. Montvale, NJ: Medical Economics Co., 1992.

3. Nittler A. **The Use of Tissue and Glandular Substances,** (booklet) undated. No publisher listed. Widely available in US health food stores.

4. Williams MH, eds. Ergogenic foods. In: **Nutritional Aspects of Human**

Physical And Athletic Performance. 2nd Ed. Springfield, IL: CC Thomas, 1985:312.

5. Chandler JV, Hawkins JD. The effect of bee pollen on physiological performance. **Med Sci Sports Exper** 1985;17:287.

6. Steben RD, Boudreaux P. The effects of pollen and pollen extracts on selected factors and performances of athletes. **J Sports Med** 1978;18:221.

7. Maughan RJ, Evans SP. Effects of pollen extract upon adolescent swimmers. **Brit J Sports Med** 1982;16:142.

8. Berger P, Sanders EH, Gardner PD, Negus NC. Phenolic plant compounds functioning as reproductive inhibitors in Microtus montanus. **Science** 1977;195:575.

9. Gorewit, RC. Pituitary and thyroid hormone responses of heifers after ferulic acid administration. **J Dairy Sci** 1983;66:624-629.

10. Cockerill DL, Bucci LR. Increases in muscle girth and decreases in bodyfat associated with a nutritional supplement program. **Chir Sports Med** 1987;1:73.

11. Bruni J. **Gamma Oryzanol: The Facts.** Long Island, NY, 1988.

12. **Physicians Desk Reference.** 44th Ed. Oradell, NJ: Medical Economics, 1990:1576.

13. **Physicians Desk Reference.** 46th Ed. Montvale, NJ: Medical Economics, 1992.

14. Tyler V. **Pharmacy International** 1986;7:203-207.

15. Morales A, et al. N Engl J Med 1981, 12 November, 1221.

16. Tyler V. **The New Honest Herbal.** New York: George F. Stickley, 1987.

17. Kucio C, et al. Does Yohimbine Act as a Slimming Drug? **Israel Journal Medical Science** 1991;27:550-556.

18. Boddy K, et al. **Lancet** 1968;7:10.

19. Sullivan LW. **N Engl J Med** 1965;272:340.

20. Stopozyk K. Xobalin. Preseglad Lekasski 1969;25:723.

21. Bessman SP, Fishbein WN. Gamma-hydroxybutyrate. A new metabolite in brain. **Fed Proc** 1963;22:334.

22. Mitoma C, Neubauer SE. Gamma-hydroxybutyric acid and sleep. **Experientia** 1968;24:12.

23. Takahara J, et al. Stimulatory effects of gamma-hydroxybutyric acid on growth hormone and prolactin release in humans. **J Clin Endocrin Metabol** 1977;44:1014.

24. Centers For Disease Control. **J Am Med Assoc** 1991;265:447-448.

25. Aviado DM. Inosine: A naturally occurring cardiotonic agent. **J Pharmacol** 1983;14(Supp III): 47-71.

26. Kipshidze NN, et al. Indications for the use of inosine in myocardial infarction; clinical and experimental study. **Kardiologiia** 1978;18:18-28.

27. Wickham JEA, et al. Inosine in preserving renal function during ishemic renal surgery. **Br Med J** 1978;2:173-174.

28. Nevins MS. Oxyhemoglobin equilibrium in ischemic heart disease. **JAMA** 1974;229:804-808.

29. Colgan M. Inosine. **Muscle & fitness** 1988;Jan:94-96, 204-206.

30. Bucci LR. In: Hickson J, Wolinsky I, eds. **Nutrition and Exercise in Sport.** Boca Raton, FL: CRC Press, 1989:157.

31. Kurtz TW, et al. Liquid chromatographic measurements of inosine, hypoxanthine, and xanthine in studies of fructose induced degradation of adenine neucleotides in humans and rats. **Clin Chem** 1986;32:782.

32. Colgan M. **Your Personal Vitamin Profile.** New York: Morrow, 1982.

33. Karpuchina YL, et al. Effect of pangamic acid on biochemical changes in the blood of athletes during performance of exercise. In: Michlin VN, ed. **Vitamin B15 (Pangamic acid). Properties Functions and Uses.** Moscow: Science Publishing, 1965: 182.

34. Dohm GL, Debanath S, Frisell WR. Effects of commercial preparations of pangamic acid (B15) on exercised rats. **Biochem Med** 1982;28:77.

35. Pipes TV. The effects of pangamic acid on performance in trained athletes. **Med Sci Sports Exer** 1980;12:98, Abstract.

36. Gray ME, Titlow LW. The effect of pangamic acid on maximal treadmill performance. **Med Sci Sports Exer** 1982;14:424-427.

37. Girandola RN, Wiswell RA, Bulbulian R. Effects of pangamic acid (B15) ingestion on metabolic response to exercise. **Med Sci Sports Exer** 1980; 12:98.

38. Bishop PA, Smith JF, Young B. Effects of N, N-dimethylglycine on physiological response and performance in trained runners. **J Sports Med Phys Fit** 1987;27:53.

39. Girondola RN, Wiswell RA, Bulbulian R. Effects of pangamic acid (B15) ingestion on metabolic response to exercise. **Biochem Med** 1980;24:218.

40. Black DG, Suec AA. Effects of calcium pangamate on aerobic endurance parameters, a double-blind study. **Med Sci Sports Exer** 1981;13:93.

41. Harpaz M, Otto RM, Smith TK. The effect of N,N-dimethylglycine ingestion upon aerobic performance. **Med Sci Sports Exer** 1985;17:287.

42. Brainum J. Lactate: does it cause muscle fatigue or is it a new energy source for bodybuilders? **Muscle & fitness** May, 1989.

43. Sahlin K. Effects of acidosis on energy metabolism and force generation in skeletal muscle. In: Knuttgen HG, Vogel H, eds. **Biochemistry of Exercise.** Champaign, IL: Human Kinetics, 1983:151-160.

44. Sahlin K, Henriksonn J. Buffer capacity and lactate accumulation in skeletal muscle of trained and untrained men. **Acta Physiol Scand**

1984;122:331-339.

45. Brooks G. The lactate shuttle during exercise recovery. **Med Sci Sports Exer** 1986;18:360-368.

46. Brooks GA. Lactate production under fully aerobic conditions: the lactate shuttle during rest and exercise. **Fed Proc** 1986;45:2924-2929.

47. Pendergast D, Leibowitz R, Wilson D, Cerretelli P. The effect of preceding anaerobic exercise on aerobic and anaerobic work. **Euro J Appl Physiol** 1983;52:29-35.

48. **Dorlands Medical Dictionary 26th Edition**. Philadelphia: WB Saunders, 1981.

49. Fahey TD, et al. The effect of ingesting polylactate or glucose polymer drinks during prolonged exercise. **Internat J Sport Nutr** 1991;1:249-256.

50. Ivy JL, et al. Influence of caffeine and carbohydrate feedings on endurance performance. **Med Sci Sports Ex** 1979;11-6-11.

51. Ivy JL, et al. Endurance improved by ingestion of a glucose polymer supplement. **Med Sci Sports Ex** 1983;15:466-471.

52. Edwards TL, Santeusanio D, Wheeler KB. Endurance of cyclists given carbohydrate solutions during moderate intensity rides. **Texas Med** 1986;82:29.

53. Snell PG, et al. **Med Sci Sports Exer** 1986;18:April (Suppl): S9.

54. Morton JF. **Atlas of Medicinal Plants of Middle America**. Springfield IL: CC Thomas, 1981.

55. Leung AY. **Encyclopedia of Common Natural Ingredients Used in Foods**. New York: John Wiley, 1980.

56. List PH, Horhammer I. **Hager's Handbuch der Pharmazeutischem Praxis**. Berlin: Springer Verlag, 1979.

57. **Washington Drug Letter** 1991;Feb 25:6.

58. Williams RJ, Lansford EM, eds. **Encyclopedia of Biochemistry**, New York: Reinhold Publishing, 1967.

59. Shutt DA. The effects of plant oestrogens on animal reproduction. Endeavour 1976;35:110-113.

60. Leavitt WW, Meismer DM. Sexual development alterd by non-steroidal oestrogens. **Nature** 1969;218:181-182.

61. Whitten PL, Russell E, Naftolin F. Effects of a normal, human-concentration, phytoestrogen diet on rat uterine growth. **Steroids** 1992; 57:98-105.

62. Chermnykh NS, et al. Effects of methandrostenolone and ecdisterone on physical endurance of animals and protein metabolism in skeletal muscle. **Farmakologiia Toksikologiia** 1988;51:6:57-60.

63. Nielsen FH. Possible future implications of ultratrace elements in human health and disease. In: Prasad AS, eds. **Essential and Toxic Trace Elements in Human Health and Disease. Current Topics in Nutrition and**

Disease. Vol 18. New York: Alan R Liss, **1988.**

64. **Recommended Dietary Allowances.** 10th Ed. Washington DC:
National Academy Press, 1989: 267.

65. Mertz W, eds. Trace elements in Human and Animal. **Nutrition** 5th
Ed. Vol 1. New York: Academic Press Inc, 1987: 275-300.

66. Tamura S, et al. A novel mechanism for the insulin-like effects of
vanadate on glycogen synthesis in rat adipocytes. **J Biol Chem** 1984;259:
6650-6658.

67. Nelson TS, Gillis MB, Peeler HT. **Poultry Sci** 1962; 41:519.

68. Underweed EJ. **Trace elements in Human and Animal Nutrition.** New
York: Academic Press, 1977.

69. Heyliger CE, Tuihiluni AG, McNeil JH. Effect of vanadate on elevated
blood glucose and depressed cardiac performance of diabetic rats.
Science 1985;227:757-759.

70. Meyerovitch JZ, et al. Oral administration of vanadate normalizes blood
glucose levels in streptozotocin treated rats. **J Biol Chem** 1987;262:6658-
6662.

71. Paulson DJ, et al. Effects of vanadate on in vivo reactivity to
norepinephrine in diabetic rats. **J Pharmacl Exp Therapy** 1987;240:
529-534.

72. Ramanadham S, et al. Oral vanadate in treatment of diabetes mellitus in
rats. **Amer J Physiol** 1989;257:H904-H911.

73. Domingo JL, Gomez M, Liobet JM, Corbella J, Keen CL. Improvement
of glucose homeostasis by oral vanadyl or vanadate treatment in diabetic
rats is accompanied by negative side effects. **Phar Toxic** 1991;68:249-253.

74. The Colgan institute who publish NUTRITION & Fitness magazine
receivedone of the letters offering to obtain advertising for colostrum
in return for printing an article about it. This letter is available for
perusal at our offices.

75. Clemmons DR, Underwood LE. Nutritional regulation of IGEI and IGF
binding proteins. **Ann Rev Nutr** 1991;11:393-412.

76. Lituka H, Naito A. **Microbial Transformation of Steroids and Alkaloids.**
State College, PA: University Park Press, 1967.

77. Duke JA. **Handbook of Medicinal Herbs.** Boca Raton, FL: CRC Press,
1985.

78. Cureton TK. **The Physiologcial Effects of Wheat Germ Oil on Humans
in Exercise**, Springfield IL: CC Thomas, 1972.

79. Saint-John M, McNaughton L. Octacosanol ingestion and its effects on
metabolic responses to submaximal cycle ergometry, reaction time,
and chest grip strength. **Int Clin Nutr Rev** 1986;6:81.

80. Levin E. Effects of octacosanol on chick comb growth. **Proc Soc Exp
Biol Med** 1963;112:331-334.

81. Norris FH, Denys EH, Fallat RJ. Trial of octacosanol in amyotrophic lateral sclerosis. **Neurology** 1986;36:1263.
82. Snider SR. Octacosanol in Parkinsonism. **Ann Neurol** 1984;16:723.
83. Ariel G, Saville W. Anabolic steroids: the physiological effects of placebos. **Med Sci Sports** 1972;4:124.
    14:1305-1365.

Chapter 32. The Anabolic Drive & Anti-catabolism

1. Daughaday WH, ed. **Endocrine Control of Growth**. New York: Elsevier, North Holland Press, 1981
2. Weigle DS. **Diabetes** 1987;36:764-775.
3. Laron Z, Butenandt O, eds. Evaluation of Growth Hormone Secretion. Basel: Karger Publishing, 1983.
4. Padh H. Vitamin C: newer insights into its biochemical functions. **Nutr Rev** 1991;49:65-70.
5. Barbeau A, Growdon JH, Wurtman RJ, eds. **Nutrition and the Brain: Vol 5**. New York: Raven Press, 1979.
6. Knaack D, et al. Ascorbic acid and acetylcholine receptor expression. **Ann New York Acad Sci** 1987;498:77-89.
7. Dorup I, Clausen T. Effects of potassium deficiency on growth and protein synthesis in skeletal muscle and the heart. **Brit J Nutr** 1989;62: 269-284.
8. Alleyne GAO. Studies on total body potassium in malnourished infants. Factors affecting potassium repletion. **Brit J Nutr** 1970;24: 205-212.
9. Flyvbjerg A, et al. Evidence that potassium deficiency induces growth retardation through reduced circulating levels of growth hormone and insulin-like growth factor I. **Metabolism** 1991;40:769-775.
10. Millward DJ, Rivers HPW. The need for indispensable amino acids: The concept of the anabolic drive. **Diabetes Metab Rev** 1989;5:191-211.
11. Schweiller E, Guler HP, Merryweather J. **Nature** 1986;323:169-171.
12. Phillips LS, Fusco AC, Unterman TG. **Metabolism** 1985;34:765-770.
13. Waterlow JC, et al. **Protein Turnover in Mammalian Tissues and the Whole Body**. Amsterdam: Elsevier-North Holland, 1978
14. Guyton AC. **Textbook of Medical Physiology: 7th Edition**. Philadelphia: WB Saunders, 1986:923-930.
15. Reiser S, et al. An insulinogenic effect of oral fructose in humans during post-prandial hyperglycemia. **Am J Clin Nutr** 1987;45:580-587.
16. Barbul A. Arginine: biochemistry, physiology, and therapeutic implications. **J Parent Ent Nutr** 1986;10:227-238.

17. Bucci Lr, et al. Ornithine supplementation and insulin release in bodybuilders. **Int J Sports Nutr** 1992;2:287-291.

18. Felig P. The glucose-alanine cycle. **Metabolism** 1973;22:179-186.

19. Felig P, Wahren J. Amino acid metabolism in exercising man. **J Clin Invest** 1971;50:2703-2708.

20. Roth E, et al. Glutamine: Anabolic effector? **J Parent Ent Nutr** 1990; 14:1305-1365.

21. Lacey J, Wilmore D. Is glutamine a conditionally essential amino acid? **Nutr Rev** 1990;48:297-309.

22. Cynobar L, et al. Action of ornithine alpha-ketoglutarate, ornithine hydrochloride and calcium alpha-ketoglutarate on plasma amino acid and hormonal patterns in healthy subjects. **J Amer Coll Nutr** 1990;9: 2-12.

23. Vaubourdolle M, et al. Action of enterally administered ornithine alpha-ketoglutarate on protein breakdown in skeletal muscle and liver of the burned rat. **J Parent Ent Nutr** 1991;15:517-520.

24. Cynobar L, et al. Action of ornithine alpha-ketoglutarate on protein metabolism in burn patients. **Nutrition** 1987;3:187-191.

25. Leander U, et al. Nitrogen sparing effects of Ornicetil in the immediate post operative state. **Clin Nutr** 1985;4:43-51.

26. Gay G, et al. Effects of ornithine alpha-ketoglutarate on blood insulin, glucagon and amino acids in alcoholic cirrhosis. **Biomedicine** 1979;30: 173-177.

27. Krassowski J, et al. The effect of ornithine alpha-ketoglutarate on insulin and glucagon secretion in normal subjects. **Acta Endocrinol** 1981;98:252-255.

28. Cynobar L, et al. Kinetics and metabolic effects of orally administered ornithine alpha-ketoglutarate in healthy subjects fed with a standardized regimen. **Amer J Clin Nutr** 1984;39:514-519.

29. Wilkerson JE, Batterson DL, Horvath SM. Exercise induced changes blood ammonia levels in humans. **Eur J Appl Physiol** 1977;37:255-263.

30. Michel H, Oge P, Bertrand L. Action de l'alpha-cetoglutarate d'ornithine sur l;hyperammoniemie du cirrhotique. **Presse Med** 1971; 19:867-868.

31. Molinard R, Charpentier C, Lemonnier F. Modifications de l'aminoacidemie des cirrhotiques sous l'influence de sels ornithine. **Ann Nutr Metab** 1982;26:25-36.

32. Harper A et al. Branched-chain amino acid metabolism. **Ann Rev Nutr** 1984;4:409-454.

33. Brooks G. Amino acid and protein metabolism during exercise and recovery. **Med Sci Sports Exer** 1987;19:Suppl:8150-8156.

34. Paul G. Dietary protein requirements of physically active individuals.

Sports Med 1989;8:154-176.

35. Cerra F, et al. Branched-chain amino acids support postoperative protein synthesis. **Surgery** 1982;92:192-199.

36. Maddrey W. Branched-chain amino acid therapy in liver disease. **J Amer Coll Nutr** 1985;4:639-650.

37. Sapir G, et al. Effects of alpha ketoisocaproate and of leucine on nitrogen metabolism in post-operative patients.**Lancet** 1983;1:1010-1014.

38. McNurian M, Garlick P. Influence of nutrient intake on protein turnover. **Diabetes Metab Rev** 1989;5:165-189.

39. Grant DB, et al. Reduced sulphation factor in undernourished children. **Arch Dis Child** 1973;48:596-600.

40. Maes M, et al. Plasma somatomedin C in fasted and re-fed rats. **J Endocrinol** 1983;87:243-252.

41. Clemmons D, Underwood LE. Nutritional regulation of IGF1 and IGF binding proteins. **Ann Rev Nutr** 1991;11:393-412.

42. Smith AT, et al. The effect of exercise on somtomedin C - insulin-like growth factor-1 concentration. **Metabolism** 1987;36:533.537.

43. Isley Wl, Underwood LE, Clemmons DR. Dietary components that regulate serum somatomedin C in humans. **J Clin Invest** 1983;71:175-182.

44. Maes M, et al. Low somatomedin C in protein deficiency. **Mol Cell Endocrinol** 1984;37:301-309.

45. Maes M, et al. Decreased serum insulin-like growth factor-1 response to GH in hypophysectionized rats fed low protein diet. **Acta Endocrinol** 1988;117:320-326.

46. Yahya Z, et al. Dietary and hormonal influences on plasma IGF levels in the rat. **J Endocrinol** 1987;Suppl:71.

47. Clemmons DR. Supplemental essential amino acids augmented the somatomedin C response in re-feeding after fasting. Metabolism 1983;34: 391-395.

48. Okajima F, Ui M. Adrenergic modulation of insulin secretion in vivo dependent on thyroid status. **Am J Physiol** 1978;234:E106-E111.

49. Millward DJ, Brown JG, Van Buren J. **J Endocrinol** 1988;118:417-422.

50. Gavin LA, Moeller M. The mechanism of recovery of hepatic T4-5" deiodinase during glucose refeeding: Role of glucagon and insulin. **Metabolism** 1983;32:543-551.

51. Millward DJ, et al. Role of thyroid insulin and cortico-steroid hormones in the physiological regulation of proteolysis in muscle. **Prog Clin Biol Res** 1985;180:531-542.

52. Millward Dj. The endocrine response to dietary protein: The anabolic drive on growth. In Barth CA, Schlimme E, eds. **Milk Proteins**. New York: Springer-Verlag, 1989;49-67.

53. Consolazio CF, et al. Comparison of nitrogen, calcium, and iodine

excretion in arm and total body sweat. **Am J Clin Nutr** 1966;18:443.

54. Barth CA, et al. Endocrine response to animal and vegetable protein. In Barth CA, Schlimme E, eds. **Milk Proteins**. New York: Springer Verlag, 1989;62-67.

55. Forsythe WA. Comparison of dietary casein or soy protein effects on plasma lipids and hormone concentrations in the gerbil. **J Nutr** 1986;116:1165-1171.

56. Cree TC, Schalch DS. Protein utilization in growth: effect of lysine deficiency on serum growth hormone somatomedins, insulin, total thyroxine (T4) and triiodothyronine, free T4 index and total corticosterone. **Endocrinology** 1985;117:667-673.

57. Stryker L. **Biochemistry 2nd Edition**. New York: WH Freeman, 1981.

58. Gilman AG, et al, eds. Goodman and Gilman's, **The Pharmacological Basis of Therapeutics, 7th Edition**. New York: Macmillan, 1986.

59. Francis C. **Speed Trap**. New York: St Martin's Press, 1990.

60. Whitten Pl, Russell E, Naftolin F. Effects of a normal human concentration phytoestrogen diet on rat uterine growth. **Steroids** 1992;57:98-106.

61. Chermnykh NS, et al. Effects of methandrostenolone and plant sterols on physcial endurance of animals and protein metabolism in skeletal muscles. **Pharm Toxicol** 1988;51:57-60.

62. Chinoy NJ, et al. Effects of vitamin C deficiency on physiology of male reproductive organs of guinea pigs. **Int J Fertil** 1986;31:322.

63. Dawson EB, et al. Effect of ascorbic acid on male fertility. In Burns JJ, et al, eds. **Third Conference On Vitamin C**. New York: New York Adcademy of Sciences, 1986;312-323.

64. Kitabshi AE. Ascorbic acid in steroidogenesis. **Nature** 1967;215:1385-1386.

65. Komindr S, et al. Bimodal effects of megadose vitamin C on adrenal steroid production in man. In Burns JJ, et al, eds. **Third Conference On Vitamin C**. New York: New York Academy of Sciences, 1986;487-490.

66. Salem SI, et al. **Ann Nutr Metab** 1984;28:44.

67. Prasad As, et al. **Am J Hematol** 1981;10:119.

68. Abassi AA, et al. **J Lab Clin Med** 1980;96:544.

69. Carli G, et al. Changes in the exercise induced hormone response to branched-chain amino acids administration. **Eur J Appl Physiol** 1992;64:272-277.

70. Kraemer WJ. Endocrine response to resistance exercise. **Med Sci Sports Exer** 1988;20,Suppl:S152-S157.

71. Li CH. Anterior pituitary hormones. **Postgrad Med** 1961;29:13.

72. Li CH, Liu WK. Human pituitary growth hormone, VIII. **Experientia** 1964;20:169.

Chapter 33. Steroids: The Real Story

1.   Alzedo L. I lied, I lied, I lied. **Sports Illustrated** 1991;8 July, Cover story.
2.   Courson S, Schreiber LR. **False Glory**. Stanford, CT: Longmeadow Press, 1991.
3.   Voy R. **Drugs Sport and Politics**. Champaign, IL: Human Kinetics, 1991.
4.   Leigh W. **Arnold: The Unauthorized Biography**. New York: Congden-Weed, 1990.
5.   Johnston R. The men and the myth. **Sports Illustrated**. 1974; 14 October:106-120.
6.   Scott J. It's not how you play the game, but what pill you take. **New York Times Magazine** 1971;17 October.
7.   Blunting steroid epidemic requires alternatives, innovative education. **J Amer Med Assoc** 1990;264:1641.
8.   Goodstadt MS. Drug education - a turn on or a turn off. **J Drug Educ** 1980;10:89-99.
9.   Bosworth E, et al. Anabolic steroids and high school athletes. **Med Sci Sports Exer** 1988;20:3.
10.   Goldberg L, et al. Use of anabolic - androgenic steroids by athletes. **N Engl J Med** 1990;322:775-776.
11.   Bosworth E, et al. Anabolic steroids and high school athletes. **Med Sci Sports Exer** 1987;20:S3-S17(Suppl).
12.   Johnston L, Bachman J, O'Malley P. **Monitoring the future: Continuing Study of the Lifestyles and Values of Youth**. Ann Arbor, Michigan: University of Michigan, 1990.
13.   Johnston L, Backman J, O'Malley P. **Monitoring the Future: Continuing Study of the Lifestyles and Values of Youth**. Ann Arbor, Michigan: University of Michigan, 1991.
14.   **National Household Survey on Drug Abuse: Population Estimates 1991**. Publication No ADM-92-1887. Rockville, MD: Department of Health and Human Services, 1991.
15.   Anderson WA, et al. A national survey of alcohol and drug use by college athletes. **Physician and Sportsmed** 1991;19:91-104.
16.   Yesalis CE, et al. Athletes' projections of anabolic steroid use. **Clin Sports Med** 1990;2:155-171.
17.   Pearson B, Hanson B. Survey of US Olympians. **USA Today** 1992;5 February:10C.
18.   **Runners World** 1987;22:12.
19.   Forbes G. Steroid users know all the tricks. **USA Today**, 8 October 1991:3C.

20. Klecko J, Fields J. Nose to Nose. **Survival in the Trenches in the NFL.** New York: Morrow, 1989

21. Yesalis CE, ed. **Anabolic Steroids in Sport and Exercise.** Champaign, IL: Human Kinetics, 1992.

22. Hendershott J. Steroids: Breakfast of champions. **Track and Field News** 1969;22:3.

23. Shahidi NT. Androgens and Erythropoiesis. **N Engl J Med** 1973;289:72.

24. Klein FC. Confessions of a steroid-abusing lineman. **Wall Street Journal.** 1992, 6 January:A12

25. Almond E, Cart J, Harvey R. Even the man who was in control regretted results of his research. **Los Angeles Times** 1984;1 February:J8

26. Le Breo D. Of MDs and muscles - lessons from two retired steroid doctors. **J Amer Med Assoc** 1990;263:1697-1705.

27. Pumped Up. **US News and World Report** 1992;1 June:55-63.

28. David K, et al. Crystalline male testes hormone (testosterone) is more active than androsterone from urine or cholesterol. **Zeitschrift Physiologische Chemie** 1935;233:281-293.

29. American Medical Association Report, Drug abuse in athletes; Anabolic steroids and human growth hormone. **J Amer Med Assoc** 1988;259:1703.

30. Arnold A, Potts GO, Beyler AL. Evaluation of the protein anabolic properties of certain orally active anabolic agents based on nitrogen balance studies in rats. **Endocrinology** 1963;72:408-417.

31. Albanese AA. Newer knowledge in the clinical investigation of anabolic steroids. **J New Drugs** 1965;5:208-224.

32. Christ DM, Stackpole PJ, Peake GT. Effects of androgenic-anabolic steroids on neuromuscular power and body composition. **J Appl Physiol** 1983;54:366-370.

33. Hervey GR, et al. Effects of methandienone on the performance and body composition of men undergoing athletic training. **Clinical Science** 1981;60:457-461.

34. Alen M, Hakkenin K, Komi PV. Changes in neuromuscular performance and muscle fiber characteristics of elite power athletes self-administering androgenic and anabolic steroids. **Acta Physiologica Scand** 1984;122: 535-544.

35. Hervey GR, et al. Anabolic effects of methandionone in men undergoing athletic training. **Lancet** 1976;2:699-702.

36. Loughton S, Ruhling R. Human strength and endurance responses to anabolic steroids and training. **J Sports Med** 1977;17:285-296.

37. Ward P. The effect of an anabolic steroid on strength and lean body mass. **Med Sci Sports Exer** 1973;5:277-283.

38. O'Shea JP. The effects of an anabolic steroid on dynamic strength levels

of weightlifters. **Nutr Rep Int** 1971;4:363-370.

39. Kuipers H, et al. Influence of anabolic steroids on body composition, blood pressure, lipid profile and liver functions in bodybuilders. **Int J Sports Med** 1991;12:413-418.

40. Mas SR. Cystolic androgen receptors in skeletal muscle from normal and dystrophic mice. **J Steroid Biochem** 1983;18:281.

41. Max SR, Toop J. Androgens enhance in vivo 2-deoxyglucose uptake by rat striated muscle. **Endocrinology** 1981;113:119.

42. Moudgil VK, ed. **Molecular Mechanism of Steroid Hormone Action.** Berlin: Walter de Gruyter, 1985.

43. Rogozkin VA. **Metabolism of Anabolic Androgenic Steroids**. Boca Raton, FL: CRC Press, 1991.

44. Dickman S. East Germany: Science in disservice of the State. **Science** 1991;254:26-27.)

45. Exner GU, Standte HW, Pette D. Isometric training of rats: effects on fast and slow muscle and modification by an anabolic hormone (nandrolone decanoate): female rats. **European J Physiol** 1973;345:1-114.

46. Coaches concede that steroids fueled East Germany's success in swim ming. **New York Times**. 3 December 1991:B15.

47. American College of Sports Medicine, Position stand on the use of anabolic-androgenic steroids in sports. **Med Sci Sports Exer** 1984;19: 13-18.

48. American College of Sports Medicine, **Sports Med Bull** 1984;19:4:1.

49. Shipe JR. Mass spectrometry instrumentation in the '90s. In:Shipe, JR, Savory J, eds. **Drugs in Competitive Athletics.** Oxford: Blackwell Scientific Publications 1991:61-68.

50. Dubin C. **Commission of Inquiry Into The Use of Drugs and Banned Practices Intended to Increase Athletic Performance**. Ottowa, Ontario: Canadian Government Publishing Center, 1990.

51. Di Pasquale M. Beating drug tests: Part 2. **Drugs in Sport** 1992;3:6-12.

52. Hamilton JB. The role of testicular secretions as indicated by the effects of castration in man and by studies of pathological conditions and the short life span associated with maleness. **Recent Progress in Hormone Res** 1948;3:257-322.

53. Matsumoto AM. Effects of chronic testosterone administration in normal men. **J Clin Endocrin Metab** 1990;70:282-287.

54. Aiache AE. Surgical treatment of gynecomastia in the bodybuilder. **Plas Reconstruct Surg** 1989;83:61-66.

55. Kochakian CD. Definition of androgens and protein anabolic steroids. **Pharmacol Ther** 1975;1:149-177.

56. Noble RL. Androgen use by athletes: A possible cancer risk. **Canadian Med Assoc J** 1984;130:549-550.

57. Larkin GL. Carcinoma of the prostate. **N Engl J Med** 1991;324:1892.

58. Roberts JT, Essenhigh DM. Adenocarcinoma of prostate in 40-year old bodybuilder. **Lancet** 1986;2:742.

59. Schally AV, Comaru-Schaly AM. Male contraception involving testosterone supplementation: Possible increased risks of prostate cancer? **Lancet** 1987;1:448-449.

60. Prat J, et al. Wilms' tumor in an adult associated with androgen abuse. **J Amer Med Assoc** 1977;21:2322-2323.

61. Alen M, Rahkila P. Anabolic-androgenic steroid effects on endocrinology and lipid metabolism in athletes. **Sports Med** 1988;6:327-332.

62. Webb OL, et al. Severe depression of high density lipoprotein cholesterol levels in weightlifters and bodybuilders by self-administered exogenous testosterone and anabolic androgenic steroids. **Metabolism** 1984;33: 971-975.

63. Alen M, Hakkinen K, Komi PV. Changes in neuromuscular performance and muscle fiber characteristics of elite power athletes self-administering androgenic and anabolic steroids. **Acta Physiol Scand** 1984;122:535-544.

64. Lenders JWM, et al. Deleterious effects of anabolic steroids on serum lipoproteins, blood pressure, and liver functions in amateur bodybuilders. **Int J Sports Med** 1988;9:19-23.

65. Lenders JW, et al. Deleterious effects of anabolic steroids on serum lipoproteins, blood pressure, and liver functions of amateur bodybuilders. **Int J Sports Med** 1988;9:19-23.

66. McKillop G, Todd IC, Ballantyne D. Increased left ventricular mass in a bodybuilder using anabolic steroids. **Br J Sports Med** 1986;20:151-152.

67. Salke RC, Rowland TW, Burke EJ. Ventricular size and function in bodybuilders using anabolic steroids. **Med Sci Sports Exerc** 1985;17: 701-704.

68. De Piccoli B, et al. Anabolic steroid use in bodybuilders: An echo-cardiographic Study of Left Ventricle Morphology and Function. **Int J Sports Med** 1991;12:408-412.

69. Longhurst JC, et al. Echocardiographic left ventricular masses in distance runners and weightlifters. **J App Physiol** 1980;48:154-162.

70. Johnson M, Ramey E, Ramwell P. Androgen mediated sensitivity in platelet aggregation. **Am J Physiol** 1977;232:H381-H385.

71. Ferenchick G, et al. Androgenic/anabolic steroid use and platelet aggregation: A pilot study in weightlifters. **Amer J Med Sci** 1992;303:78-82.

72. Everly RS, et al. Severe cholestasis associated with stanozolol. **Brit Med J** 1987;294:612-613.

73. Lin GC, Erinoff L, eds. **Anabolic Steroid Abuse**. Washington, DC: Government Printing Office, 1990.

74. Knuth VA, Maniera H, Nieschlag E. Anabolic steroids and semen

parameters in bodybuilders. **Acta Endocrinologica** 1989;120:(Suppl): 121-122.

75. World Health Organization, Methods for the regulation of male fertility. **Lancet** 1990;336:955-959.

76. Michna H. Tendon injuries induced by exercise and anabolic steroids in mice. **Int Orthop** 1987;11:157-162.

77. Michna H. Organization of collagen fibrils in tendon changes induced by anabolic steroid: I and II. **Virchows Arch** 1986;52:75-89.

78. Wood TO, Cooke PH, Goodship AE. The effect of exercise and anabolic steroids on the mechanical properties and crimp morphology of the rat tendon. **Am J Sports Med** 1988;16:153-158.

79. Laseter JT, Russell JA. Anabolic steroid induced tendon pathology: A review of the literature. **Med Sci Sports Exer** 1991;23:1-3.

80. Udry JR, et al. Serum androgenic hormones motivate sexual behavior in adolescent boys. **Fertility and Sterility** 1985;43:90.

81. Rada RT, Laws DR, Kellner R. Plasma testosterone levels in the rapist. **Psychosomatic Medicine** 1976;38:257.

82. Ehrenkranz JE, Bliss E, Sheard MH. Plasma testosterone: correlation with aggressive behavior and social dominance in man. **Psychosomatic Medicine** 1974;36:469.

83. Scaramella TJ, Brown WA. Serum testosterone and aggressiveness in hockey players. **Psychomatic Medicine** 1978;40:262.

84. Bahrke MS, Yesalis II CE, Wright JE. Psychological and behavioral effects of endogenous testosterone levels and anabolic-androgenic steroids among males: a review. **Sports Medicine** 1990;10:303.

Chapter 34. Testosterone Tales

1. Forbes GB, et al. Sequence of Changes in Body Composition Induced by Testosterone and Reversal of Changes After Drug is Stopped. **J Amer Med Assoc** 1992;267:397-399.

2. Kochakian CD, ed. **Handbook of Experimental Pharmacology Vol 43. Anabolic-Androgenic Steroids.** New York: Springer Verlog, 1976.

3. Padron RS, et al. Prolonged Biphasic Response of Plasma Testosterone to Single Intramuscular Injections of Human Chorionic Gonadotropin Administration in Normal Men. **J Clin Endocrinol Metab** 1980;50:190-192.

4. Voy R. **Drugs Sport and Politics.** Champaign, IL: Human Kinetics, 1991:19.

5. US Olympic Committee Drug Education and Control Policy. Colorado Springs: USOC, 1988.

6. For example, see Brooks RV, et al. Proceedings 12th International

Congress of Clinical Chemistry. **Rev Bras Anal Chem** 1984;6:109.

7. Wilson H, Lipsett MB. **J Clin Endocrinol** 1966;26:902-914.

8. Brooks RV, et al. Detection of the administration of natural androgens. **Drugs in Competitive Athletics.** Oxford, Blackwell Scientific Publications, 1991:29-32.

9. Southam GJ, et al. Possible indices for the detection of the administration of dihydrotestosterone in athletes. **J Steroid Biochem Mol Biol** 1992;42:87-94.

10. MacCann J. Testosterone patches boost hormone levels and improve function in elderly. **Medical Tribune** 1992;33:3.

11. McClure RD, Oses R, Ernest ML. Hypogonadal impotence treated by transdermal testosterone. **Urology** 1991;37:224-228.

Chapter 35. Human Growth Hormone

1. **Physicians Desk Reference.** 44th Edition. Oradell, NJ: Medical Economics Co, 1990.

2. A new biosynthetic human growth hormone. **The Medical Letter** 1987;29:(745), 73.

3. Gilbert D. Smith Barney data reported in US News and World Report. March, 1992.

4. Phone communication between Colgan Institute and Eli Lilly, 25 March 1992.

5. Voy R. **Drugs, Sport and Politics.** Champaign, IL: Human Kinetics, 1991:61.

6. Brown P, et al. Potential epidemic of Creutzfeldt-Jacob disease from human growth hormone therapy. **N Engl J Med** 1985;313:718.

7. **Science News** 1990;138:356.

8. **Physicians Desk Reference 46th Edition.** Montvale, NJ: Medical Economics, 1992:1266.

9. Rosenfeld RG, et al. Methionyl human growth hormone and oxandrolone in Turners syndrome. **J Pediatr** 1986;109:936.

10. Gerner JM, et al. Renewed catch-up growth with increased replacement doses of human growth hormone. **J Pediatr** 1987;110:425.

11. Rudman D, et al. Effects of human growth hormone in man over 60 years old. **N Engl J Med** 1990;323:1-6.

12. Crist DM, et al. Body composition response to exogenous GH during training in highly conditioned adults. **J Appl Physiol** 1988;65:579-584.

13. Florini JR, et al. Somatomedin-C levels in healthy young men: relation to peak and 24-hour integrated levels of growth hormone. **J Gerontology**

1985;40:2-7.

14. Goldman B. **Death in the Locker Room.** South Bend, IN: Icarus Press, 1984.

15. Todd T. The use of human growth hormone poses a grave dilemma. **Sports Illustrated** 1984;60:8-12.

16. Picket JB, et al. Neuromuscular complications of acromegaly. **Neurology** 1975; 25:638-645.

17. Macintyre JG, Growth hormone and athletes. **Sports Med** 1987;4:129-142.

18. **Lancet** 1991;337:1131-1132.

19. Daugheday WH. The anterior pituitary. **Williams Textbook of Endocrinology 7th Ed.** Philadelphia: WB Saunders 1985:577-611.

20. Linfoot JA, Acromegaly and giantism. In: Daughaday WH, ed. **Endocrine Control of Growth.** New York: Elsevier, 1981.

Chapter 36. Beta-Blockers: Beta-Boosters

1. Voy R. **Drugs Sport and Politics.** Champaign, IL; Leisure Press, 1991:53.

2. US Olympic Committee. **Drug Free.** Colorado Springs, CO: USOC, 1989.

3. Gilman AG, ed. **The Pharmacological Basis of Therapeutics.** 7th Edition. New York: Macmillan, 1985.

4. Reeds PJ, et al. The effect of beta-agonists and antagonists on muscle growth and body composition of young rats. **Comp Biochem Physiol** 1988;89C:337-341.

5. MacLennan P, Edwards HT. Effects of clenbuterol and propanolol on muscle mass. **Biochem J** 1989;264:573-579.

6. Emery PW, et al. Chronic effects of B_2 adrenergic agonists on body composition and protein synthesis in the rat. **Bioscience Reports** 1984;4:83-91.

Chapter 37. Cocaine: Manco Cepac's Revenge

1. Voy R. **Drugs, Sport and Politics.** Champaign, IL: Human Kinetics, 1991.

2. Wadler GI, Hainline B. **Drugs and the Athlete.** Philadelphia: F.A. Davis, 1989.

3. Cocaine: an unpredictable killer. **Harvard Heart Letter 1992;2:6-8.**

4. Cocaine deaths reported for century or more. **J Amer Med Assoc.** 1992;267:1045-1046.

5. Haddad LM. Cocaine abuse. **Int Med Specialist** 1986;7:67.

6.   Bozarth M, Wise R. Toxicity associated with long-term heroin and cocaine self-administration in the rat. **J Amer Med Assoc** 1985;254:81.

7.   Van Dyke C, Byck R. Cocaine. **Scientific Amer** 1982;246:128.

8.   Karch S. **Hum Pathol** 1989;20:1037-1039.

9.   Fairbanks DN, Fairbanks GR. Cocaine uses and abuses. **Primary Ear, Nose and Throat** 1986;2:2.

10. Resnick RB, Resnick EB. Cocaine abuse and its treatment. **Psychiat Clin N Amer** 1984;7:713.

11   Washton AM, et al. "Crack" early report of a new drug epidemic. **PostgradMed** 1986;80:52.

12. Spitz HI, Rosecan JS, eds. **Cocaine Abuse**. New York: Brunner/Mozel, 1987.

13. Freud S. **Cocaine Papers**. (R Byck, ed). New York: Stonehill Publishing, 1974.

14. **Sports Illustrated**. March 16, 1987.

15. Kirkman D. Coke even hurts best athletes. **Newsday** 1986, 24 April.

Chapter 38. Speed Kills

1.   Lake CR, Quirk RS. CNS stimulants and the look-alike drugs. **Psychiatr Clin N Am** 1984;7:689.

2.   Voy R. **Drugs Sport and Politics**. Philadelphia: FA Davis, 1989.

3.   Smith GM, Beecher HK. Amphetamines sulfate and athletic performance: Objective effects. **JAMA** 1959;170:542-557.

4.   Wadler GI, Hainline B. **Drugs and the Athlete**. Philadelphia: FA Davis, 1989, Chapter 6.

5.   Laties VG, Weiss B. The amphetamine margin in sports. **Fed Proc** 1981;40:2689.

6.   Chandler J, Blair S. The effect of amphetamines on selected physiological components related to athletic success. **Med Sci Sports Exer** 1980; 12:65-69.

7.   Stone E. Swim-stress-induced inactivity: Relation to body temperature and brain nor-epinephrine and effects of d-amphetamine. **Psychosom Med** 1970;32:32-51.

8.   Estler C, Gabrys M. Swimming capacity of mice after prolonged treatment with psychomotor stimulants. Psychopharmacology, 1979;60: 173-176.

9.   Gilman AG, et al, eds. **The Pharmacological Basis of Therapeutics 7th Edition.** New York: Macmillan, 1985.

10. Evans M, et al. Effects of dextroamphetamine on psychomotor skills.

Clin Pharmacol Ther 1976;19:777-781.

11. Belleville J, Dorey F. Effect of nefopan on visual tracking. **Clin Phamacol Ther** 1979;26:457-463.

12. Mandell AL, et al. The Sunday Syndrome: From kinetics to altered conciousness. **Fed Proc**, 1981;49:2693.

13. Hanley DF. Drug and sex testing: Regulations for international competition. **Clin Sports Med** 1986;2:13.

14. Harrington H, et al. Intracerebral hemorrhage and oral amphetamine. **Arch Neurol** 1983;40:503-507.

15. Caplan LR, Hier DB, Banks G. Current concepts of cerebrovascular disease - stroke: Stroke and drug abuse. **Stroke** 1982;13:869.

16. Gawin FH, Willinwood EH. Cocaine and other stimulants; actions, abuse and treatment. **N Engl J Med** 1988;318:1173.

17. Puffer J. The use of drugs in swimming. **Clin Sports Med** 1986;5:77.

Chapter 39. Erythropoietin: Blood Dope

1. Graber SE, Krantz SB. Erythropoietin and the control of red cell production. **Ann Rev Med** 1978;29:51-66.

2. Miyake T, Kung CKH, Goldwasser E. Purification of human erythropoietin. **J Biol Chem** 1977;252:5558-5564.

3. Jacobs K, et al. Isolation and characterization of genomic and CDNA clones of human erythropoietin. **Nature** 1985;313:806-810.

4. Egrie JC, et al. Characterization and biological effects of recombinant human erythropoietin. **Immunobiol** 1986;72:213-224.

5. **Physicians Desk Reference 46th Edition**. Montvale, NJ: Medical Economics Press, 1992, 1647.

6. Higden H. Blood doping among endurance athletes; rationalizations, results, and ramifications. **Am Med News** 1985;27 September:37.

7. Williams MH, et al. The effect of induced erythrocythemia upon 5-mile treadmill time. **Med Sci Sports Exer** 1981;13:169.

8. Brien AJ, Simon TL. The effects of red blood cell infusion on 10 km race time. **JAMA** 1987;257:2761.

9. Colgan M, Fielder S, Colgan LA. Micronutrient status of endurance athletes affects hematology and performance. **J Applied Nutrition** 1991;43:16-30.

10. Parr RB, Bachman LA, Moss RA. Iron deficiency in female athletes. **Physician and Sports Med** 1984;12:81-86.

11. **New York Times** 1991, 19 May.

12. Burke ER, EPO: Heart-stopping performance. **Winning** 1990;

October:86.

13. Cyclists deaths linked to erythropoietin. **Physicians and Sportsmed** 1990;18:48.

Chapter 40. Grab Bag of Ergogenic Drugs

1. **Physicians Desk Reference 46th Edition.** Montvale, NJ: Medical Economics, 1992.

2. Nielsen B, et al. Physical work capacity after dehydration and hyperthermia. **Scand J Sports Sci** 1981;3:2.

3. Caldwell JE, et al. Differential effects of sauna, diuretic, and exercise induced hypohydration. **J Appl Physiol** 1984;57:1018.

4. Pentel P. Toxicity of over-the-counter stimulants. **J Amer Med Assoc** 1984;252:1898.

5. Martin WR, et al. Physiological, subjective, and behavioral effects of amphetamine, methamphetamine, ephedrine, phenmetrazine and methylphenidate in man. **Clin Pharmacol Ther** 1971;12:245.

6. Woolverton WL, et al. Behavioral and neurochemical evaluation of phenylpropanolamine. **Pharmacol Exp Ther** 1986;237:926.

7. Sidney KH, Lefcoe WM. The effects of ephedrine on the physiological and psychological responses to submaximal and maximal exercises in man. **Med Sci Sports** 1977;9:95.

8. Cornelius JR, et al. Paranoià, homicidal behavior and seizures associated with phenylpropanolamine. **Am J Psychiat** 1984;141:120.

9. Wooter MR, et al. Intracerebral hemorrhage and vasculitis related to ephedrine abuse. **Ann Neurol** 1983;13:337.

10. Dulloo AG, Miller DS. Ephedrine, caffeine, and aspirin: over-the-counter drugs that interact to stimulate thermogenesis in the obese. **Nutrition** 1989;5:7.

11. Astrup A, etal. The effect of ephedrine/caffeine mixture on energy expenditures and body compostion in obese women. **Metabolism** 1992; 41:886-888.

12. Astrup A, et al. The effect and safety of an ephedrine/caffeine compound compared with ephedrine, caffeine, and placebo in obese subjects on an energy restricted diet. **Int J Obesity** 1992;16:269-277.

13. Dulloo AG, Miller DS. The thermogenic properties of ephedrine/ methizanthine mixtures; human studies. **Int J Obesity** 1986;10:467-481.

14. Bedi JF, Gong H, Horvath SM. Enhancement of exercise performance with inhaled albuterol. **Can J Sports Med** 1988;13:144-148.

15. Oota I, Nagal T. Effects of catecholamines on excitation contraction

coupling in frog single twitch fiber. **Japanese J Physiol** 1975;27:195-213.

Chapter 41. Your Personal Sports Nutrition Program

1.   Millman D. **The Way of the Peaceful Warrior**, Tiburon CA: HJ Kramer, 1989.
2.   Hyams J. **Zen in the Martial Arts**, Los Angeles: JP Tarcher, 1979
3.   Allen M. **Total Triathlete**, New York: Contemporary Books, 1988.

Chapter 42. Strength Program To Beat Steroids

1.   Morehouse LE, Miller AT. **Physiology of Exercise 7th Edition**, St Louis: CV Mosby, 1976.
2.   Davis EC, Logan GA, McKinney WC. **Biophysical Values of Muscular Activity**, Iowa: Wm C Brown, 1965
3.   Gambetta V, ed. **Track and Field Coaching Manual**, West Point NY: Leisure Press, 1981.
4.   Pearl B. **Keys to the Inner Universe, Vol 1**. Phoenix OR: Bill Pearl Enterprises, 1982.

Index

A

Acerola vitamin C 213
Acetylcholine 370
Acidity 281
Acromegaly 429
ACTH 363
Addisons disease 74
Additives 213
Adenosine triphosphate (ATP) 95, 234
Adrenal glandulars 336
Adrenal glands 74,386
Adrenal-pituitary axis 445
Adrenalin 386
Aids 448,449
Aikens, Willie 437
Air pollution 55
    antioxidant protection 62
    carbon monoxide 57, 59
    how to avoid 61
    Los Angeles Basin 55, 58,61
    lung damage 55,62
    ozone 55,57,58
Alanine 162,376,377
Albacore 47
Albumin 200
Albuterol 455
Alice in Wonderland 68
Allen, Mark 29,464
Allithiamins 212
Aloe vera 363
17-alpha alkylated steroids 411
Alpha-2-macroglobin 200
Alpha-2-receptor agonists 343
Alpha-amidating monooxygenase 370
Alpha-galactosidase 50

Alpha-ketoglutarate 276-277,377
Aluminum 69
    and brain degeneration 70
    in foods 72
Alza Pharmaceuticals 423
Alzedo, Lyle 395
American College of Sports
    Medicine 29,293,408
American Heart Association 79
American Journal of Clinical Nutrition 242
American Journal of Psychiatry 301
American Medical Association 444
Amgen Inc 448
Amino acids
    blood/brain barrier and 325-327
    classification 326
    essential 5,6
    growth hormone and athletes' requirements 334
    large neutral 369
Ammonia 153,282,377
Amphetamines 402
    aerobic exercise and 445
    anaerobic exercise and 445
    dosage 444,445,446
    downside of 445,446
Anabolic drive 323,365-391,461
    program for 469
    rules to maximize 391
    schematic 367
Anabolic Steroids Control Act 398, 451
Anabolic steroids, see Steroids
Anaerobic threshold 447
Anavar 402
Anderson, Richard 315
Androgenic 402
Androstenedione 387
Annals of Internal Medicine 127
Anti-catabolic nutrients 366
Antibiotics, in meat 42
Antioxidants

B

C

G

H

N

P

T

V

W